Tendon and Ligament Injuries of the Foot and Ankle

AF393509

Jarrett D. Cain • MaCalus V. Hogan

Editors

Tendon and Ligament Injuries of the Foot and Ankle

An Evidence-Based Approach

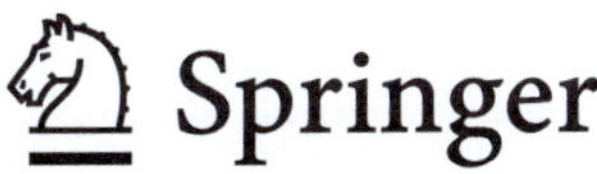

Springer

Editors
Jarrett D. Cain
Department of Orthopaedic Surgery
University of Pittsburgh School of Medicine
Pittsburgh, PA, USA

MaCalus V. Hogan
Department of Orthopedic Surgery
University of Pittsburgh School of Medicine
Pittsburgh, PA, USA

ISBN 978-3-031-10492-3   ISBN 978-3-031-10490-9   (eBook)
https://doi.org/10.1007/978-3-031-10490-9

© Springer Nature Switzerland AG 2022
This work is subject to copyright. All rights are reserved by the Publisher, whether the whole or part of the material is concerned, specifically the rights of translation, reprinting, reuse of illustrations, recitation, broadcasting, reproduction on microfilms or in any other physical way, and transmission or information storage and retrieval, electronic adaptation, computer software, or by similar or dissimilar methodology now known or hereafter developed.
The use of general descriptive names, registered names, trademarks, service marks, etc. in this publication does not imply, even in the absence of a specific statement, that such names are exempt from the relevant protective laws and regulations and therefore free for general use.
The publisher, the authors, and the editors are safe to assume that the advice and information in this book are believed to be true and accurate at the date of publication. Neither the publisher nor the authors or the editors give a warranty, expressed or implied, with respect to the material contained herein or for any errors or omissions that may have been made. The publisher remains neutral with regard to jurisdictional claims in published maps and institutional affiliations.

This Springer imprint is published by the registered company Springer Nature Switzerland AG
The registered company address is: Gewerbestrasse 11, 6330 Cham, Switzerland

Foreword

It was during my foot and ankle fellowship, with Dr. Roger Mann, that my research and clinical interests gravitated to tendon injuries of the foot and ankle. In the 1980s, orthopedic traumatologists started to emphasize the critical importance of soft tissue management in complex fracture management. This kindled my career-long interest in Achilles tendon and posterior tibial tendon ruptures and dysfunction. The pathophysiology, clinical diagnosis, and treatment options for soft tissue injuries of the foot and ankle in the 1980s were by today's standards uncharted and on a significant scale, anecdotal.

In 2013, the groundbreaking research in Achilles tendon regeneration by Dr. Hogan was acclaimed by his colleagues with the bestowing of the AOFAS J. Leonard Goldner Award. The continuation of his forward-thinking research has led to his team being viewed as international leaders in tendon research.

Dr. Hogan and Dr. Cain are to be applauded for having gathered a dream team of contributors to provide the practicing foot and ankle surgeon the knowledge base in soft tissue, ligament, and tendon injuries essential to providing the best care for our patients. The contributors have created an evidence-based, comprehensive, and cohesive foundation for the further expansion of our knowledge of soft tissues injuries of the foot and ankle. This is the book I wish was available at the beginning of my foot and ankle career.

George B. Holmes
Department of Orthopaedic Surgery
Rush University Medical Center
Chicago, IL, USA

Preface

Understanding the anatomy and biomechanics of the foot and ankle is required to make the appropriate diagnosis of any pathology. Acute injury symptoms appear immediate while chronic injuries tend to persist for days, months, and even years. Diagnosis and treatment, whether operative or non-operative, requires attention to the factors that contribute to the patient returning to symptom-free activity.

While each approach varies depending on the nature of the pathology, whether acute or chronic, the overall goal remains to provide a functional foot and ankle that allows patient to return to daily activities. Overtime, with the evolution of technology that improves our diagnosis acumen, management of pathology is also impacted by published literature that reflect the latest advancements.

To that end, it is our pleasure to present *Tendon and Ligament Injuries of the Foot and Ankle: An Evidence-Based Approach*. This book is written for the foot and ankle specialists in mind with the intention of providing an approach to diagnosis of acute and chronic injuries through the lens of evidence-based medicine. Each chapter of the textbook provides an evidence-based algorithm that is based on the latest knowledge and advancements in various tendon and ligament injuries of the foot and ankle.

In order to achieve this task, our international experts provide a consensus for management of the various tendon and ligament pathologies. The experts provided evaluation of long-term studies that decrease the chance of misdiagnosis and an algorithm that avoids ineffective treatments that are not substantiated by the evidence. We acknowledge, with gratitude and appreciation, the experts' time and commitment to help accomplish this objective. We also like to thank the team at Springer Publishing, especially Kristopher Spring and Eugenia Judson, for the opportunity to share this knowledge with the foot and ankle community. Finally, we thank the readers of the textbook, who we hope will be inspired and challenged to take this information to their patient population. Our goal is to serve them with the acquisition and application of the evidence-based knowledge that improves their care.

Pittsburgh, PA	Jarrett D. Cain
Pittsburgh, PA	MaCalus V. Hogan

Contents

Imaging of Soft Tissue Injuries of the Foot and Ankle

1

Carol L. Andrews, Don D. Williams, and Lorraine Boakye

Introduction

Imaging for evaluation of tendon and ligament injuries includes a wide variety of techniques as the foot and ankle are some of the most challenging anatomic structures to image. This is accounted for, in part, by the fact that the transition from the leg to the foot is an acute angle, the multiple curved osseous surfaces as well as the mediolateral and anteroposterior arches of the midfoot, and the alignment of the multiple individual joints of the forefoot.

Imagers consider the ankle and hindfoot [tibiotalar, subtalar, as well as talonavicular and calcaneocuboid (Chopart) joints] separately from the midfoot [intertarsal and tarsometatarsal (Lisfranc) joints] and the forefoot (metatarsophalangeal and interphalangeal joints) (Fig. 1.1). This becomes important in both the consideration of the clinical question and the focused, dedicated imaging of each region to allow the appropriate assessment of pathology.

Large field of view (FOV) imaging, with any modality, allows the impression of comprehensive imaging but, in fact, may result in decreased conspicuity of relevant structures, thus limiting diagnostic interpretation. In radiographic imaging, this may mean improved ability to see alignment but decreased likelihood of identifying subtle cortical avulsions or more complex injuries that include or affect the function of the tendons and ligaments. Focused multiplanar imaging of the ankle comprises the tibiotalar and subtalar joints to include the proximal portion of the midfoot. Midfoot imaging includes imaging from the Chopart to the Lisfranc joints, and

C. L. Andrews (✉) · D. D. Williams
Department of Radiology, University of Pittsburgh, Pittsburgh, PA, USA
e-mail: andrewscl3@upmc.edu; williamsdd5@upmc.edu

L. Boakye
Department of Orthopaedic Surgery, University of Pittsburgh, Pittsburgh, PA, USA
e-mail: boakyela@upmc.edu

© Springer Nature Switzerland AG 2022
J. D. Cain, M. V. Hogan (eds.), *Tendon and Ligament Injuries of the Foot and Ankle*,
https://doi.org/10.1007/978-3-031-10490-9_1

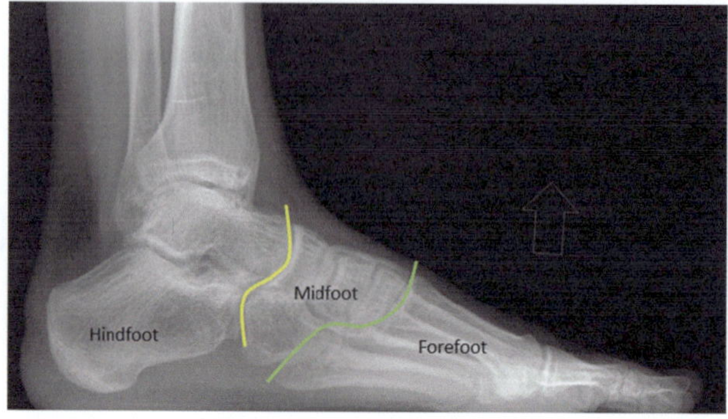

Fig. 1.1 Normal lateral radiograph. The ankle and foot are considered as the hindfoot divided from the midfoot by the Chopart joint (yellow line) and the forefoot divided from the midfoot by the Lisfranc joint (green line)

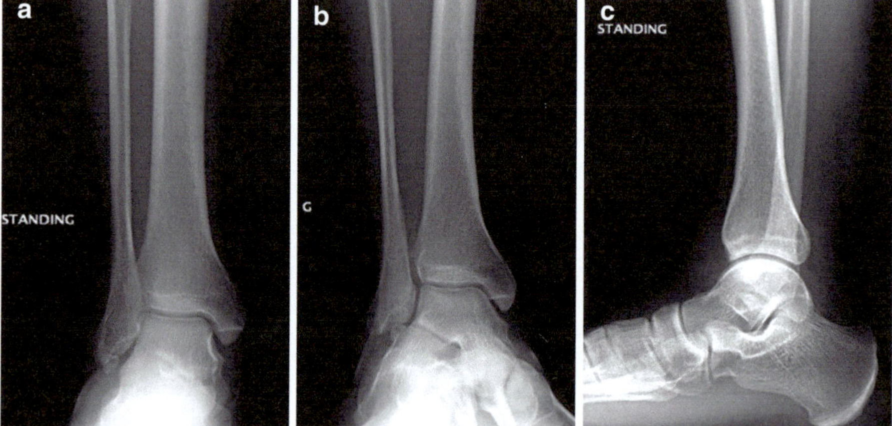

Fig. 1.2 Normal weight-bearing radiographs of the ankle. (**a**) Anteroposterior (AP), (**b**) mortise oblique, and (**c**) lateral

forefoot imaging includes from the Lisfranc joint through the toes. Dedicated small FOV imaging allows high spatial resolution of the area of interest [1].

Weight-bearing is an important tool in foot and ankle imaging. It allows direct assessment of alignment and, thus, an indirect measure of the integrity of the supporting soft tissues (Figs. 1.2 and 1.3). Stress views can be employed to confirm and accentuate particular osseous and soft tissue pathology. Gross injury, such as dislocation, is readily seen with non-weight-bearing imaging, but subtle subluxations could easily be missed (Figs. 1.4 and 1.5).

This is easily accomplished in radiographic imaging but is less commonly used in multiplanar imaging such as computed tomography or magnetic resonance imaging. Cone-beam computed tomography (CT) technology now provides the opportunity to evaluate ankle and foot alignment, allowing functional information of joint biomechanics [2, 3]. Weight-bearing magnetic resonance imaging (MRI) is also proposed. Attempts to simulate weight-bearing have been less than successful over the years. It is essential that the patient be able to remain still throughout MR imaging to assure adequate acquisition of the images. A weight-bearing position is difficult to maintain

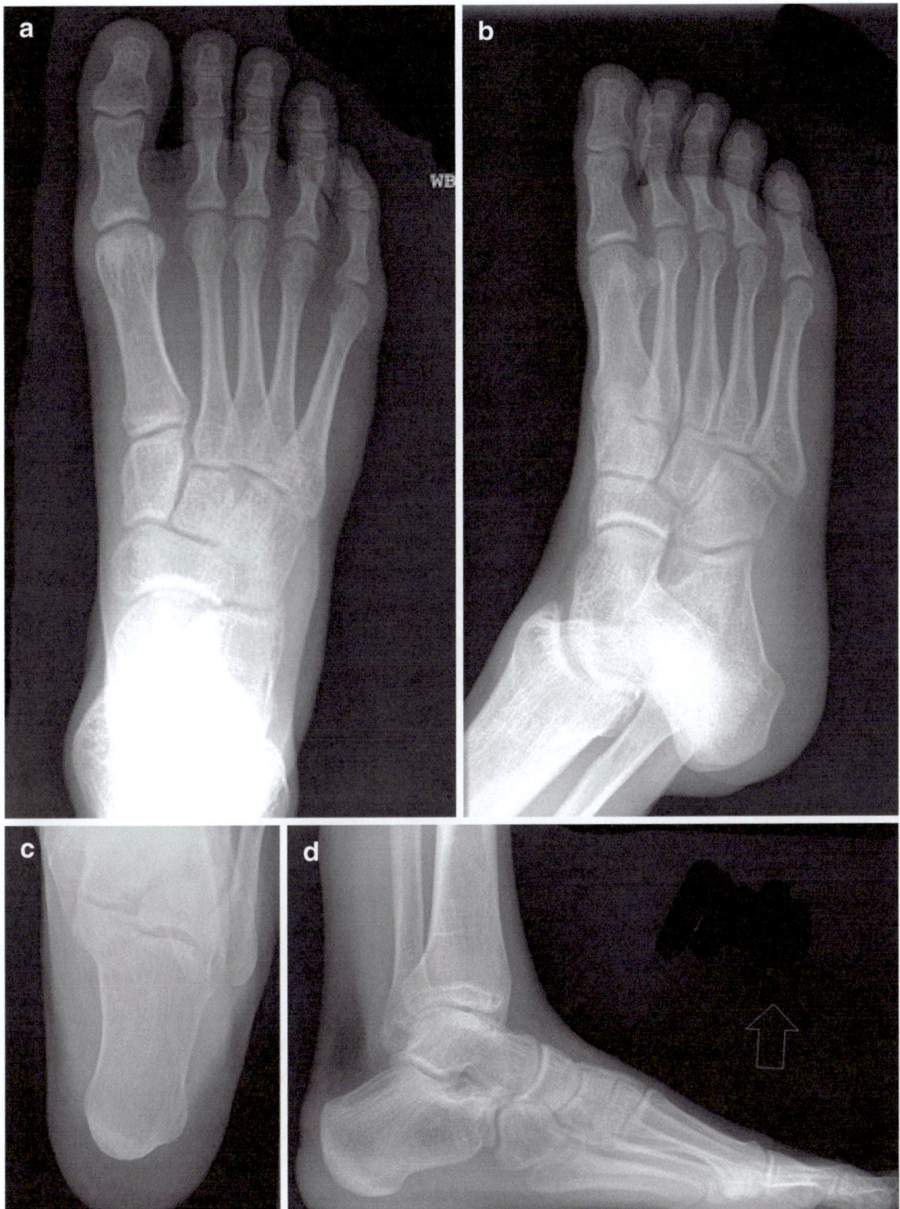

Fig. 1.3 Normal weight-bearing foot radiographs. (**a**) AP, (**b**) oblique, (**c**) Harris-Beath axial, and (**d**) lateral

without micromotion, and the weight-bearing position is often a painful position which limits patient stillness as well. Weight-bearing MRI may be accomplished in open low-field strength scanner with a tilt table that allows the patient to weight-bear during imaging. These units are not in widespread use at this time [2].

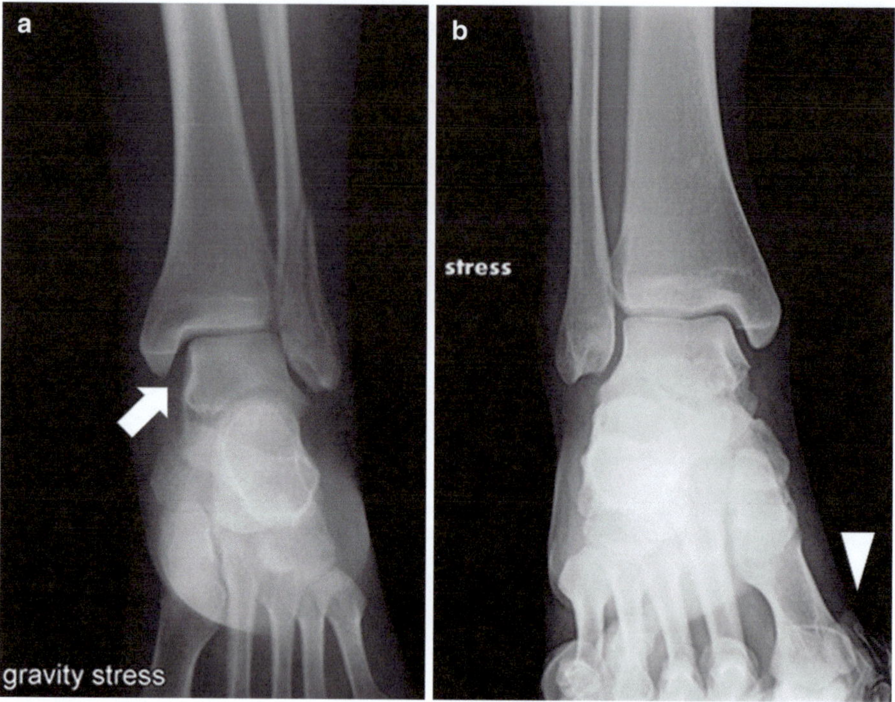

Fig. 1.4 Stress radiographs. (**a**) Gravity stress view of the ankle in patient with Weber B fracture (white arrow) demonstrates widening of the medial tibiotalar joint, indicating ankle instability. (**b**) Manual stress view demonstrates no change in the symmetric ankle mortise. Note the fingers of the person applying stress (white arrowhead). Manual stress views should be undertaken with protection against radiation

The majority of ankle and foot imaging does not warrant intravenous or intraarticular contrast. Intravenous contrast has been suggested in the evaluation of soft tissue impingement as synovitis/synovial hypertrophy is vascular and will enhance. It is also useful in the setting of possible soft tissue infection. It does not assist in the evaluation of acute or chronic tendon or ligament abnormalities [4].

Arthrography with MRI is useful in the evaluation of osteochondral lesions and may be useful in evaluation of the postoperative ankle presenting with ongoing pain [5] but is not routinely employed in evaluating of soft tissue injuries of the foot and ankle.

Specific Modalities

Radiography provides a baseline for quality of bone, alignment and assessment of acute trauma, residual from prior trauma, presence of arthritis and presence of soft tissue swelling, masses or calcification, as well as evidence of prior surgeries. Radiographs are useful for serial imaging over time. Radiographs do not provide direct visualization of tendons, other than the Achilles tendon and the

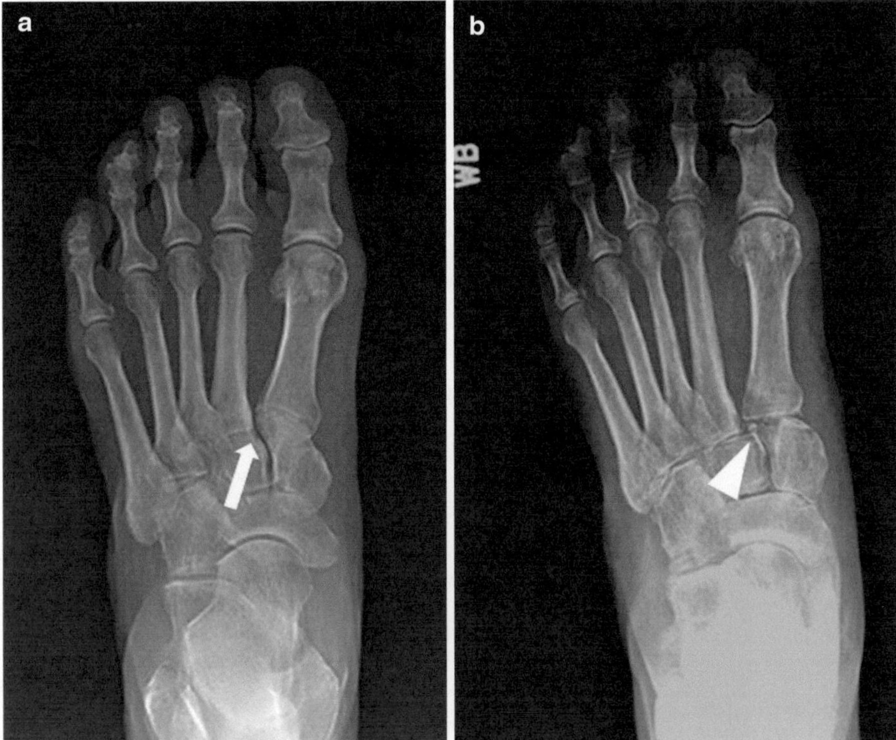

Fig. 1.5 Midfoot Lisfranc ligament injury. (**a**) Non-weight-bearing radiograph demonstrates subtle widening of the medial and middle cuneiforms but no clear malalignment at the medial Lisfranc joint (white arrow). (**b**) Weight-bearing radiograph reveals fracture fragment and lateral subluxation of the first and second tarsometatarsal joints (white arrowhead)

plantar fascia, but they provide indirect information regarding alignment related to the integrity of the tendons and ligament restraints. Weight-bearing imaging provides further information about the dynamic integrity of normal alignment [6]. This chapter is not meant to provide an exhaustive summary of the many measurements about the foot and ankle. That information can be acquired elsewhere.

Ultrasound is an extremely useful tool for identifying and interrogating regions of pain. It is operator dependent, requiring extensive practice to acquire the technical skill needed in concert with the professional understanding of the anatomy and pathology of the structures imaged [7–9]. Adequate evaluation requires high-frequency transducer (15–18 MHz) and a small footprint to adequately assess the accessible ligaments and tendons (Fig. 1.6). It can delineate the anatomy and pathology of the superficial structures including tendons and superficial ligaments but is less effective with deeper soft tissue structures, especially if surrounded by bone. It is a dynamic imaging method, allowing visualization of a structure through its range of motion such as evaluation of the peroneal tendons when transient tendon subluxation is suspected (Fig. 1.7) [7–9].

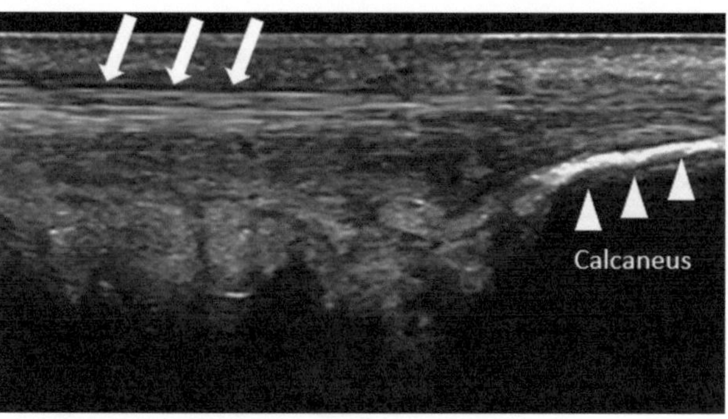

Fig. 1.6 Normal Achilles tendon. Longitudinal ultrasound demonstrated the organized striated appearance of the intact tendon fibers (white arrows) as the tendon approached its insertion on the calcaneus (white arrowheads)

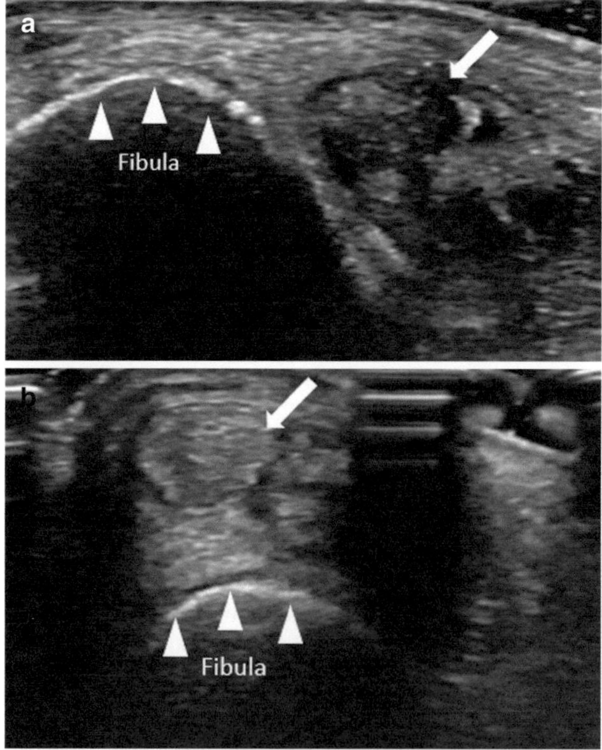

Fig. 1.7 Peroneal tendon dislocation. (**a**) Transverse ultrasound of the distal fibula demonstrates the peroneal tendons (white arrow) in normal position dorsal to the fibula (white arrowhead). (**b**) Transverse ultrasound during dynamic manipulation of the ankle shows the peroneal tendons (white arrow) dislocated lateral to the fibular retromalleolar groove (white arrowhead)

Computed tomography may be useful for evaluation of fractures associated with tendon and ligament disruption and may, on occasion, allow for direct visualization of soft tissue injury, especially when imaging in a delayed fashion as region edema often limits reasonable assessment of the ligaments and partial tendon injury (Fig. 1.8).

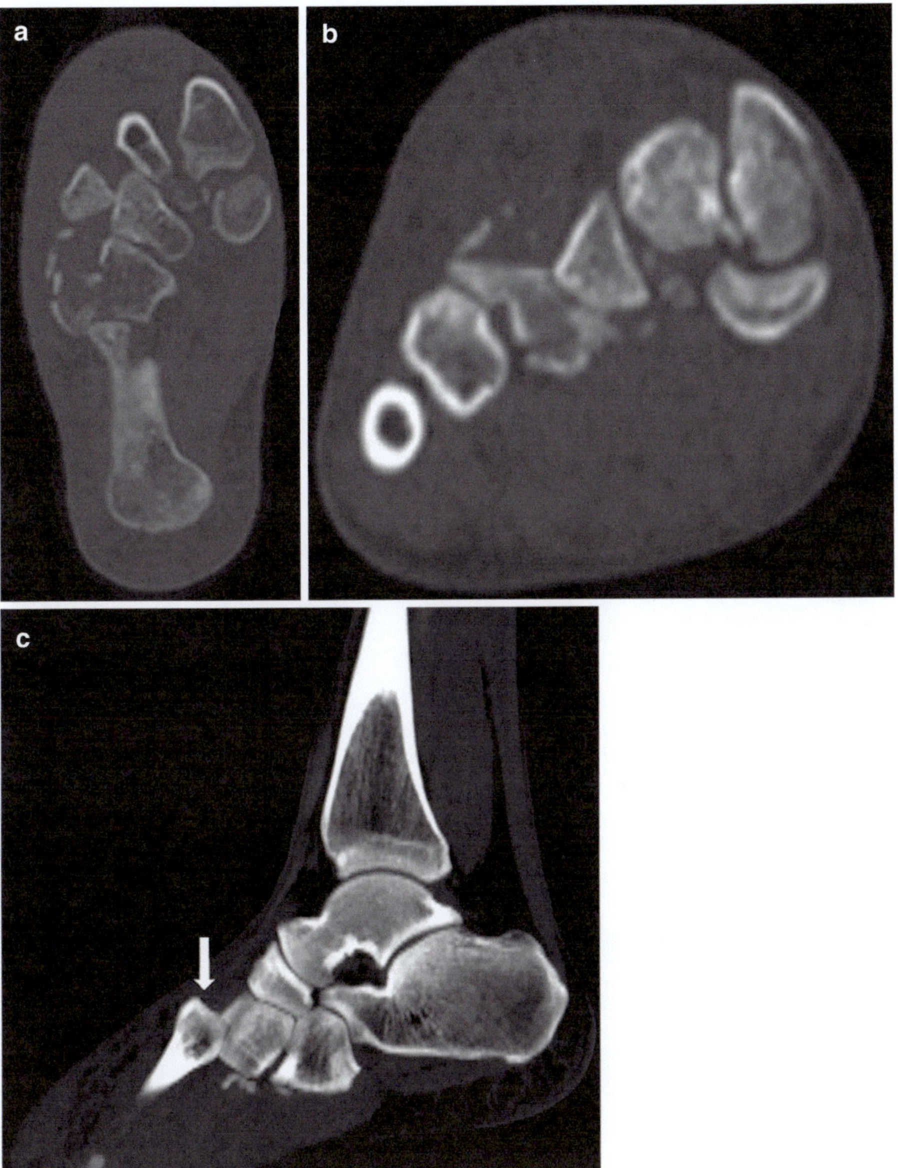

Fig. 1.8 Lisfranc fracture dislocation. Short-axis CT imaging demonstrates marked comminution of the tarsometatarsal joints with disruption of multiple joints at the (**a**) Lisfranc joint with fracture of the cuneiforms and cuboid as well as more distally at the (**b**) fractured metatarsal bases. (**c**) Sagittal reconstruction shows the malalignment with dorsal dislocation of the third metatarsal base (white arrow)

MRI is widely accepted as an excellent method of assessing the soft tissue structures of the ankle and foot. There are a myriad of options available with this tool to maximize the information yielded by a given study including the strength of the magnetic field (1.5 and 3.0 Tesla are the most common in clinical use today), various coils ranging from surface coils (widely available and in common use) to dedicated micro-coils (limited availability), variable FOV with large FOV being less detail-oriented and small FOV for detailed assessment, and a wide range of pulse sequences to choose from to allow evaluation of a specific tissue type or structure [1, 10]. Protocols vary depending on the preferences of the supervising radiologist, scanner type, and strength and available coils and software. Sample protocols from three different institutions are included (Table 1.1). All three planes are used at each institution, and each includes PD and PD fat suppression (FS) sequences to provide

Table 1.1 Sample protocols for MR imaging of the foot and ankle [1, 10]

	Institution 1	Institution 2	Institution 3
	Ankle		
Patient position	Prone with ankle in plantar flexion	Supine with foot held in position of comfort	Supine with foot held in position of comfort
FOV	160 mm	160	180
Axial oblique	PD, T2FS		
Axial	PD	PD, STIR	PD
Coronal	T2FS	PD, PDFS	PD
Sagittal	T1, T2FS	PD, PDFS	PD, STIR
	Midfoot		
Patient position	Supine with foot held in position of comfort	Supine with foot held in position of comfort	Supine with foot held in position of comfort
FOV	160 mm	120	160
Axial (short axis)	T1, PDFS	PDFS	PD
Coronal (long axis	T1, PDFS	PD, PDFS	PD, STIR
Sagittal	T1, STIR	PDFS	PD
	Forefoot		
Patient position	Supine with foot held in position of comfort		Supine with foot held in position of comfort
FOV	120 mm		160
Axial (short axis)	T1, T2FS		PD
Coronal (long axis l	T1, PDFS		PD, STIR
Sagittal	T1, STIR		PD
	Toes		
Patient position	Supine with foot held in position of comfort	Supine with foot held in position of comfort	
FOV	80 mm	80 mm	
Axial (short axis)l	T1, T2FS	PD, PDFS	
Coronal (long axis l	T1, PDFS	PD, PDFS	
Sagittal	T1, STIR	PD, PDFS	

FOV field of view, *PD* proton density, *FS* fat suppression, *STIR* short tau inversion recovery

the best spatial resolution, signal-to-noise ratio, and contrast, allowing assessment of bone, cartilage, ligaments, and tendons. The orientation of the coronal and axial planes can be somewhat confusing as some institutions define the plane orientation with reference to the foot, while other institutions with reference to the ankle. To avoid confusion, these planes may be referred to as short-axis (providing imaging that is transverse to the forefoot structures) and long axis (allowing a view similar to an AP foot radiograph) [1].

Comprehensive summary of the technical factors of various imaging modalities is beyond the scope of this text. An understanding of the histopathology of acute and chronic injury to tendons and ligaments yields specific imaging appearances, and a summary of these findings will be reviewed.

Tendons

Tendons are formed with taut parallel collagen fibers of uniform slightly flattened fibrocytes, resulting in uniform organization. Degeneration of the tendon results in disruption of this organization with tearing of individual fibers and subsequent ingrowth of fibrovascular reparative tissue. Tendon injury is graded as minimal fiber disruption (grade 1 strain), partial tendon tear (grade 2 strain), and complete tendon tear (grade 3 strain). These injuries may occur proximally, distally, or in midsubstance. In the more chronic setting of tendinosis, the tendon tenocytes are more rounded with increased cell numbers and an increase in larger hydrophilic proteoglycans, resulting in increased bound water and tendon thickening, fibrillar disorganization, and infiltration of blood vessels and accompanying nerves [9, 11–14]. The paratendinous soft tissues including the tendon sheath and bursae will often demonstrate inflammatory changes as well [9, 13, 15]. The Achilles tendon serves as an excellent representation of process (Fig. 1.9).

The organization of the tendon fibers is well demonstrated on ultrasound with a slightly hyperechogenic fibrillar pattern [9]. Disruption of this continuity of fibers may be seen within or along the surface of the tendon. Progressive fiber disruption correlates with increasing grade of tendon strain. Partial or intrasubstance tears may be fusiform and thickened (Fig. 1.10). As the tearing progresses continues, the tendon contour becomes more attenuated and thinned. Complete tear shows fiber discontinuity demonstrated as hypoechoic or anechoic echotexture (Fig. 1.11). In tendinosis, the tendon echotexture is disrupted and appears hypoechoic and thickened without a discrete tear. Doppler studies will often reveal increased vascularity (Fig. 1.12) [9].

Care must be taken to assure that the probe is directly parallel with the tendon fibers to avoid the major pitfall of anisotropy, a mimic of partial of intrasubstance tearing. Anisotropy occurs when evaluating linear structures such as tendons and ligaments. If the transducer is not parallel to the structure being evaluated, there will be a loss of the normal echotexture of the structure that can be fiber tearing (Fig. 1.13) [8, 9].

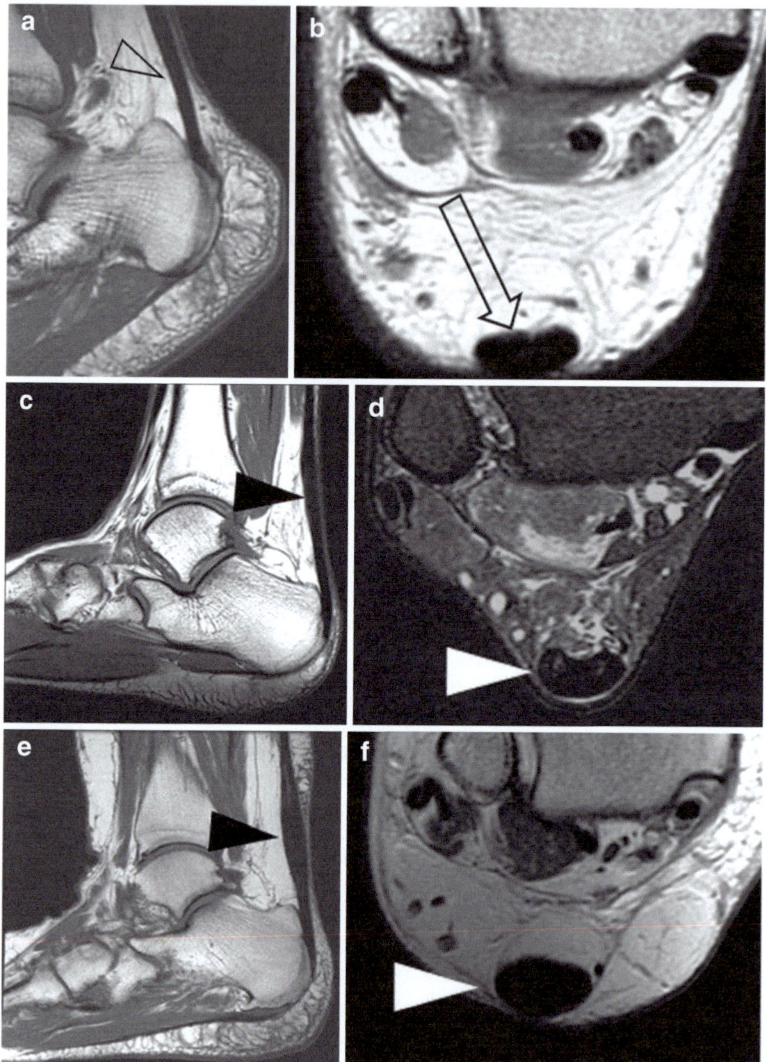

Fig. 1.9 Achilles tendon strain grades. (each axial image corresponds to the level of the black arrowhead seen on the sagittal images). (**a**) Sagittal T1-weighted MR shows the taut straight margin of the Achilles tendon throughout its course (black open arrowhead). (**b**) Axial T1-weighted MR shows the tendon uniform low signal intensity with a semilunar contour (black open arrow). (**c**) Grade 1 strain. Sagittal T1-weighted imaging shows midsubstance tendon strain with minimal tendon thickening (black arrowhead), while (**d**) axial T2 fat-suppressed imaging shows the normal concave contour of the tendon with punctate focal areas of high signal representing scattered disrupted tendon fibers (white arrowhead). (**e**) Grade 2 strain. Sagittal T1-weighted imaging shows more bulbous contour (black arrowhead) with (**f**) axial T1-weighted imaging showing the rounded contour of the tendon in transverse perspective (white arrowhead). (**g**) Grade 2 strain. Sagittal T1-weighted imaging shows marked tendon thickening (black arrowhead) with (**h**) axial T1-weighted imaging showing the large gaps in the tendon fibers with progressive intrasubstance tearing (white arrowhead). (**i**) Grade 3 strain. Sagittal STIR imaging shows complete tendon disruption (black arrowhead) with (**j**) axial T1-weighted imaging revealing complete disruption of the tendon fiber integrity with extensive soft tissue swelling (white arrowhead)

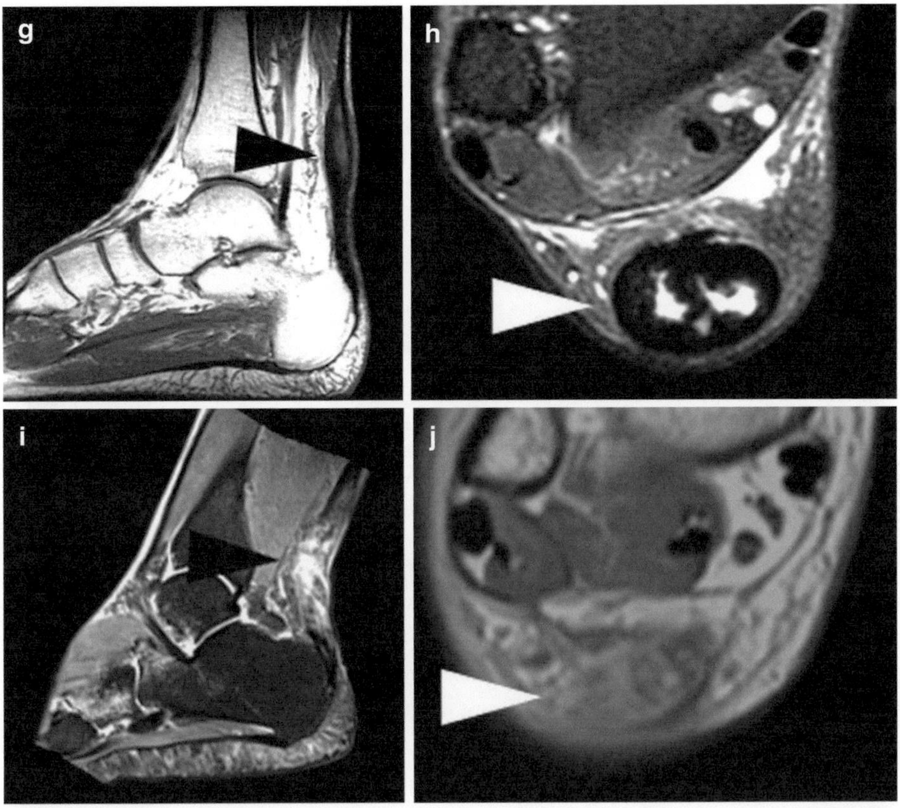

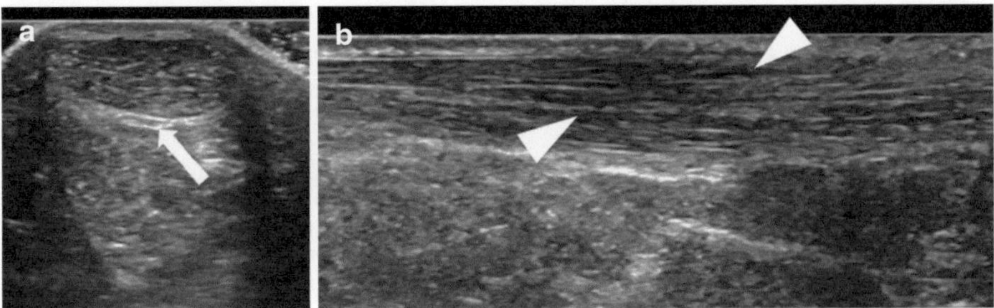

Fig. 1.9 (continued)

Fig. 1.10 Mild Achilles tendinosis. (**a**) Short-axis ultrasound of mild Achilles tendinosis demonstrates (**a**) mild disorganization of the normally straight and taut fibers with increased intrasubstance fluid, resulting in a bulbous thickening (white arrow) of the mid-tendon. (**b**) Long-axis imaging shows the increased interstitial fluid between the thickened tendon fibers (white arrowheads)

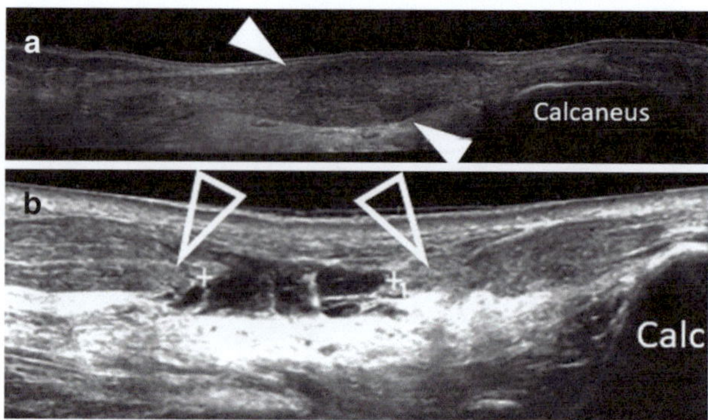

Fig. 1.11 Severe Achilles tendinosis and complete tendon tear. (**a**) Large FOV long-axis imaging demonstrates the fusiform shape (white arrowheads) of a moderately severe tendinosis through the length of the tendon from the myotendinous junction to the calcaneal insertion. (**b**) Large FOV long-axis imaging reveals a complete midsubstance Achilles tear with retraction of the torn fibers (white open arrowheads), resulting in an anechoic gap

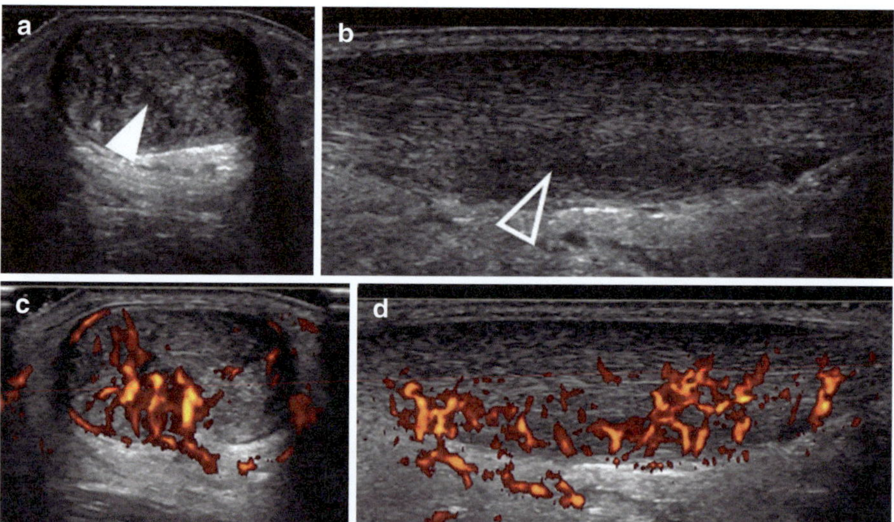

Fig. 1.12 Severe Achilles tendinosis. (**a**) Short-axis imaging demonstrates the increased anechoic areas (white arrowhead) interdigitating with the thickened irregular fibers which appear very punctate on short-axis imaging. (**b**) Long-axis imaging also shows the anechoic gaps (white open arrowhead) in this severe tendinosis. The application of power Doppler reveals the anechoic regions with increased vascularity in the (**c**) short and (**d**) long-axis views of the tendon

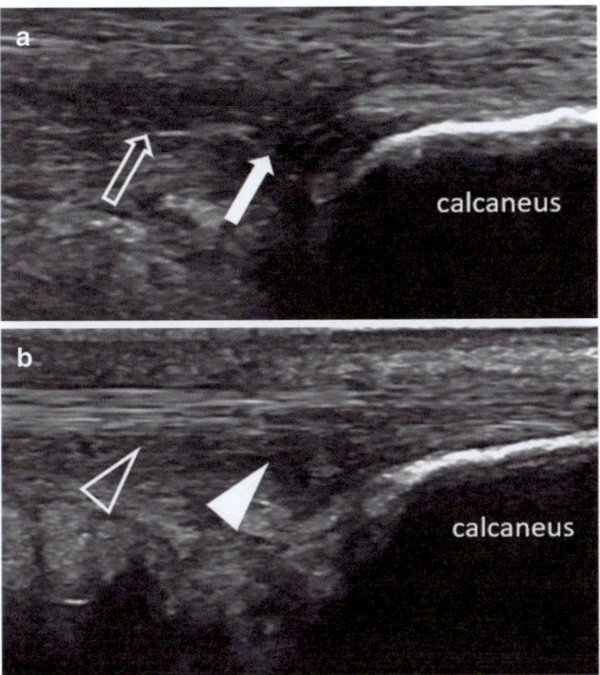

Fig. 1.13 Anisotropy of the Achilles tendon. (**a**) Long-axis ultrasound near the Achilles calcaneal insertion shows a lack of organized tendon fibers (white open arrow) with a more hypoechoic region (white arrow) near the calcaneus. This represents artifact because of the off-angle transducer position. This could easily be mistaken for tendinosis and tendon tear. (**b**) With realignment of the ultrasound transducer to a position parallel to tendon fibers, the organized striated appearance of the normal tendon is evident (white open arrowhead). The area near the calcaneus did improve in appearance but shows a hypoechoic area in the fibers along the deep surface of the tendon representing a small partial tear of the tendon (white arrowhead)

MRI is an excellent method of assessing the integrity of a tendon (Figs. 1.14, 1.15, 1.16, 1.17, and 1.18) [9, 12]. Understanding the variable contour of the tendons is important as the tendon may appear slightly different in signal and contour throughout its course. The tendons widen slightly as they insert on their respective osseous attachments and that the signal and shape may vary as they pass over osseous prominences. For example, the posterior tibialis tendon should not be mistakenly called as a tear as it widens to insert on the medial navicular. Peroneal tendons are typically slightly flattened as they pass behind the fibular retromalleolar groove [9].

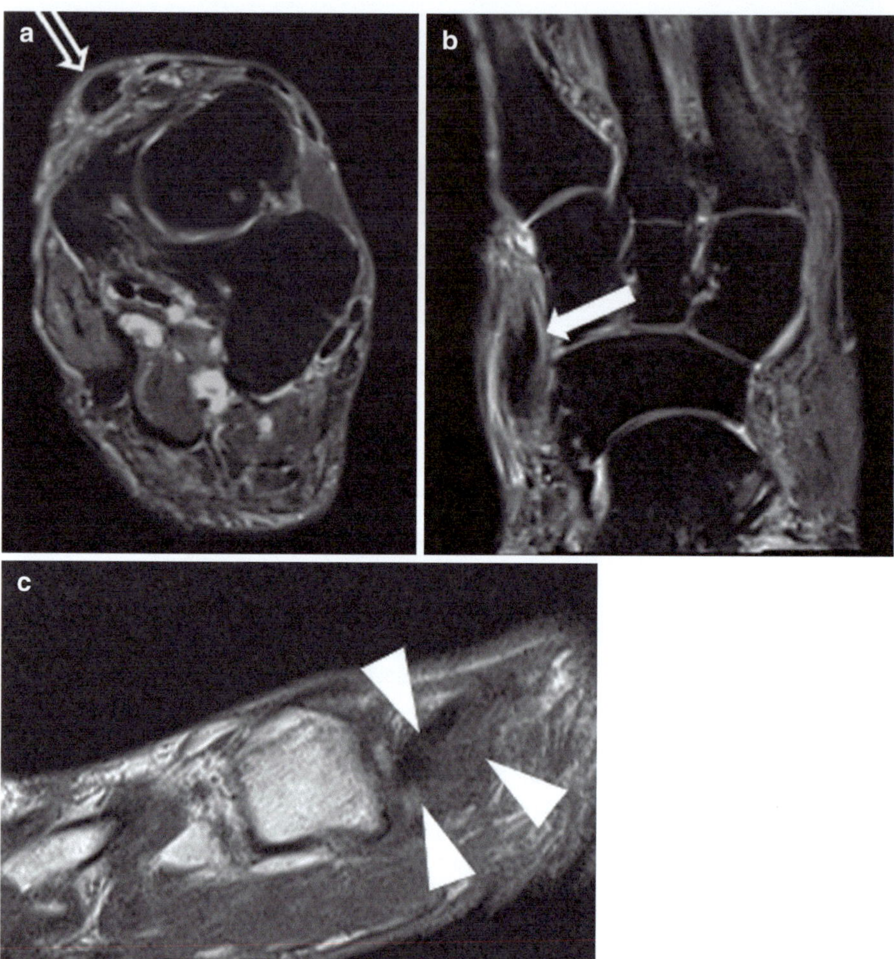

Fig. 1.14 Distal anterior tibial tendinosis – grade 2. A 72-year-old male runner presents with a painful mass in his medial midfoot. (**a**) Short-axis STIR demonstrates a focal mass corresponding to the enlarged anterior tibialis tendon (white open arrow). (**b**) Long-axis T2 fat-suppressed imaging reveals the thickened, striated appearance of the distal 4 cm of the tendon (white arrow) just at and distal to the inferior extensor retinaculum. (**c**) Long-axis PD-weighted imaging at the medial cuneiform anterior tibialis insertional site demonstrates the intermediate signal (white arrowheads) in an area where the tendon would normally be uniformly low signal

The tendons have to make the 90-degree turn from the leg and ankle into the foot. This results in the tendons going through a complex angle and creates a pitfall known as magic angle effect in which the organized tendon collagen bundles are oriented 55° relative to the static magnetic induction field, resulting in apparent increased intrasubstance signal in the tendon on T1-weighted and proton density pulse sequences. This signal phenomenon is less evident on T2 and short tau inversion recovery (STIR) sequences (Fig. 1.19). This may mistakenly be interpreted as tendinosis [1, 9, 16, 17].

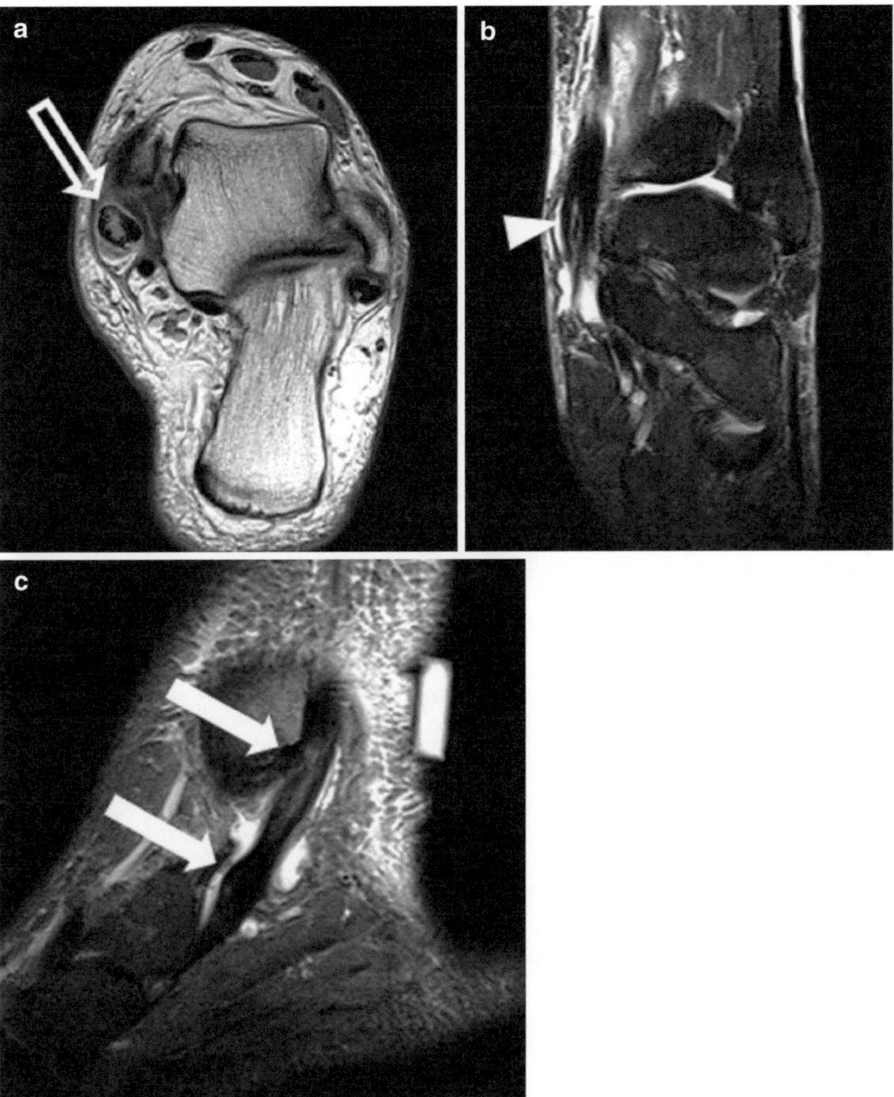

Fig. 1.15 Posterior tibialis tendon intrasubstance tear. (**a**) Short-axis T1-weighted imaging demonstrates the enlarged contour of the posterior tibialis tendon with extensive intrasubstance tearing (white open arrow), while the adjacent flexor tendons are normal in caliber. (**b**) Coronal STIR demonstrates the slightly striated appearance (white arrowhead) of the intrasubstance tear with associated tenosynovitis. (**c**) Sagittal T2 fat-suppressed imaging reveals the length of this pathology in the tendon (white arrow) with the fluid in the adjacent tendon sheaths

Radiographs are not considered a primary direct visualization tool for tendons. The Achilles tendon is an exception to that rule. The tendon is outlined by surrounding subcutaneous fat and Kager's fat pad, and its contour is clearly visualized (Fig. 1.20). The radiographic assessment of tendon health is based on its contour, normally straight and thin. It may become diffusely thickened or focally bulbous,

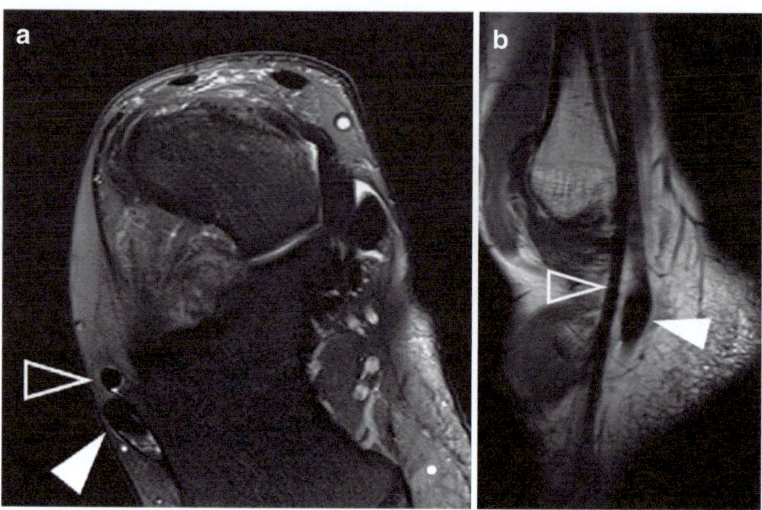

Fig. 1.16 Peroneal longus focal tendinosis. (**a**) Axial T2 fat-suppressed and (**b**) sagittal T1-weighted imaging reveals the normal taut slender uniform appearance of the normal peroneus brevis tendon (white open arrowhead), while the peroneus longus focal tendinosis (white arrowhead) is evident as bulbous swelling in the tendon just at and distal to the peroneal tubercle

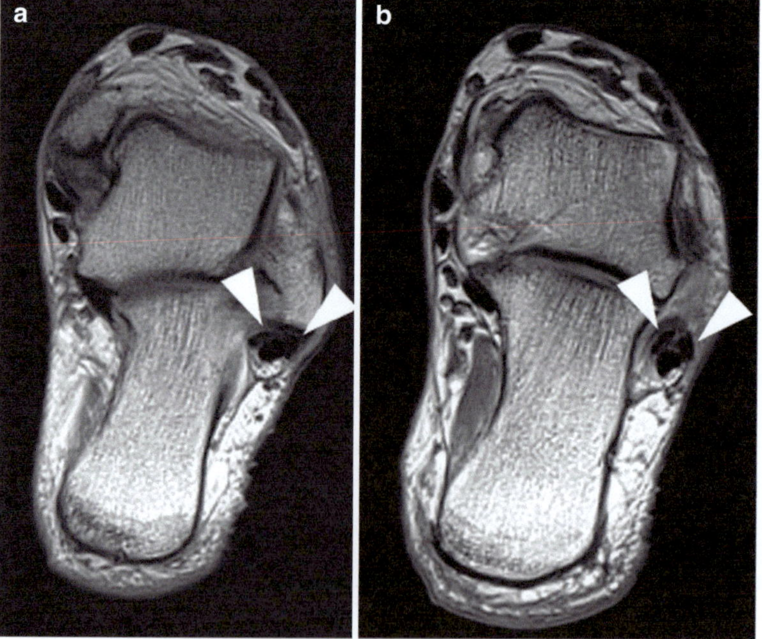

Fig. 1.17 Peroneus brevis split tear. (**a**) and (**b**) Short-axis PD-weighted imaging reveals the two distinct peroneus brevis hemi-tendons (white arrowheads) resulting from a split tear as the peroneal tendons pass dorsal to the retromalleolar groove, resulting from the microtrauma of the peroneus longus tendon crowding the peroneus brevis against the distal fibular cortex

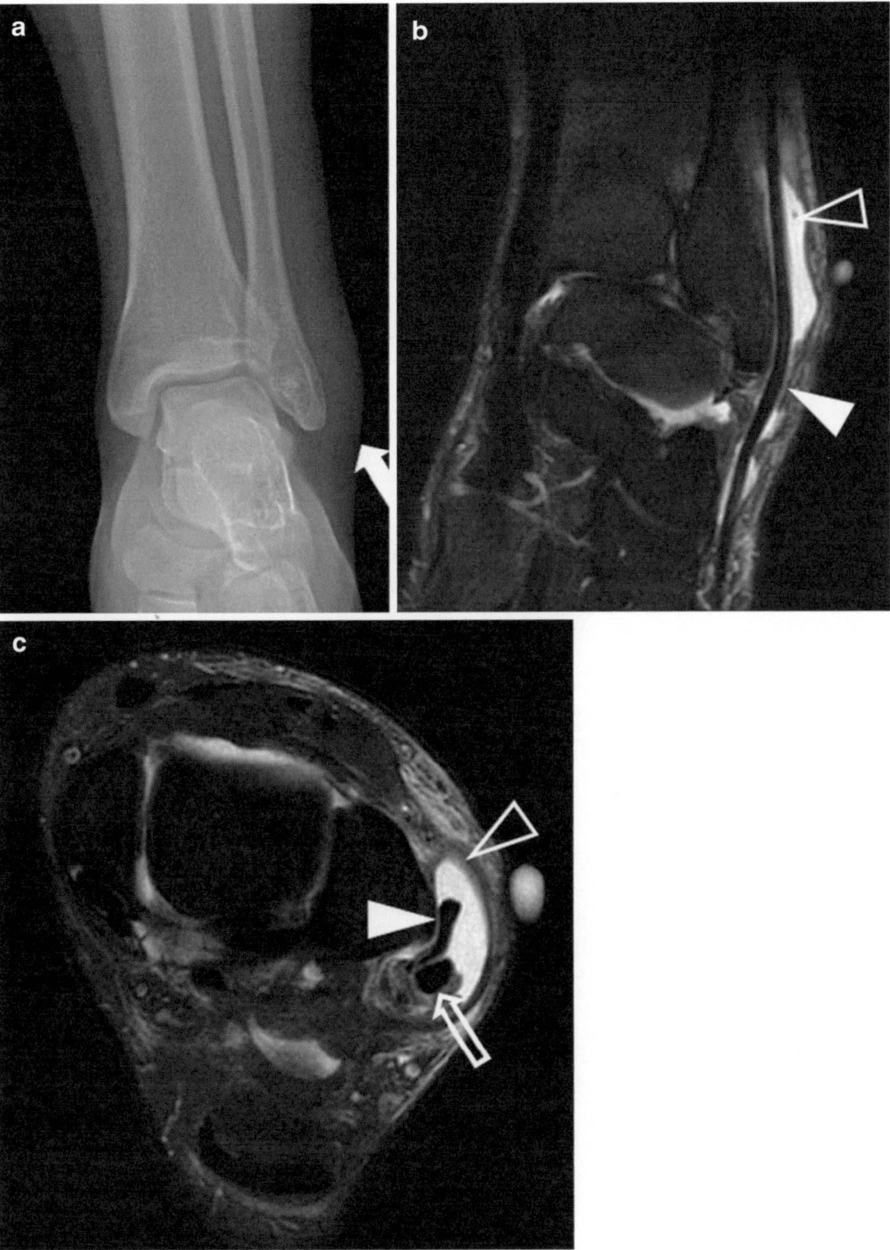

Fig. 1.18 Peroneal brevis dislocation with tenosynovitis. (**a**) AP radiograph demonstrates significant lateral soft tissue swelling (white arrow) and correlates with the (**b**) coronal STIR image. The peroneus brevis tendon overlies the lateral aspect of the fibular (white arrowhead) with associated tenosynovitis (white open arrowhead). (**c**) Axial T2 fat-suppressed imaging reveals the elongate comma-shaped deformity of the peroneus brevis (white arrowhead) with lateral subluxation. The peroneus longus tendon is normal in contour and caliber. The tendon sheath is markedly distended with fluid (white open arrowhead)

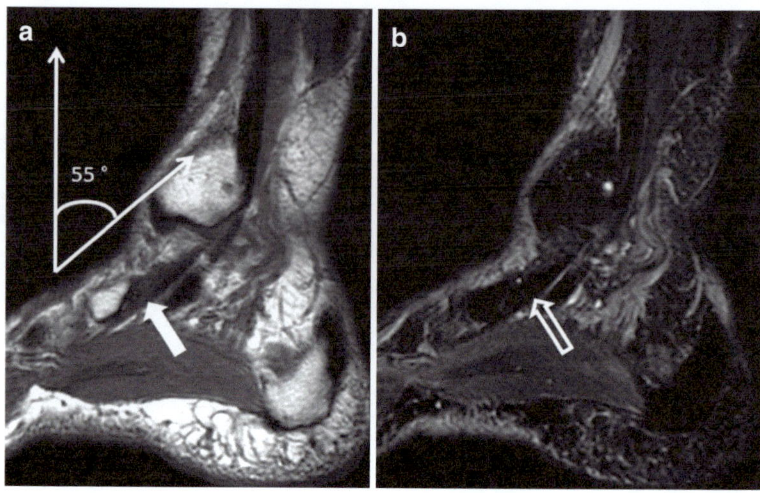

Fig. 1.19 Magic angle artifact. (**a**) Sagittal T1-weighted imaging demonstrates the magic angle phenomenon in the distal posterior tibialis tendon as it approaches the navicular insertion (white arrow). The normal tendon demonstrates intermediate signal in the segment of the organized tendon fibers at 55° angle from the long axis of the magnet. (**b**) When the same area is imaged with a sagittal STIR, the intermediate signal disappears, and the normal low tendon signal is evident

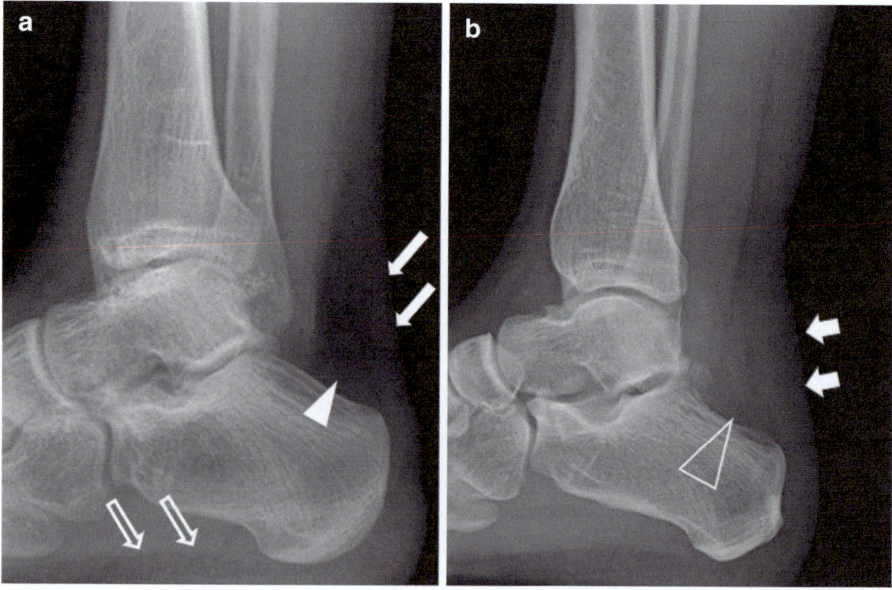

Fig. 1.20 The Achilles tendon appearance without and with tendinopathy. (**a**) Lateral radiograph shows the taut straight Achilles tendon (white arrow) outlined by the thin skin surface superficially and Kager's fat pad along its deep surface (white arrowhead). The plantar margin of the fascia is evident against the plantar fat pad (white open arrow). (**b**) Lateral radiograph demonstrates the fusiform thickening of the tendon in the setting of severe tendinopathy (white arrow). The Kager's fat pad is effaced by the significant tendon swelling (white open arrowhead)

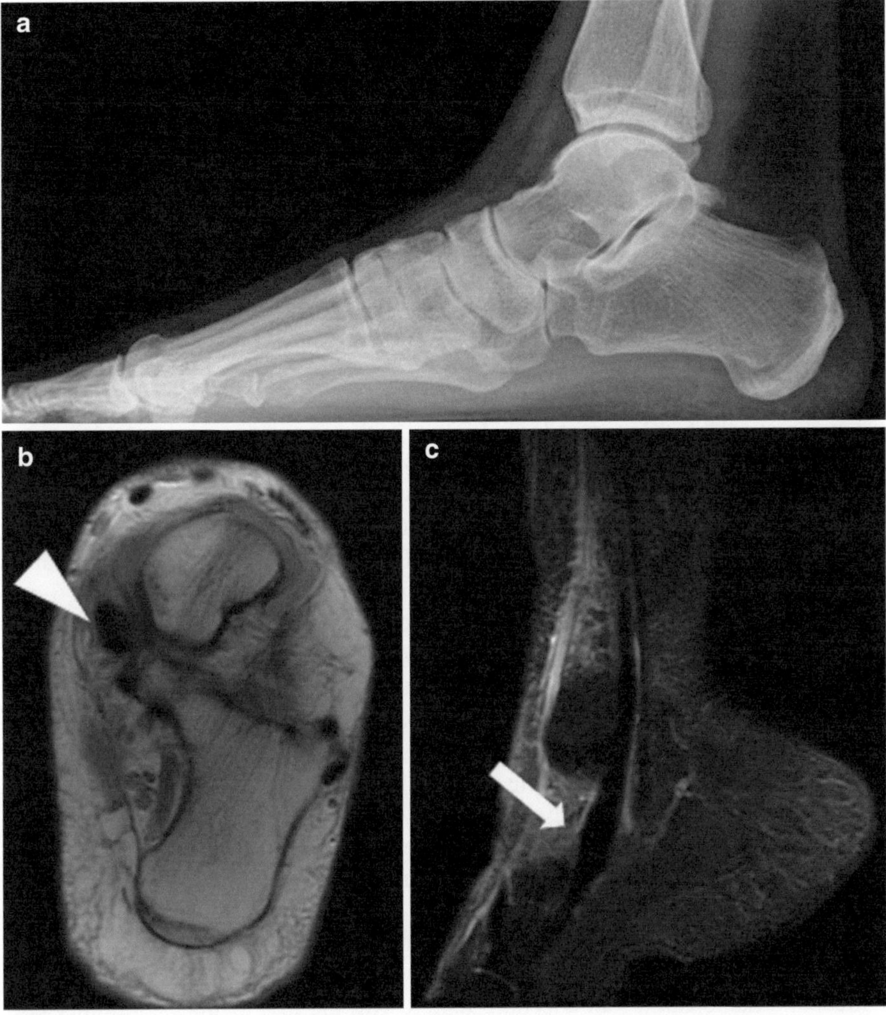

Fig. 1.21 Painful flatfoot deformity. (**a**) Lateral weight-bearing radiograph reveals a mild pes planus alignment. (**b**) Short-axis T1-weighted imaging reveals mild enlargement of the posterior tibialis tendon contour (white arrowhead). (**c**) This is confirmed on sagittal T2-weighted imaging, which demonstrates the bulbous enlargement of the posterior tibialis tendon just as it passes the medial malleolar tip (white arrow)

representing progressive tendinosis. There may be associated dystrophic calcification. It may demonstrate focal attenuation, typical of partial tear, or marked soft tissue with limited tendon visualization in complete tear [18].

Secondary effects of tendon injury can be demonstrated radiographically. Soft tissue swelling and osseous malalignment are secondary indicators of tendon pathology. For example, a weight-bearing image in a 55-year-old female will demonstrate the pes planus alignment and hindfoot valgus as a consequence of posterior tibialis dysfunction (Fig. 1.21) [11, 19].

Ligaments

Understanding the anatomy of the specific ligament in question is key to imaging evaluation. Each ligament has its own unique orientation and structure, composed of a variable number of individual bundles such as the deep and superficial deltoid ligament [20], dorsal intermediate and plantar bands of the tarsometatarsal ligaments [21], and the interrelation of plantar plate, the deep intermetatarsal ligaments, and the adjacent collateral ligaments [22, 23].

Ligament injury may be graded with grade 1 sprain demonstrated as periligamentous edema with otherwise intact fibers, grade 2 as partial tear of the ligament fibers, and grade 3 as complete tear. As the ligament heals, it initially forms ill-defined edematous fibrovascular tissue. This will continue to evolve over time with a decrease in the edema and degree of ligament thickening [7, 10]. This healing process may take 6–12 months (Fig. 1.22).

Radiographs do not directly visualize the ligaments, but radiographs can be used to assess as well as concomitant injury such as avulsion fractures and assess the abnormal alignment resulting from ligament injury. Soft tissue swelling with a concomitant tibiotalar effusion may be the only sign of ligamentous injury. Subtle malalignment such as widening of the tibiofibular clear space (greater than 6 mm measured 1 cm above the tibiotalar joint), seen in syndesmotic ligament disruption [4, 10, 24], widening of the medial ankle joint space, indicating deltoid ligament injury, or widening of the interspace between the first and second metatarsal bases, seen in Lisfranc ligament disruption (Fig. 1.23) [21, 25]. Weight-bearing imaging remains a key to assessment of anatomic alignment, and stress views may be used, especially in the hindfoot and ankle.

CT provides detail to the alignment and associated bone injuries such as the Weber B distal fibular fracture commonly seen associated with syndesmosis ligament injuries or the multiple smaller avulsion fractures along the plantar aspect of the remaining tarsometatarsal joints [21].

Ultrasound can directly demonstrate superficial ligament injury [8]. The normal ligament is mildly echogenic with a fibrillar architecture (Fig. 1.24) [8–10]. Ultrasound demonstrates an anechoic region with the loss of fiber continuity corresponding to the area of acute tear. There is often some redundancy and retraction of the proximal and distal ligament fibers. As the ligament heals, the ultrasound will demonstrate an evolution of ligament thickening, persistent ill-defined echogenicity, and increased vascularity, consistent with the fibrovascular healing process [5, 9, 10]. Ultrasound can be used in evaluating joint stability in ligament injury when imaged without and with applied stress to the associated joint.

Some ligaments are more accessible than others for evaluation with ultrasound. For example, the anterior talofibular ligament is easily imaged, while the calcaneofibular ligament is more difficult to image. Additionally, ultrasound is extremely operator dependent with great attention to the orientation of the ultrasound transducer to avoid anisotropy (Fig. 1.25). Additionally, imaging small parts requires specialized small, high megahertz transducer that is essential to adequately evaluate the ligaments [7, 9].

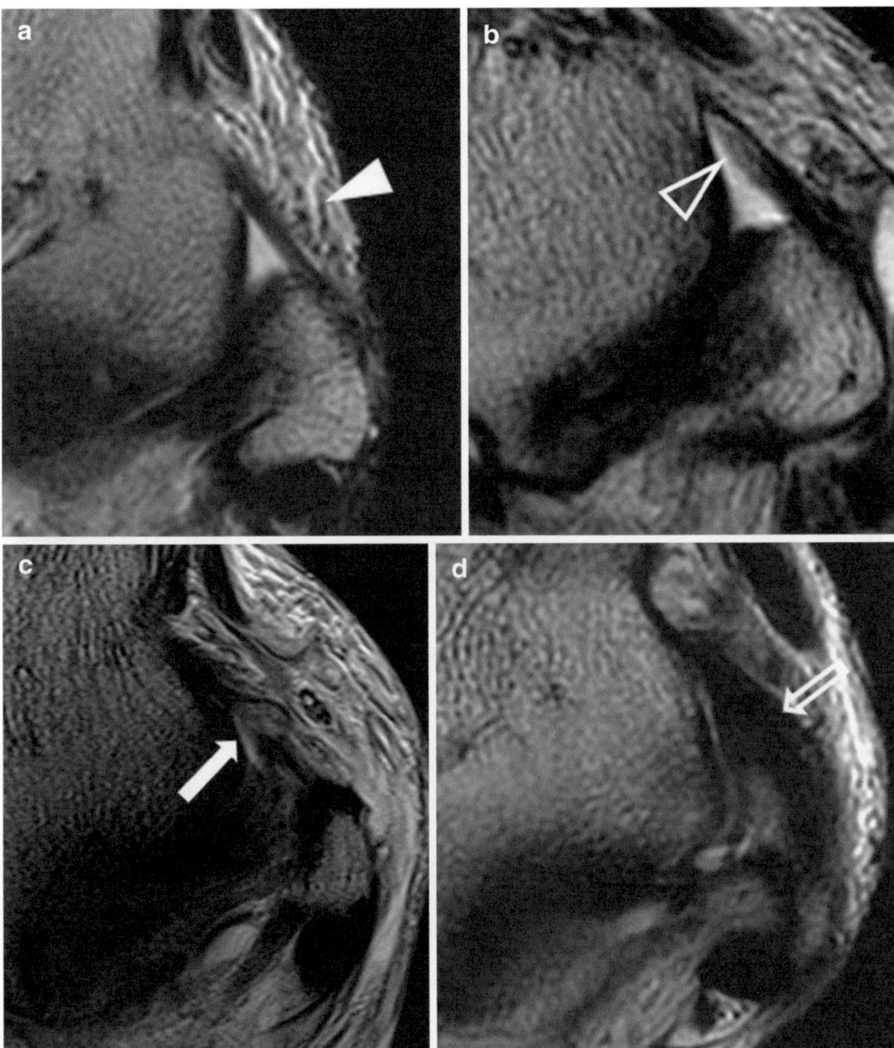

Fig. 1.22 Anterior talofibular ligament (ATFL) sprain. Short-axis PD-weighted imaging demonstrates (**a**) a normal contoured ATFL with adjacent soft tissue edema (white arrowhead) and a small joint effusion, representing a grade 1 sprain. (**b**) A partial (grade 2) ATFL tear is present near the talar attachment (white open arrowhead). (**c**) A complete (grade 3) ATFL tear is present at the talar attachment with ligament fiber retraction (white arow). (**d**) ATFL demonstrates uniform ligament thickening (white open arrow) without adjacent soft tissue edema, consistent with changes related to prior injury

MR imaging clearly delineates the various ligaments in and around the complex osseous anatomy of the ankle and foot [4, 10, 20, 21, 24, 26]. Attention to the patient position and the orientation of the scanner planes will clearly demonstrate the complex anatomy. A wide selection of coils, patient position, and pulse

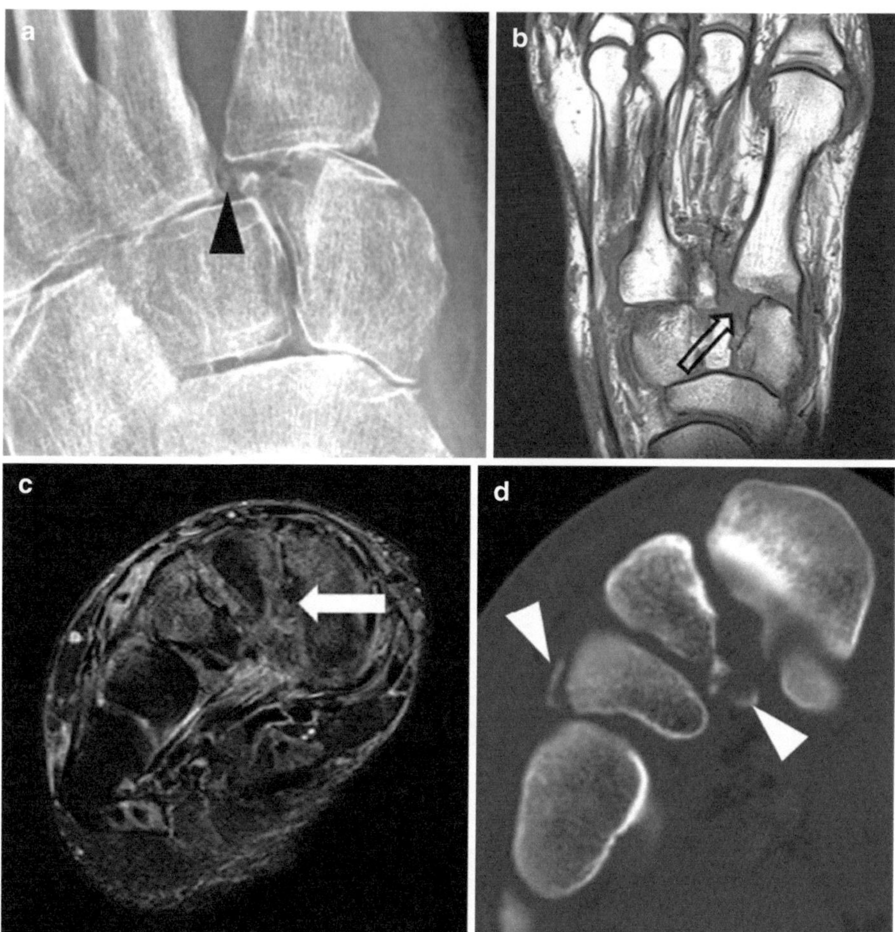

Fig. 1.23 Lisfranc fracture subluxation with fleck sign. (**a**) AP weight-bearing radiograph demonstrates lateral subluxation of at the Lisfranc join. A small cortical avulsion fracture (black arrowhead) is seen just medial to the second metatarsal base, sometimes referred toa a "fleck" sign. (**b**) Long-axis T1-weighted imaging allows direct visualization of the disrupted Lisfranc ligament (black open arrow). (**c**) Short-axis T2 fat-suppressed imaging shows the extensive bone and soft tissue edema with complete disruption of the Lisfranc ligament. (**d**) Short-axis CT demonstrates the multiple small fracture fragments not readily seen on other imaging modalities (white arrowheads)

sequences can be employed to accomplish the assessment. One must consider that the ligaments take on a different orientation and appearance depending on whether the patient is in plantar flexion or dorsiflexion, particularly in the hindfoot. The appearance of the ligament will also depend on the timing from injury in which it is imaged.

Fig. 1.24 Normal ATFL with effusion. Short-axis ultrasound imaging of the ATFL reveals the normal caliber (white arrowhead) and fine fibrillar appearance of the ligament. The ligament is well seen against a small joint effusion (white open arrow)

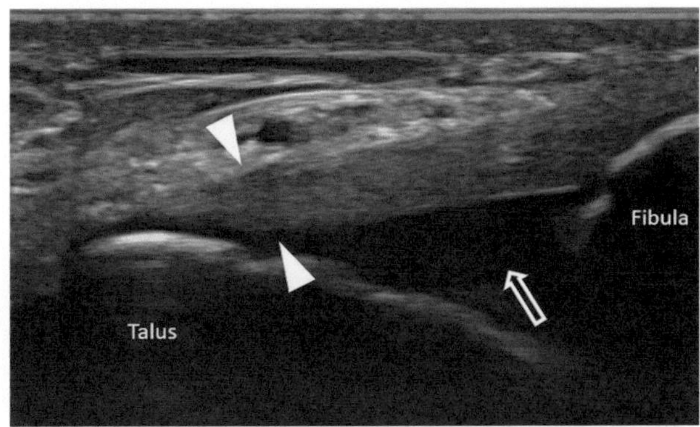

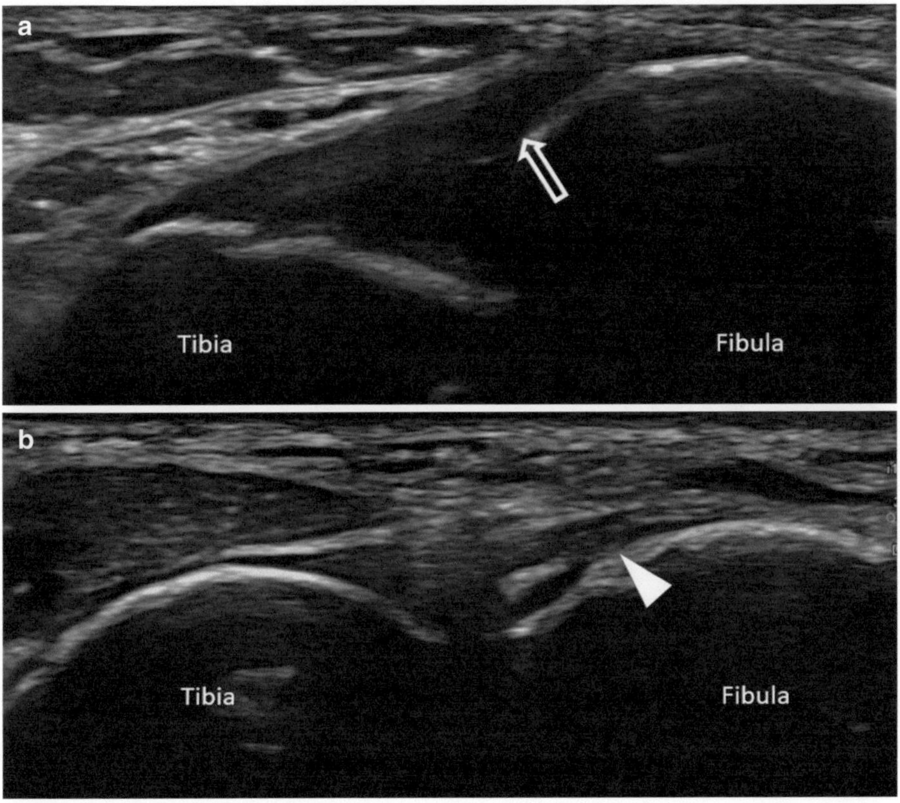

Fig. 1.25 Anisotropy. (**a**) Short-axis scanning at the anteroinferior tibiofibular ligament (AITFL) demonstrates a focal anechoic region (white open arrow) representing artifact related to scanning technique. The organized fibers of the ligament at being scanned out of plane which creates the apparent loss of signal that could be misinterpreted as an area of ligament disruption. (**b**) Correction of the orientation of the transducer reveals the ligament to be fully intact (white arrowhead)

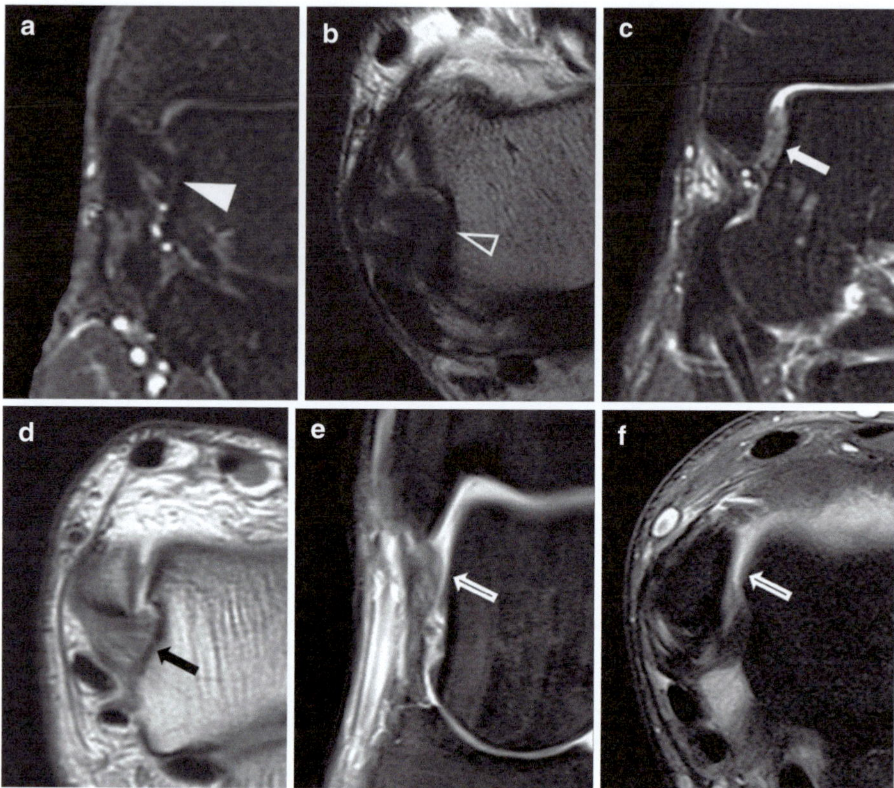

Fig. 1.26 Deltoid ligament sprain. (**a**) Coronal STIR imaging demonstrated the uniform low signal of the normal deep deltoid ligament (white arrowhead). (**b**) Short-axis PD-weighted imaging through this normal deep deltoid ligament (white open arrowhead). (**c**) Coronal T2-weighted imaging shows a grade 2 partial tear of the deep tibiotalar component of the deltoid ligament (white arrow). (**d**) Short-axis T1-weighted imaging of the same grade 2 sprain reveals a striated intermediate signal (black arrow). (**e**) Coronal T2 fat-suppressed and (**f**) axial T2 fat-suppressed imaging reveals a complete disruption of the anterior tibiotalar component of the deep deltoid ligament (white open arrow)

The normal ligament is uniformly low signal on all pulse sequences. Acute injury to the ligament will be demonstrated as intermediate to high intrasubstance signal on proton density, and fluid-sensitive sequences with higher grade injuries demonstrate increasing fiber disorganization and thickening of the ligament fibers.

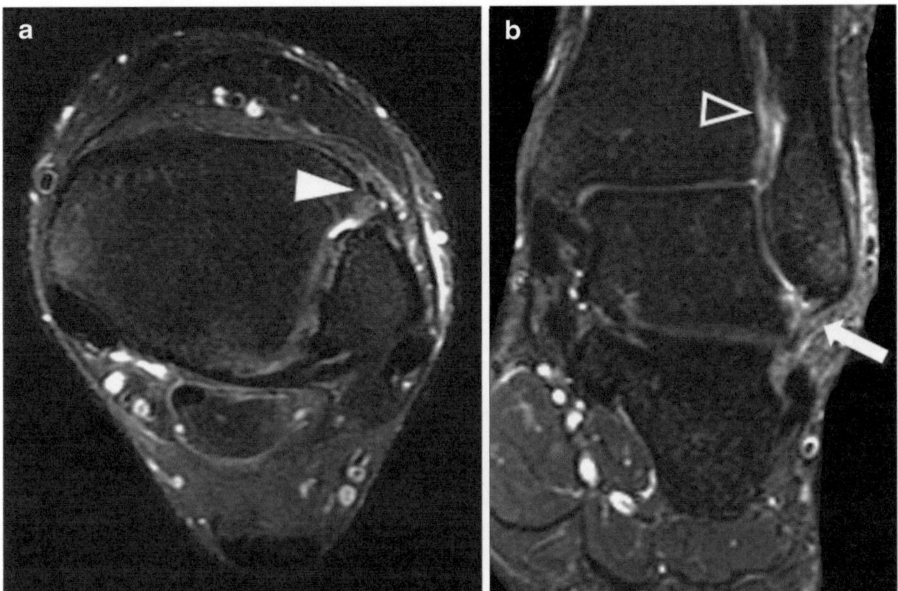

Fig. 1.27 High ankle sprain. (**a**) Axial T2 fat-suppressed imaging demonstrates grade 2 sprain of the anterior tibiofibular ligament with intermediate signal in the ligament (white arrowhead). Adjacent soft tissue swelling is present. (**b**) Coronal T2 fat-suppressed imaging demonstrates the tear of the inferior interosseous ligament with fluid extending proximally into the defect created by the ligament loss (white open arrowhead). Note the disruption of the ATFL (white arrow) as well as marrow contusion of the distal fibular tip

Complete tears are often accompanied by retraction and irregularity of the ligament fibers (Fig. 1.26) [5, 20, 21]. As the ligament begins to heal, the ligament contour is thickened with loss of defined ligament fibers and typically with peri-ligamentous edema. This tends to evolve over time with decrease in ligament contour and decrease in ligament signal [10]. Associated bone marrow contusions may be present in addition to the soft tissue injuries (Fig. 1.27).

In the forefoot, the complexity of the capsule and pericapsular ligaments requires a detailed knowledge of that anatomy regardless of the modality (Fig. 1.28). Attention to the orientation of the specific joint in question requires attention to three dimensions to maximize anatomic detail, and a very focused small FOV will yield the needed detail [22, 23, 27, 28].

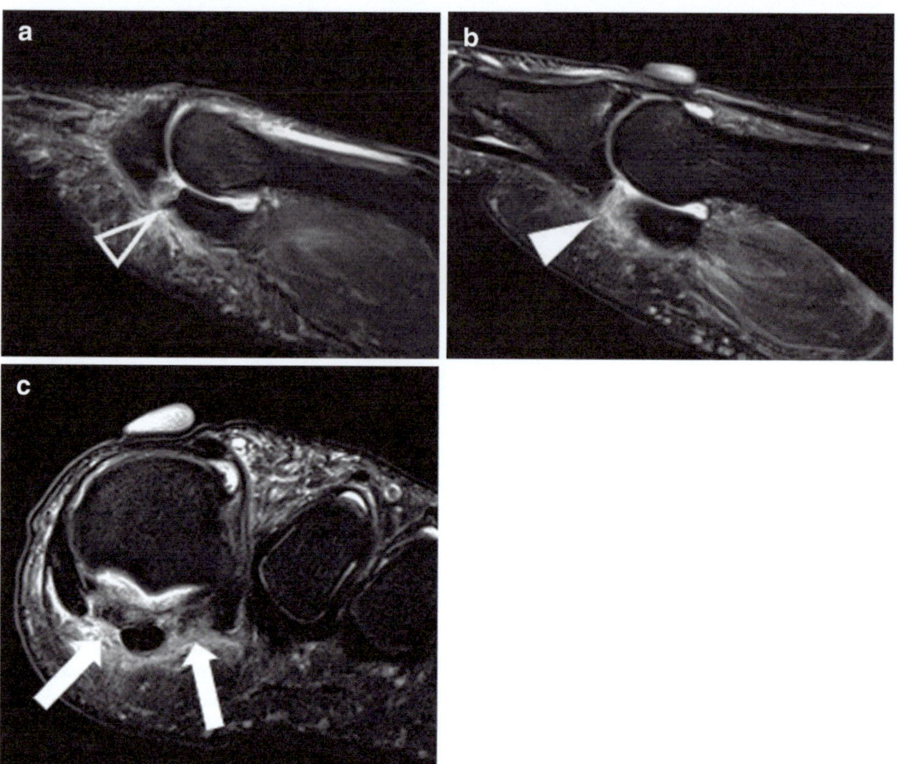

Fig. 1.28 Turf toe. Sagittal T2 fat-suppressed imaging through the (**a**) medial sesamoid and (**b**) lateral sesamoid demonstrates complete disruption of the medial (white arrowhead) and lateral (white open arrowhead) plantar plate. (**c**) Short-axis T2 fat-suppressed imaging demonstrates the soft tissue edema and disruption of the sesamoid-phalangeal ligaments (white arrows)

Summary

Understanding of normal anatomy of the tendons and ligaments and the histopathology of acute and chronic injury facilitates selection and interpretation of diagnostic imaging. Each imaging modality plays a specific role in the assessment of injuries of the ankle and foot. Radiographs provide information about alignment and bone injury with indirect information about the soft tissues. CT demonstrates detailed osseous information. Ultrasound demonstrates detailed anatomic information about ligaments and tendons, and while it is operator dependent, it is the one tool that provides dynamic information. MRI serves as excellent data regarding acute and chronic soft tissue injury as well as subtle bone injury.

References

1. Sofka CM. Technical considerations: best practices for MR imaging of the foot and ankle. Magn Reson Imaging Clin N Am. 2017;25(1):1–10. https://doi.org/10.1016/j.mric.2016.08.001.
2. Bruno F, Arrigoni F, Palumbo P, Natella R, Splendiani A, Di Cesare E, Guglielmi G, Masciocchi C, Barile A. Weight-bearing MR imaging of knee, ankle and foot. Semin Musculoskelet Radiol. 2019;23(6):594–602. https://doi.org/10.1055/s-0039-1697940.
3. Tuominen EKJ, Kankare J, Koskinen SK, Mattila KT. Weight-bearing CT imaging of the lower extremity. AJR Am J Roentgenol. 2013;200(1):146–8. https://doi.org/10.2214/AJR.12.8481.
4. Kellett JJ, Lovell GA, Eriksen DA, Sampson MJ. Diagnostic imaging of ankle syndesmosis injuries: a general review. J Med Imaging Radiat Oncol. 2018;62(2):159–68. https://doi.org/10.1111/1754-9485.12708.
5. Cao S, Wang C, Ma X, Wang X, Huang J, Zhang C. Imaging diagnosis for chronic lateral ankle ligament injury: a systemic review with meta-analysis. J Orthop Surg Res. 2018;13(1):122–35. https://doi.org/10.1186/s13018-018-0811-4.
6. Krahenbuhl N, Horn-Lang T, Hintermann B, Knupp M. The subtalar joint: a complex mechanism. EFORT Open Rev. 2017;2(7):309–16. https://doi.org/10.1302/2058-5241.2.160050.
7. Alves T, Dong Q, Jacobson J, Yablon C, Gandikota G. Normal and injured ankle ligaments on ultrasonography with magnetic resonance imaging correlation. J Ultrasound Med. 2019;38(2):513–28. https://doi.org/10.1002/jum.14716.
8. Sconfienza LM, Orlandi D, Lacelli F, Serafini G, Silvestri E. Dynamic high-resolution US of ankle and midfoot ligaments: normal anatomic structure and imaging technique. Radiographics. 2015;35(1):164–78. https://doi.org/10.1148/rg.351130139.
9. Taljanovic MS, Alcala JA, Gimber LH, Rieke JD, Chilvers MM, Latt DL. High-resolution US and MR imaging of peroneal tendon injuries. Radiographics. 2015;35(1):179–99. https://doi.org/10.1148/rg.351130062.
10. Linklater JM, Hayter CL, Vu D. Imaging of acute capsuloligamentous sports injuries in the ankle and foot: sports imaging series. Radiology. 2017;283(3):644–62. https://doi.org/10.1148/radiol.2017152442.
11. Flores DV, Mejía Gómez C, Fernández Hernando M, Davis MA, Pathria MN. Adult acquired flatfoot deformity: anatomy, biomechanics, staging, and imaging findings. Radiographics. 2019;39(5):1437–60. https://doi.org/10.1148/rg.2019190046.
12. Albano D, Martinelli N, Bianchi A, Romeo G, Bulfamante G, Galia M, Sconfienza LM. Posterior tibial tendon dysfunction: Clinical and magnetic resonance imaging findings having histology as reference standard. Eur J Radiol. 2018;99:55–61. https://doi.org/10.1016/j.ejrad.2017.12.005.
13. Docking SI, Ooi CC, Connell D. Tendinopathy: is imaging telling us the entire story? J Orthop Sports Phys Ther. 2015;45(11):842–52. https://doi.org/10.2519/jospt.2015.5880.
14. Kahn KM, Cook JL, Bonar F, Harcourt P, Astrom M. Histopathology of common tendinopathies. Update and implications for clinical management. Sports Med. 1999;27(6):393–408. https://doi.org/10.2165/00007256-199927060-00004.
15. Varghese A, Bianchi S. Ultrasound of tibialis anterior muscle and tendon: anatomy, technique of examination, normal and pathologic appearance. J Ultrasound. 2013;17(2):113–23. https://doi.org/10.1007/s40477-013-0060-7.
16. Lee MH, Chung CB, Cho JH, Mohana-Borges AV, Pretterklieber ML, Trudell DJ, Resnick D. Tibialis anterior tendon and extensor retinaculum: imaging in cadavers and patients with tendon tear. AJR Am J Roentgenol. 2006;187(2):W161–8. https://doi.org/10.2214/AJR.05.0073.
17. Rosenberg ZS, Beltran J, Bencardino JT. MR imaging of the ankle and foot. Radiographics. 2000;20:S153–79. https://doi.org/10.1148/radiographics.20.suppl_1.g00oc26s153.
18. Wijesekera NT, Calder JD, Lee JC. Imaging in the assessment and management of Achilles tendinopathy and paratendinitis. Semin Musculoskelet Radiol. 2011;15(1):89–100. https://doi.org/10.1055/s-0031-1271961.

19. Lin YC, Mhuircheartaigh JN, Lamb J, Kung JW, Yablon CM, Wu JS. Imaging of adult flatfoot: correlation of radiographic measurements with MRI. AJR Am J Roentgenol. 2015;204(2):354–9. https://doi.org/10.2214/AJR.14.12645.
20. Crim J, Longenecker LG. MRI and surgical findings in deltoid ligament tears. AJR Am J Roentgenol. 2015;201(1):W63–9. https://doi.org/10.2214/AJR.13.11702.
21. Siddiqui NA, Galizia MS, Almusa E, Omar IM. Evaluation of the tarsometatarsal joint using conventional radiography, CT, and MR imaging. Radiographics. 2014;34(2):514–31. https://doi.org/10.1148/rg.342125215.
22. Yamada AF, Crema MD, Nery C, Baumfeld D, Mann TS, Skaf AY, Fernandes ADRC. Second and third metatarsophalangeal plantar plate tears: diagnostic performance of direct and indirect MRI features using surgical findings as the reference standard. AJR Am J Roentgenol. 2017;209(2):W100–8. https://doi.org/10.2214/AJR.16.17276.
23. Nery C, Baumfeld D, Umans H, Yamada AF. MR imaging of the plantar plate: normal anatomy, turf toe, and other injuries. Magn Reson Imaging Clin N Am. 2017;25(1):127–44. https://doi.org/10.1016/j.mric.2016.08.007.
24. Walter WR, Hirschmann A, Alaia EF, Tafur M, Rosenberg ZS. Normal anatomy and traumatic injury of the midtarsal (Chopart) joint complex: an imaging primer. Radiographics. 2018;39:136–52. https://doi.org/10.1148/rg.2019180102.
25. Sripanich Y, Weinberg MW, Krahenbuhl N, Rungprai C, Milles MK, Saltzman CL, Barg A. Imaging Lisfranc injury: a systematic literature review. Skelet Radiol. 2020;49(1):31–53. https://doi.org/10.1007/s00256-019-03282-1.
26. Ablimit A, Ding HY, Liu LG. Magnetic resonance imaging of the Lisfranc ligament. J Orthop Surg Res. 2018;13(1):282–5. https://doi.org/10.1186/s13018-018-0968-x.
27. Duan X, Li L, Wei DQ, Liu M, Yu X, Xu Z, Long Y, Xiang Z. Role of magnetic resonance imaging versus ultrasound for detection of plantar plate tear. J Orthop Surg Res. 2017;12(1):14–21. https://doi.org/10.1186/s13018-016-0507-6.
28. Cran JM, Phancao JP. Imaging of a turf toe. Radiol Clin N Am. 2016;54(5):969–78. https://doi.org/10.1016/j.rcl.2016.04.010.

Turf Toe Injuries

2

Craig C. Akoh, Rishin Kadakia, and Selene G. Parekh

Introduction

Turf toe is a broad term used to describe injuries to the capsuloligamentous complex of the first metatarsophalangeal joint (MTPJ). Turf toe injuries represent a common forefoot injury in athletes [1, 2]. Bowers first described turf toe injuries in a case series of West Virginia football players in 1976, reporting an incidence of 5.4 cases of turf toe injuries per year [2]. In 1978, Coker et al. found an incidence of 6.0 cases per year at the University of Arkansas [1]. Clanton et al. in 1986 reported an incidence of 3.8 turf toe cases per year at Rice University [3]. Rodeo et al. reported that turf toe injuries occur in up to 45% of National Football League (NFL) players [4]. Most recently, Hunt et al. found that the overall incidence of turf toe injuries in National Collegiate Athletics Association (NCAA) foot players was 0.062 per 1000 athlete-exposures [5].

The mechanism of turf toe injuries is commonly due to a hyperflexion of the first MTPJ, leading to disruption of the plantar capsular structures of the great toe [4]. Less commonly, sand toe injuries can be caused by hyperflexion of the first MTPJ as a dancer lands from a jeté (leap) or landing while playing volleyball, leading to dorsal capsule disruption [6, 7]. Traumatic hallux valgus and traumatic varus injuries can occur from angular injury forces [8]. Other risk factors for sustaining turf toe injuries include flexible shoe wear and participating in sporting activities on artificial surfaces [1, 2, 4, 5]. Hunt et al. found that there was an 85% higher risk for sustaining turf toe injuries on third-generation artificial grass surfaces (longer grass fibers and a sand/rubber infill) compared to natural grass surfaces [5]. Turf toe injuries can affect one's ability to perform high-end running and cutting during athletic activities, leading to substantial time missed from sporting activities [3, 9].

C. C. Akoh (✉) · R. Kadakia · S. G. Parekh
Department of Orthopaedic Surgery, Duke University, Durham, NC, USA
e-mail: craig_akoh@rush.edu; rkadaki@emory.edu

© Springer Nature Switzerland AG 2022
J. D. Cain, M. V. Hogan (eds.), *Tendon and Ligament Injuries of the Foot and Ankle*,
https://doi.org/10.1007/978-3-031-10490-9_2

Anatomy/Biomechanics

The hallux MTPJ capsuloligamentous complex is a complex structure composed of both static and dynamic stabilizers. The first MTPJ bears 40–60% of one's body weight during ambulation [10]. Additionally, the first MTPJ absorbs up to eight times of one's body weight during running and jumping activities [11]. The most important static stabilizer of the hallux MTPJ is the plantar plate apparatus, which is a fibrocartilaginous rectangular confluence of the plantar capsule and periosteum of the metatarsal bone [12]. Lucas et al.'s cadaveric study showed that the hallux plantar plate originates 17.29 mm proximal to the MTPJ on the metatarsal head and inserts 0.33 mm distal to the MTPJ onto the base of the proximal phalanx [13]. The footprint of the distal insertion of the plantar plate is 6.33 mm in the sagittal plane. The main function of the plantar plate is to resist dorsal subluxation of the proximal phalanx. The sesamoid-ligamentous complex is imbedded within the plantar plate, and it is comprised of the tibial/fibular sesamoid bones, medial/lateral collateral ligaments, medial/lateral phalangeal-sesamoid ligaments, and intersesamoid ligament (Fig. 2.1) [12, 14]. The larger tibial sesamoid is separated from the smaller fibula sesamoid by the sesamoid crista. The sesamoid complex serves as a fulcrum for the flexor digitorum brevis muscles to generate more power during active plantarflexion of the hallux MTPJ [15]. The medial and lateral collateral ligaments provide valgus and varus stabilization to the first MTPJ, respectively. The bony structures of the shallow concave proximal phalanx articular base and biconvex metatarsal head also provide some static stability.

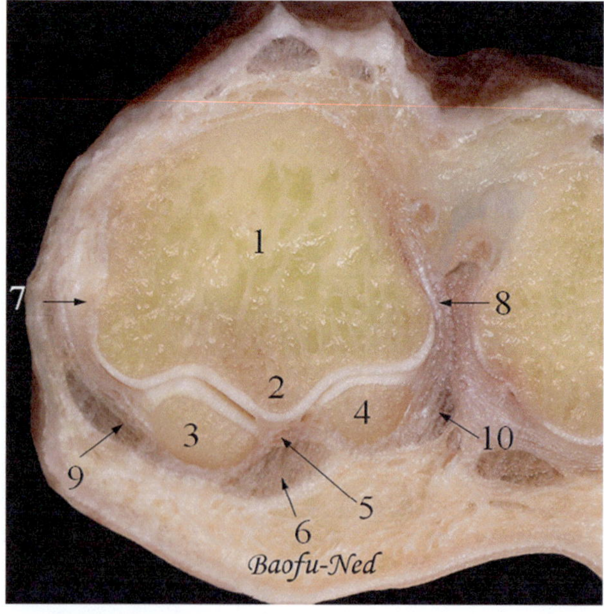

Fig. 2.1 Anatomy of the sesamoid capsuloligamentous complex. Cross-sectional view of the first metatarsophalangeal joint (images provided by Baofu Wei and Ned Amendola): metatarsal head (1), crista (2), tibial sesamoid (3), fibular sesamoid (4), plantar plate (5), flexor hallucis longus (6), medial collateral ligament (7), lateral collateral ligament (8), abductor hallucis (9), adductor hallucis (10)

There are also several dynamic stabilizers of the hallux MTPJ. The flexor hallucis brevis tendon splits into two tendons and inserts onto the sesamoids and plantar plate. The adductor hallucis and abductor hallucis tendons insert into the lateral and medial aspects of the first MTPJ, respectively. The flexor hallucis longus tendon traverses between the tibial and fibula sesamoids, inserting onto the plantar distal phalanx. The flexor hallucis longus tendon provides minimal support to the first MTPJ.

Diagnosis/Clinical Evaluation

Tuft toe injuries present with vague pain and minimal swelling around their first MTPJ that is usually elicited with pushing off the great toe during ambulation. Hallux alignment should also be assessed for hallux valgus and hallux varus deformities that are often found in chronic cases as the lateral and medial capsular structures become contracted, respectively. Physical exam includes testing the stability of the MTPJ with dorsal and plantar drawer tests as well as varus and valgus stress testing [11]. Flexor tendon strength should also be evaluated by holding the interphalangeal joint (IPJ) in neutral and having the patient plantarflex against the examiner's finger as it resists the proximal phalanx.

Severe ecchymosis and dorsomedial skin dimpling can signify an irreducible great toe MTPJ [16]. A prominent plantar metatarsal head along with hyperflexed proximal phalanx can indicate a dorsal MTPJ dislocation that requires urgent reduction. Patients with plantar MTPJ dislocation of the first toe may have a dorsal metatarsal head that is less prominent than dorsal MTPJ dislocations [17].

Classification/Imaging

Weight-bearing plain radiographs of the great toe should include three orthogonal foot views (AP, lateral, and oblique) to assess for MTPJ reduction, avulsion injuries of the MTPJ, impaction injuries, and proximal sesamoid retraction from the MTPJ. The distal sesamoid-MTPJ distance should be no greater than 3 mm for the tibial sesamoid and 2.7 mm for the fibular sesamoid [18]. A distal sesamoid-MTPJ distance greater than 10.4 mm on the tibial sesamoid or 13.3 mm for the fibular sesamoid is 99% predictive of a plantar plate rupture (Fig. 2.2) [19]. If no sesamoid diastasis is seen and a plantar plate injury is suspected, then a dorsiflexion lateral first MTP stress test can be utilized to assess for proximal sesamoid migration [11]. Waldrop et al. showed that 3.04 mm proximal retraction of the sesamoids occurs during lateral dorsiflexion stress radiographs when three out of four plantar structures were injured (i.e., medial/lateral collateral ligament and medial/lateral phalangeal-sesamoid ligaments were injured) [14]. When all four ligaments are disrupted, 6.96 mm of proximal retraction of the sesamoid bones can be seen on stress radiographs. Sesamoid axial views of the great toe are used to assess for diastasis which is indicative of disruption of the intersesamoid ligament. Bilateral standing

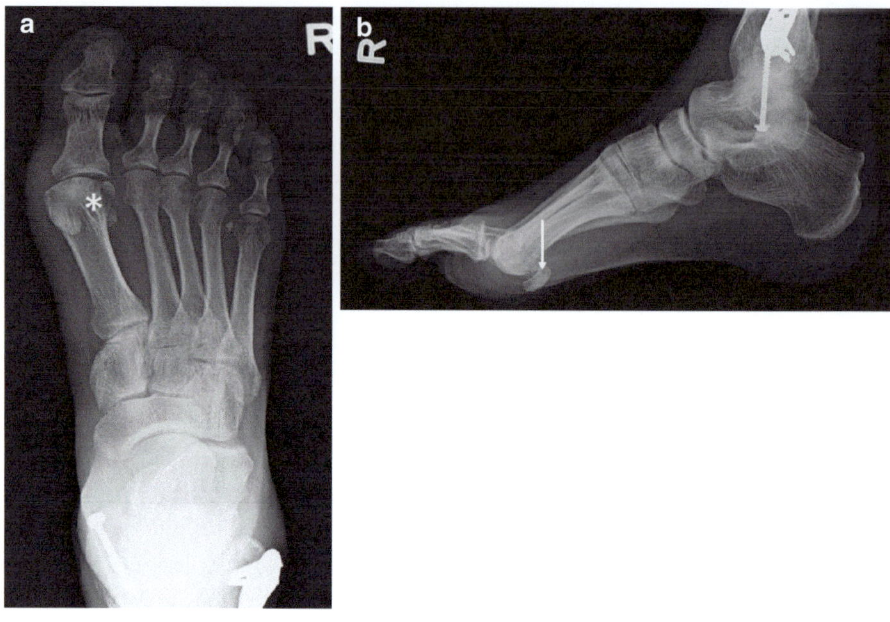

Fig. 2.2 Grade III turf toe injury. AP (**a**) and lateral (**b**) plain radiographs of a patient with a grade 3 turf toe injury with associated fibular sesamoid fracture. Sesamoid fracture (white asterixis), proximal sesamoid retraction (white arrow)

Fig. 2.3 MRI imaging of plantar plate rupture. T2 sagittal image of the hallux MTPJ reveals complete disruption of the proximal attachment of the plantar plate (asterisks)

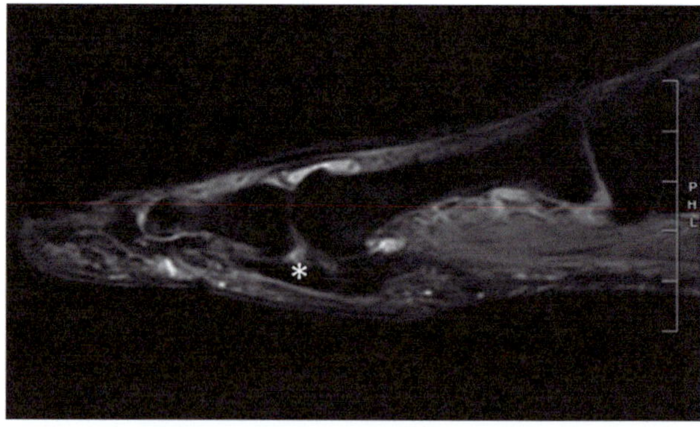

foot radiographs are utilized for evaluation of presence of bipartite sesamoid diastasis, which is also seen in 14.3% of turf toe injuries [20]. Sesamoid diastasis greater than 2.0 mm is concerning for a turf toe injury. Magnetic resonance imaging (MRI) can be used in higher-grade injuries to assess for plantar plate disruption, chondral injuries, and sesamoid edema (Fig. 2.3) [21].

Turf toe injuries can occur as a continuum of injury from a mild sprain to fracture dislocation of the first MTPJ complex (Table 2.1). Clanton et al. described a classification system that was later modified by Anderson et al. for turf toe injuries [3, 11]. Grade 1 injuries include mild sprains with localized plantar pain and minimal swelling. Grade 2 injuries are partial tears of the capsuloligamentous structures with

Table 2.1 Classification of turf toe injuries

Mechanism of injury	Grade	Description
Hyperextension (turf toe)	1	1. Stretching of the plantar complex
		2. Localized tenderness, minimal swelling, no ecchymosis
	2	1. Partial plantar plate tear
		2. Diffuse swelling, ecchymosis, restricted ROM
	3	1. Complete tear
		2. Severe tenderness and ecchymosis
		3. Positive anterior drawer test
		4. Sesamoid injuries (retraction, fracture, bipartite diastasis)
	4A	1. Traumatic hallux valgus
	4B	1. Traumatic hallux varus
Hyperflexion (sand toe)	N/A	
Dislocation	I	1. Dislocation of the hallux with the sesamoids entrapped in the MTPJ
		2. No disruption of the intersesamoid ligament
		3. Usually irreducible
	IIA	1. Associated disruption of intersesamoid ligament.
		2. Usually reducible
	IIB	1. Sesamoid fracture
		2. Usually reducible
	IIC	1. Complete disruption of intersesamoid ligament or sesamoid fracture
		2. Usually reducible

Adapted from Anderson [27]

associated swelling and restricted range of motion. Grade 3 injuries are complete tears of the capsuloligamentous complex with diffuse swelling and dorsal pain. Patients with grade 3 turf toe injuries usually have the inability to bear weight on their medial foot. We proposed additional grade 4 injuries to represent traumatic angular injuries. Grade 4A injuries include traumatic hallux valgus, while grade 4B injuries represent traumatic hallux varus deformities.

Severe turf toe injuries can also present with plantar [17], dorsal [22], or lateral [23–25] first MTPJ dislocations. Jahss described a classification system for traumatic dorsal first MTPJ dislocations. Type I dislocations involve disruption of the plantar plate from the metatarsal head. The metatarsal head buttonholes plantarly through the capsular defect, and the sesamoids become entrapped dorsally over the metatarsal head. Type I injuries are often irreducible and require surgery [22, 26]. Type II dislocations involves disruption of the intersesamoid ligament, leading to wide diastasis of the sesamoid (type IIA) or sesamoid fracture (type IIB). Type II injuries are usually reducible. Type IIC dislocations are a variant of both IIA and IIB first MTP dislocations [27].

Treatment

Nonoperative

Treatment for turf toe injuries is dictated by the severity of injury and level of activity of the patient [28]. Nonoperative treatment includes a period of rest, ice, immobilization in plantarflexion, and activity modification [18, 29]. Buddy tapping the great toe to the adjacent digit can provide adequate stability and pain relief during ambulation for low-grade turf toe injuries. Rigid soled shoes, orthotics, and anti-inflammatory medications should also be utilized to limit first MTPJ hyperdorsiflexion and reduce inflammation [29]. Lidocaine-only injections have been shown to be a pregame diagnostic tool for turf toe injuries of in-season athletes of turf toe injuries. Clanton et al.'s original algorithm recommended 1–2 days of rest and early range of motion for grade 1 injuries, grade 2 injuries required up to 2 weeks of rest, and grade 3 injuries required 3–6 weeks of rest [3, 29]. In some cases, severe turf toe injuries can take up to 6 months before full recovery occurs [30]. Patients with grade 3 injuries should exhibit 50–60 degrees of painless passive dorsiflexion of the first MTPJ before return to high-impact activity. Unsuccessful nonoperative treatment of severe turf toe injuries can lead to decreased first MTPJ dorsiflexion and higher peak hallux pressures during ambulation [9]. Long-term sequalae from turf toe injuries include persistent pain, hallux rigidus, traumatic hallux valgus, and traumatic hallux varus [3, 4, 30].

Operative

Operative treatment for turf toe injuries is reserved for unstable injuries [5, 31, 32]. Anderson et al. stated that the indications for surgery include grade 3 injuries with significant sesamoid retraction, large capsular avulsions with an unstable MTPJ, bipartite sesamoid diastasis, sesamoid fracture, chondral injury, loose bodies, and persistent pain despite conservative treatment (Table 2.2) [11, 28]. We also proposed that patients with traumatic hallux valgus and hallux varus injuries represent an unstable injury pattern and should also undergo surgical intervention with the goal of treatment is to restore anatomy, optimize return to play, and prevent the sequalae of inadequate treatment of turf toe injuries. For direct plantar plate repair, the patient is placed in the supine position, and two surgical approaches can be utilized for surgical treatment of tuft toe injuries. A medial L-shaped is made longitudinal over the hallux and transversely at the plantar aspect of the MTPJ joint (Fig. 2.4) [33]. Another option is to perform dual incisions, with a medial hallux and plantar first web space incision [11]. Care is taken to protect the plantar digital nerve

Table 2.2 Indications for surgical treatment of turf toe injury

1. Grade III injuries with significant sesamoid retraction
2. Large capsular avulsions with an unstable hallux MTPJ
3. Bipartite sesamoid diastasis
4. Displaced sesamoid fracture
5. Chondral injury
6. Loose body
7. Traumatic hallux valgus deformity
8. Traumatic hallux varus deformity
9. Persistent pain despite conservative treatment

Adapted from McCormick and Anderson [10]

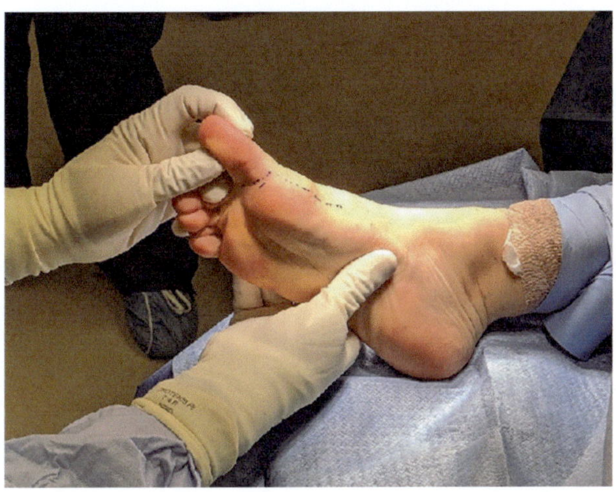

Fig. 2.4 L-shaped incision for plantar plate repair

and dorsomedial nerves. A longitudinal capsulotomy is made at the interval between the metatarsal head and the sesamoid complex. The sesamoid complex is inspected thoroughly for concomitant injuries. A primary repair can be performed with non-absorbable suture if adequate plantar plate tissue is available. In chronic cases with attenuated tissue, a plantar plate reconstruction may be required involving decorticating the base of the proximal phalanx, placing a suture anchor, and advancing the plantar plate into the base of the proximal phalanx with several nonabsorbable mattress sutures. The plantar plate is advanced and fixed with the MTPJ in slight plantarflexion. After fixation of the plantar plate, an anterior-posterior MTPJ drawer test is performed to ensure the stability of the MTPJ is reestablished. In cases of a displaced sesamoid fracture or bipartite sesamoid with diastasis, fixation with a mini-fragment screw or sesamoidectomy is indicated [30, 31]. Clanton [30] and later Anderson [28] described performing an interposition of the abductor hallucis into the sesamoidectomy defect to restrain dorsiflexion of the hallux MTPJ.

In cases of traumatic hallux valgus injuries, the medial stabilizing structure is injured, and a medial longitudinal incision is made along the hallux MTPJ (Fig. 2.5) [34]. Upon dissection onto the capsule, the surgeon will encounter disrupted medial collateral ligament and flexor hallucis brevis tendon injury. A medial capsulotomy is performed, and the sesamoid complex is evaluated. Resection of the medial eminence (Silver's bunionectomy) is performed to allow for the medial capsule to be imbricated in order to restore the balance of the hallux. If possible, the flexor hallucis brevis is repaired to augment the medial stability. A separate longitudinal dorsal incision is made along the first web space in order to perform a modified McBride procedure to pie crust the lateral collateral ligament and the adductor hallucis tendon [18, 34]. Partial release of the lateral structures aids in the restoration of the soft tissue balance of the hallux MTPJ.

The treatment of traumatic hallux varus injuries involves stabilizing the injured lateral structures of the MTPJ (Fig. 2.6). A dorsal longitudinal incision is made along the first web space. The adductor tendon is identified, and it is often torn along with the lateral collateral ligament and flexor hallucis brevis tendon. A formal

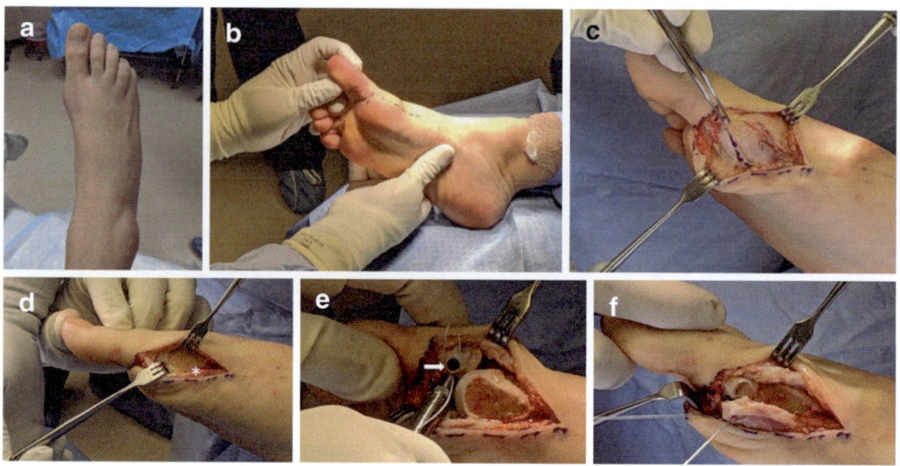

Fig. 2.5 Traumatic hallux valgus correction. Preoperative alignment showing hallux valgus (**a**). Planned L-shaped incision to address the plantar plate injury (**b**). A longitudinal medial capsulotomy is made just plantar to midline to access the sesamoid complex and collateral ligament injuries (**c**). The medial eminence of the metatarsal head is resected using a small sagittal saw (white asterisks) (**d**). Two Sonic Anchors (Stryker, New Jersey) were placed at the base of the medial proximal phalanx (**e**). Repair of the abductor hallucis tendon and collateral ligament to the proximal phalanx anchors (**f**)

lateral longitudinal capsulotomy is performed. The base of the proximal phalanx is decorticated, and an anchor is placed laterally. The lateral structures are repaired onto the lateral anchors. The medial capsule and medial collateral ligament are pie crusted to reestablish the soft tissue balance of the hallux. Intraoperative fluoroscopic images are taken to confirm hallux alignment. Another treatment option is to perform an extensor hallucis brevis (EHB) tenodesis as described by Myerson [35]. A dorsal longitudinal incision is made over the first web space, and the EHB tendon is divided at the myotendinous junction. The EHB tendon is then routed plantar to the transverse metatarsal ligament and attached to the metatarsal shaft under tension.

Postoperatively, the foot is immobilized in a short leg splint with the great toe in plantarflexion for 4 weeks. Protected weight-bearing in a postoperative shoe or CAM boot is initiated from 4–8 weeks post-operation, along with gentle passive plantarflexion range of motion. At 8 weeks, the patient can weight bear as tolerated in a carbon fiber insert (Fig. 2.7). Gradual sporting activities are initiated at 3 months with buddy tapping and graphite insoles to limit dorsiflexion. Normal shoe wear without an insole is allowed at 6 months. Serial plain radiographs should be obtained during the postoperative course to assess for sesamoid retraction and hallux MTP arthritis.

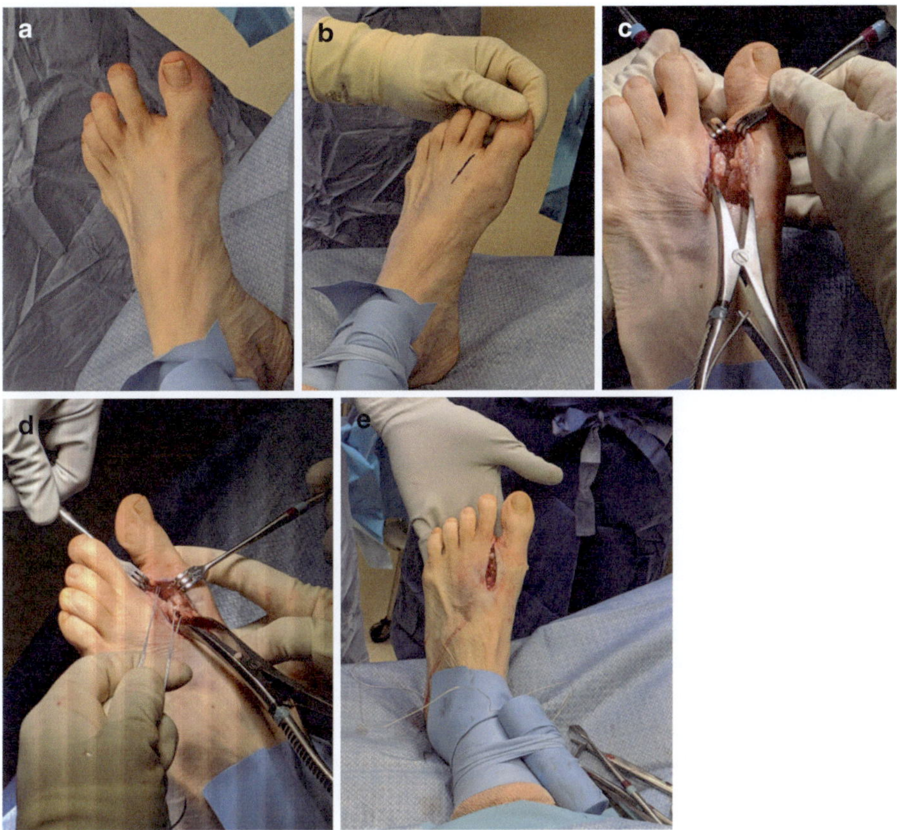

Fig. 2.6 Traumatic hallux valgus correction. Preoperative alignment showing hallux varus deformity (**a**). Planned dorsal longitudinal incision over the first web space to address the lateral plantar plate injury (**b**). Dorsal dissection at the first web space reveals significant disruption of the lateral collateral ligament structures (**c**). One Sonic Anchors (Stryker, New Jersey) were placed at the base of the medial proximal phalanx and metatarsal head (**d**). Intraoperative alignment showing improved hallux alignment after repair of the lateral collateral ligament, flexor digitorum brevis, and medial capsule pie crusting (**e**)

Hallux MTP Dislocation Treatment

Individuals that present with a frank first MTP joint dislocation require urgent reduction to reduce vascular compromise and to relieve pressure on tented skin [16]. Reduction is achieved by recreating the deformity (i.e., dorsiflex the first MTPJ for dorsal dislocation) followed by translating the proximal phalanx plantarly to reduce

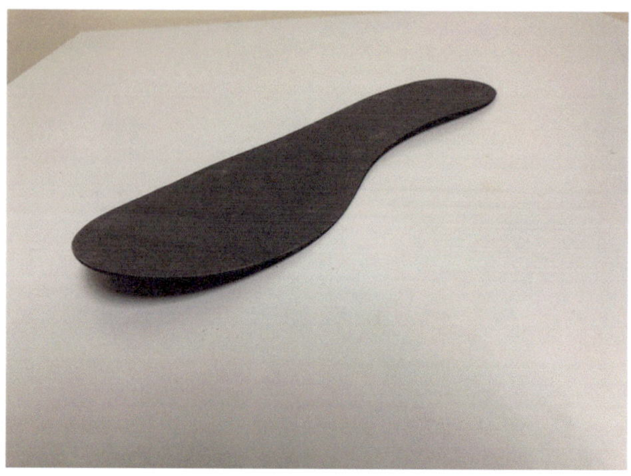

Fig. 2.7 Carbon sole insert

the joint. Postreduction plan radiographs should be obtained to confirm reduction of both the first MTPJ and sesamoid complex. Incarcerated sesamoid or irreducible joint can undergo a trial of MTPJ saline insufflation and reduction [36]. Usually, irreducible MTPJ dislocations require open reduction, where a dorsal longitudinal incision is often utilized to avoid damaging displaced plantar neurovascular structures and for ease of access of dorsal MTPJ dislocations [22, 37]. A mid-axial medial approach can also be utilized to access plantar and dorsal structures if needed. The dorsal capsule should be dissected, and any entrapped structures such as the adductor hallucis tendon or deep transverse metatarsal ligaments should be removed in order to achieve a concentric reduction [22].

Surgical Complications

Complications from the surgical treatment of turf toe injuries include transient neuritis of the plantar digital nerve, stiffness with prolonged immobilization, re-rupture of the plantar plate with aggressive rehabilitation, cock-up hallux deformity, and sesamoid retraction [28]. Persistent pain and subsequent hallux rigidus can also occur [3].

Evidence Base/Critical Appraisal of the Literature

A comprehensive literature search was performed, with no time limit to maximize the pool of work available, conforming to the PRISMA statement. The databases used were PubMed, CINAHL, and EMBASE computerized literature databases. Searches were executed comprising all years, from database inception through October 2021. The following search terms were utilized: turf toe, traumatic hallux varus, traumatic hallux valgus, metatarsophalangeal joint sprain, death toe, and metatarsophalangeal joint dislocation in human studies. This resulted in 886 articles. Excluded articles included abstracts not involving humans, review articles, case reports, non-English articles, and studies lacking clinical outcomes. The search found a literature review of turf toe injuries, which provided further articles that were included, providing eight studies available for analysis. This included 126 patients (135 feet) (Table 2.3).

Nonoperative

Turf toe injuries alter normal foot biomechanics and can lead to significant limitations in running, cutting, and other sporting activities [2, 9]. Bowers et al. were the first to publish a case series of 27 turf toe injuries in collegiate football athletes at West Virginia University [2]. He found that from 1970 to 1974, there were 5.4 low-grade turf toe injures per year in a population of 570 football players. Injured players were treated with immediate ice and protective taping. Players were allowed to progress their return to play in stiff sole shoes after symptoms resolved. The authors concluded that flexible shoe wear and artificial grass predisposed players to turf toe injuries.

Coker et al. published a prospective study at the University of Arkansas from 1972 to 1974 [1]. They reported on 18 turf toe low-grade and high-grade injuries during a 3-year period compared to 74 ankle sprains. Nonoperative treatment included ice, compression, and immobilization depending on the severity of the injury. Operative treatment was performed for chronic injuries with capsular ruptures. Operative treatment included plantar plate repair, debridement, and loose body removal. Once case of a sesamoid fracture underwent an isolated sesamoidectomy. Return to play included progression from running in place to cutting activities with a spring steel shoe insert. Turf toe injuries missed a total of 92 practices and 7 games during the study period. Return to play was highly variable in the study cohort, occurring anywhere from 3 weeks to several months. Demographic information was not reported in this study.

Clanton et al. reported on 62 forefoot injuries in 53 athletes at Rice University from 1971 to 1985 [3]. Injuries varied from mild sprains to avulsion fracture plantar plate injuries. Approximately 96% of forefoot injuries occurred in football players, with over 80% of injuries involving the hallux MTPJ. Approximately 60% of hallux injuries were from hyperextension injuries, while 4% occurred during plantarflexion. Treatment included ice, taping, anti-inflammatory, and gradual return to sports. At 5 years of follow-up, 95% of players returned to sports, missing an average of 6 days of athletic participation. There was one case of an avulsion fracture of the base of the proximal phalanx that underwent surgical intervention, subsequently missing 56 days of athletic activities. Although follow-up was incomplete, at around 10-year follow-up, two players developed progressive hallux valgus deformities as well as several cases of stiffness and hallux rigidus.

Rodeo et al. performed a questionnaire study on 80 active NFL players that sustained turf toe injuries [4]. The authors compared one team that played on artificial

Table 2.3 Systematic literature review of the treatment of turf toe injuries

Author	Study design	Level of evidence	Year	No. of patients (feet)	Demographics	Grade of injury (N)	Mean follow-up (month)	Treatment	Outcomes	Mean return to sports
Coker [1]	Case series	4	1978	18	18 University of Arkansas football players	Cases reported: II (3) III (4)	48	Nonoperative (PRICE), cast if needed, 0.51 mm spring steel splint once ambulating Operative plantar plate repair and loose body removal	Injured patients missed a total of 92 practices and 7 games	44.6 weeks
Clanton [3]	Case series	4	1986	53 (62)	Collegiate football players at Rice University	N/A	60	– Nonoperative: Ice, taping, NSAIDS, contrast therapy, cortisone injection, gradual return to sports – Operative: One player with a proximal phalanx avulsion fracture	– 95% of players return to sports, missing a mean of 6 days – The one operative case missed 56 days of athletic activity – Two players developed progressive hallux valgus deformity	0.9 weeks

Rodeo [46]	Case series	4	1990	4 (4)	Collegiate football players (2)	II (4)	46.5	Medial longitudinal approach, plantar plate repair, sesamoid excision (3), sesamoid repair (1)	– All players returned to play without pain at a minimum of 18 months follow-up – All players had a loss of plantarflexion motion – Mean postop plantarflexion 2.5°, mean dorsiflexion 30°	7 weeks
					Professional football players (2), mean age 22.75 yo					
Anderson [28]	Case series	4	2002	9 (9)	Collegiate and professional athletes 8 males, 1 female	III (9)	Minimum follow-up of 1 year	Plantar plate repair via medial J-shaped incision	7 out of 9 return to sports	N/A
								Concomitant procedures: One fibular sesamoidectomy, three tibial sesamoidectomies with abductor hallucis tendon transfer	One player had persistent pain with toe off One patient developed DJD of the first MTPJ	

(continued)

Table 2.3 (continued)

Author	Study design	Level of evidence	Year	No. of patients (feet)	Demographics	Grade of injury (N)	Mean follow-up (month)	Treatment	Outcomes	Mean return to sports
Faltus[40]	Case series	4	2014	5 (5)	– Collegiate football players	II (1)		– Nonoperative treatment: Plantarflexion bunion taping with CAM boot, NWB 2.5 weeks, progression to WBAT at week, running 10 weeks, agility drills 12 weeks, full contact play 18 weeks		Nonoperative: Mean 13 weeks. One player RTP 2 months, one player RTP 18 weeks
					– 3 out of 5 players underwent operative treatment	III (4)		– Operative – One player underwent a plantar plate repair 5 months post-injury – One player underwent plantar plate repair, intersesamoid ligament repair, and abductor tendon repair 10 days post-injury – One player underwent direct repair of the plantar plate and excision of proximal phalanx avulsion injury		Operative: Mean 25 weeks RTP at 5 months for two players, 10 weeks for one player

| Drakos [39] | Case series | 4 | 2015 | 3 (3) | – Collegiate football players

– Mean age 20.3 years | III (3) | N/A | Nonoperative: One player treated with a plantarflexion cast for 6 weeks, then CAM boot
Operative: One player with plantar plate repair via dual medial and lateral incision and nonabsorbable 2-0 suture
One player with medial incision and plantar plate repair with pinning | – | 26.1 weeks |
| Covell[34] | Case series | 4 | 2017 | 19 (19) | – 12 NFL players, 6 collegiate football players, 1 high school player
– Mean age 24.4 years
– Mean time to surgery was 4.5 months | III (19) | Minimum 6 months | – Operative: Medial incision and modified McBride bunionectomy
– Concomitant procedures: Tibial sesamoidectomy (3), tibial sesamoid bone graft (1), FHB reconstruction with abductor hallucis tendon transfer (8), cheilectomy (6), chondroplasty (1) loose body removal (1) | Mean recovery time 3.4 months
14 out of 19 (74%) of players return to preinjury play
5 out of 14 players that return to play subsequently retired
FHL tendinitis (1) | 14.7 weeks |

(continued)

Table 2.3 (continued)

Author	Study design	Level of evidence	Year	No. of patients (feet)	Demographics	Grade of injury (N)	Mean follow-up (month)	Treatment	Outcomes	Mean return to sports
Smith [32]	Case series	4	2018	15 (15)	– Football players: 1 professional, 9 division I NCAA, 2 division III NCAA, 3 high school players—mean age 19.3 yo, BMI 32.3	III (15)	27.5	Open repair with medial J-shaped incision, side to side repair or 2.4 mm suture anchor	– Mean dorsiflexion 42.3°, mean AOFAS hallux score was 91.3, mean VAS 0.7	16.5 weeks

grass versus another team that played on natural grass. They found a 45% incidence of turf toe injuries and that 85% of injures were due to hyperextension injures. Interestingly, there was no significant difference between artificial and natural grass playing surfaces. Significant risk factors included age (27.4 vs. 24.7 years), greater number of years in the league (5.2 vs. 3.0 years), and greater preinjury ankle dorsiflexion (13.3° vs. 7.87°). Post-injury plantarflexion at the MTPJ was significantly decreased on the affected side (22.1°) compared to the unaffected side (30.78°).

Parekh reported on the outcomes of turf toe injuries in 67 NFL players (71 injuries) from 2011 to 2014 [38]. The average age at the time of injury was 26.4 years with 40.8% of injuries occurring on natural grass, 40.8% occurring on artificial turf, and 18.4% on an unidentified surface. The cohort averaged 3.2 games missed, with 8 out of 67 (11.9%) players placed on injured reserve and 9 out of 67 (13.4%) of players required surgical intervention. The average power rating pre-injury (7.3 per game) and post-injury (8.1 per game) was not significantly different. The authors concluded that NFL players had similar performance after treatment of turf toe injuries.

Operative

Operative treatment is rare and is typically reserved for unstable injury patterns [28, 32]. George et al. performed a retrospective database study from the NCAA Injury Surveillance System from 2004 to 2005 and 2008 to 2009 [5]. They found that only 1.7% of turf toe injuries required surgical intervention. Direct plantar plate repair can be performed in the acute setting when adequate plantar plate tissue is present [39, 40]. If the plantar plate tissue is attenuated, then plantar plate advancement to the proximal phalanx with bone tunnels [33] or anchors [32] can be utilized. Sesamoidectomy can performed for sesamoid fractures or bipartite sesamoids with significant diastasis [30, 31].

Lee et al. retrospectively reported on 32 patients that underwent isolated tibial sesamoidectomies for sesamoiditis [41]. There was a 62.5% follow-up at an average of 62 months postoperatively. At follow-up, there was no significant change in clinical alignment, range of motion, or radiographic differences in hallux MTPJ alignment. There were no significant differences in plantar pressures at the hallux MTPJ or plantarflexion push-off strength. Similarly, Ford et al. reported on 87 patients that underwent isolated fibular sesamoidectomies for sesamoiditis, avascular necrosis, and nonunion [42]. At a minimum of 2-year follow-up, there was no significant difference in clinical or radiographic hallux alignment. Additionally, 70% of patients were very satisfied with their surgery.

Easley et al. [40] performed a retrospective case series on five collegiate football players that sustained turf toe injuries. On MRI imaging, three out of the five patients sustained high-grade plantar plate injuries. One offensive redshirt senior underwent surgical intervention after completing his senior year due to persistent symptom returned to football activities at 5 months and was able to participate in professional football camps without restrictions. A freshman wide receiver underwent plantar plate repair, intersesamoid ligament repair, and abductor tendon repair 10 days post-injury. He was able to return to football activities at 12 weeks and returned to competition the following football season. A junior fullback sustained an unstable turf toe injury with complete plantar plate rupture and underwent direct repair. He returned to football activities at 12 weeks and returned to full playing activities at 18 weeks postoperatively. He did continue to have discomfort with terminal hallux MTPJ dorsiflexion.

Smith and Waldrop conducted a short-term retrospective study on 15 competitive football players with grade 3 acute (67%) or chronic (33%) turf toe injuries from 2012 to 2016 [32]. Surgical intervention included repair of the phalangeal-sesamoid ligament distal to the sesamoids. If a bipartite sesamoid or sesamoid fracture was encountered, a sesamoidectomy was performed in conjunction with an abductor tendon transfer. The average age of the cohort was 19.3 years old with a body mass index (BMI) of 32.3. Surgery was performed at an average time of 9.5 weeks post-injury. There was a 93% follow-up rate at an average of 27.5 months. The average time missed from athletic activity was 16.5 weeks, with 78.6% of the cohort returning to football activities. Dorsiflexion range of motion at the hallux MTPJ was 42.3, the average AOFAS hallux score was 91.3, and visual analog score (VAS) was 0.7 at the time of final follow-up. There was one player that underwent reoperation.

Covell et al. performed a retrospective study of 19 male elite athletes that underwent operative treatment of traumatic hallux valgus deformities from 2006 to 2015 [34]. The cohort included 12 NFL players, 6 collegiate athletes, and 1 high school athlete with an average age of 24.4 years old. All injured players underwent a first MTPJ medial collateral ligament repair and McBride bunionectomy. Concomitant procedures included three tibial sesamoidectomies, one tibial sesamoid bone grafting, eight flexor hallucis brevis reconstructions with abductor hallucis tendon transfers, six cheilectomies, one first metatarsal head chondroplasty, and one loose body removal. There was a 74% return to preinjury activity at an average time of 3.4 months postoperatively. Five of the 14 athletes that went on to return to play postoperatively subsequently retired. One NFL player retired after six seasons, one after three seasons, one after two seasons, and one after one season of play postoperatively. A collegiate baseball player retired after one season of play.

The most common cause of hallux varus is iatrogenic after bunion correction [43]. However, the surgical treatment of traumatic hallux varus deformities is limited to case reports [44, 45]. Cheung et al. published their case report on a 68-year-old female that sustained a traumatic hallux varus deformity after stubbing her left great toe on a door laterally [45]. She was seen 5 weeks after her injury, and plain radiographs revealed an avulsion fracture of the lateral base of the proximal phalanx. She underwent delayed traumatic hallux valgus repair 5 months post-injury. An arthroscopic evaluation revealed synovitis without cartilage damage. A minimally invasive extensor digitorum brevis tenodesis of the hallux MTPJ and subperiosteal medial capsule release were performed. And plantar plate tenodesis of the second MTPJ was performed. The patient was non-weight-bearing for 4 weeks and

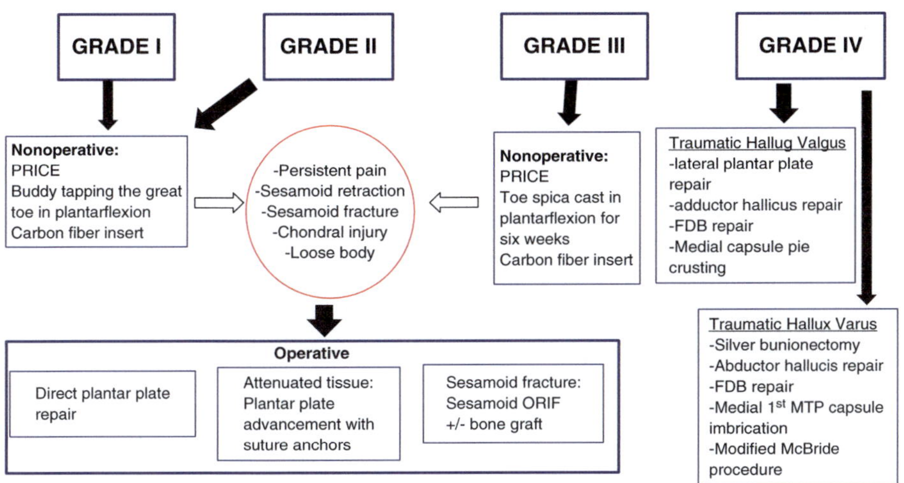

Fig. 2.8 Evidence-based turf toe treatment algorithm

then progressed to normal shoe wear by 2 months postoperatively. At 31 months follow-up, the patient had no pain and had maintained their hallux varus correction. Barp et al. published a case report of a 33-year-old male that sustained a left traumatic hallux varus deformity after sustaining a pivoting injury to his great toe. MRI imaging revealed a rupture of the adductor hallucis tendon at the base of the proximal phalanx without any fracture. The patient underwent suture augmentation of the lateral MTPJ structures. The patient was made non-weight-bearing for 2 weeks and then progressed to full weight-bearing by 4 weeks postoperatively. At 3 years clinical follow-up, the patient had maintained his correction and had good hallux MTPJ range of motion.

Final Treatment Algorithm (Fig. 2.8)

Grade 1

- **Conservative treatment**
  - We recommend rest, ice, NSAIDS, and activity modification to avoid hyper-dorsiflexion of the hallux.
  - Buddy tapping the great toe to the adjacent digit can provide adequate stability and pain relief during ambulation.
  - Rigid-soled shoes and orthotics to limit first MTPJ hyper-dorsiflexion.
  - Lidocaine-only injection can be utilized for in-season athletes right before competition.
  - Return to play is usually 1–2 days after symptoms resolve.

Grade 2

- **Nonoperative Treatment**
  - We recommend nonoperative treatment for 2 weeks (see grade 1 algorithm above).
- **Surgical treatment**
  - We recommend surgical treatment in high-level athletes for chronic injuries with recalcitrant to conservative treatment.
  - Our recommended surgical approach is to perform an L-shaped incision or dual incisions (medial mid-axial and plantar first web space).
  - Direct plantar plate repair can be performed with nonabsorbable suture if good cuff of tissue is present.
  - Plantar plate advancement should be performed if plantar plate is attenuated. The plantar plate is advanced by placing suture anchors into the proximal phalanx, and the plantar ligament complex is advanced.

Grade 3

- **Nonoperative treatment**
  - We recommend nonoperative treatment with immobilization in a toe spica cast with the hallux MTPJ in plantarflexion for 6 weeks (see grade 1 algorithm above).
- **Acute operative treatment**
  - We recommend acute operative treatment in patients with significant hallux MTPJ instability, chondral injury, loose body, sesamoid fracture, bipartite sesamoid diastasis, or sesamoid retraction.
  - Our recommended surgical approach is to perform an L-shaped incision or dual incisions (medial mid-axial and plantar first web space).
  - Direct plantar plate repair can be performed with nonabsorbable suture if good cuff of tissue is present.
  - Plantar plate advancement should be performed if plantar plate is attenuated. The plantar plate is advanced by placing suture anchors into the proximal phalanx, and the plantar ligament complex is advanced.
  - Sesamoid fracture can be fixed with small mini-fragment screws or excised.

Grade 4

- **Traumatic valgus deformity (4A)**
  - Our recommended surgical approach is to perform an L-shaped incision or dual incisions (medial mid-axial and plantar first web space).
  - We recommend performing a Silver bunionectomy, abductor hallucis repair, medial plantar plate repair, and flexor digitorum brevis repair utilizing anchor placement.

- In order to improve soft tissue balancing of the hallux MTPJ, we imbricate the medial capsule and partially release the lateral capsule.
- **Traumatic varus deformity (4B)**
  - Our recommended surgical approach is to perform a longitudinal first dorsal web space incision.
  - We utilize anchor placement at the base of the proximal phalanx and metatarsal head for adductor hallucis, lateral collateral ligament, lateral plantar plate repair, and FDB repairs.
  - We perform a partial release of the medial capsule via pie crusting to reestablish soft tissue balance at the hallux MTPJ.

Summary

Turf toe represents a continuum of injury to the capsuloligamentous complex of the hallux MTPJ, commonly affecting athletes. Risk factors for sustaining turf toe injuries include flexible shoe wear and artificial playing surface. Nonoperative treatment for low-grade injuries includes a period of rest, ice, immobilization in plantarflexion, and activity modification. Nonoperative treatment of high-grade injuries can lead to significant dysfunction and games missed. Indications for surgery include unstable injuries, associated fractures, and angular deformities. Surgical treatment of turf toe injuries leads to satisfactory clinical outcomes.

References

1. Coker TP, Arnold JA, Weber DL. Traumatic lesions of the metatarsophalangeal joint of the great toe in athletes. Am J Sports Med. 1978;6(6):326–34.
2. Bowers KD Jr, Martin RB. Turf-toe: a shoe-surface related football injury. Med Sci Sports. 1976;8(2):81–3.
3. Clanton TO, Butler JE, Eggert A. Injuries to the metatarsophalangeal joints in athletes. Foot Ankle. 1986;7(3):162–76.
4. Rodeo SA, O'Brien S, Warren RF, Barnes R, Wickiewicz TL, Dillingham MF. Turf-toe: an analysis of metatarsophalangeal joint sprains in professional football players. Am J Sports Med. 1990;18(3):280–5.
5. George E, Harris AH, Dragoo JL, Hunt KJ. Incidence and risk factors for turf toe injuries in intercollegiate football: data from the national collegiate athletic association injury surveillance system. Foot Ankle Int. 2014;35(2):108–15.
6. Sammarco GJ, Miller EH. Forefoot conditions in dancers: part II. Foot Ankle. 1982;3(2):93–8.
7. Frey C, Andersen GD, Feder KS. Plantarflexion injury to the metatarsophalangeal joint ("sand toe"). Foot Ankle Int. 1996;17(9):576–81.
8. Mullis DL, Miller WE. A disabling sports injury of the great toe. Foot Ankle. 1980;1(1):22–5.
9. Brophy RH, Gamradt SC, Ellis SJ, Barnes RP, Rodeo SA, Warren RF, et al. Effect of turf toe on foot contact pressures in professional American football players. Foot Ankle Int. 2009;30(5):405–9.
10. Stokes IA, Hutton WC, Stott JR, Lowe LW. Forces under the hallux valgus foot before and after surgery. Clin Orthop Relat Res. 1979;142:64–72.
11. McCormick JJ, Anderson RB. Rehabilitation following turf toe injury and plantar plate repair. Clin Sports Med. 2010;29(2):313–23. ix

12. Sarrafian S. Ligaments of metatarsophalangeal joints and proximal phalangeal apparatus. In: Anatomy of the foot and ankle: descriptive, topographic. Philadelphia: Lippincott Company; 1993. p. 211–6.
13. Lucas DE, Philbin T, Hatic S 2nd. The plantar plate of the first metatarsophalangeal joint: an anatomical study. Foot Ankle Spec. 2014;7(2):108–12.
14. Waldrop NE 3rd, Zirker CA, Wijdicks CA, Laprade RF, Clanton TO. Radiographic evaluation of plantar plate injury: an in vitro biomechanical study. Foot Ankle Int. 2013;34(3):403–8.
15. Aper RL, Saltzman CL, Brown TD. The effect of hallux sesamoid resection on the effective moment of the flexor hallucis brevis. Foot Ankle Int. 1994;15(9):462–70.
16. Berkowitz M, Sanders R. Metatarsophalangeal joint dislocations. In: Mann's surgery of the foot and ankle. 9th ed. Philadelphia: Mosby Elsevier; 2014. p. 1905–72.
17. Biyani A, Sharma JC, Mathur NC. Plantar panmetatarsophalangeal dislocation—a hyperflexion injury. J Trauma. 1988;28(6):868–9.
18. Clough TM, Majeed H. Turf toe injury—current concepts and an updated review of literature. Foot Ankle Clin. 2018;23(4):693–701.
19. Schein AJ, Skalski MR, Patel DB, White EA, Lundquist R, Gottsegen CJ, et al. Turf toe and sesamoiditis: what the radiologist needs to know. Clin Imaging. 2015;39(3):380–9.
20. Favinger JL, Porrino JA, Richardson ML, Mulcahy H, Chew FS, Brage ME. Epidemiology and imaging appearance of the normal bi−/multipartite hallux sesamoid bone. Foot Ankle Int. 2015;36(2):197–202.
21. Tewes DP, Fischer DA, Fritts HM, Guanche CA. MRI findings of acute turf toe. A case report and review of anatomy. Clin Orthop Relat Res. 1994;304:200–3.
22. Lewis AG, DeLee JC. Type-I complex dislocation of the first metatarsophalangeal joint--open reduction through a dorsal approach. A case report. J Bone Joint Surg Am. 1984;66(7):1120–3.
23. Gale DW. Lateral dislocation of the first metatarsophalangeal joint, a radiographic indicator of reducibility. Injury. 1991;22(3):230.
24. Vosoughi AR, Rippstein PF. Rare lateral dislocation of the first metatarsophalangeal joint: a case report and review of the literature. J Foot Ankle Surg. 2017;56(2):375–8.
25. Pietu G. Lateral dislocation of the first metatarsophalangeal joint: report of two cases. J Trauma. 2005;58(3):640–2.
26. Ando Y, Yasuda M, Okuda H, Kamano M. Irreducible dorsal subluxation of the first metatarsophalangeal joint: a case report. J Orthop Trauma. 2002;16(2):134–6.
27. Copeland CL, Kanat IO. A new classification for traumatic dislocations of the first metatarsophalangeal joint: type IIC. J Foot Surg. 1991;30(3):234–7.
28. Anderson RB. Turf toe injuries of the hallux metatarsophalangeal joint. Tech Foot Ankle Surg. 2002;1(2):102–11.
29. Clanton T, Waldrop N. Forefoot sprains. In: Mann's surgery of the foot and ankle. 9th ed. Philadelphia: Mosby Elsevier; 2014. p. 1649–57.
30. Clanton TO, Ford JJ. Turf toe injury. Clin Sports Med. 1994;13(4):731–41.
31. Richardson EG. Injuries to the hallucal sesamoids in the athlete. Foot Ankle. 1987;7(4):229–44.
32. Smith K, Waldrop N. Operative outcomes of grade 3 turf toe injuries in competitive football players. Foot Ankle Int. 2018;39(9):1076–81.
33. Doty JF, Coughlin MJ. Turf toe repair: a technical note. Foot Ankle Spec. 2013;6(6):452–6.
34. Covell DJ, Lareau CR, Anderson RB. Operative treatment of traumatic hallux valgus in elite athletes. Foot Ankle Int. 2017;38(6):590–5.
35. Myerson MS, Komenda GA. Results of hallux varus correction using an extensor hallucis brevis tenodesis. Foot Ankle Int. 1996;17(1):21–7.
36. Bohl DD, Hamid KS, Walton DM. Incarcerated plantar dislocation of the first metatarsophalangeal joint: reduction using intra-articular saline injection. Foot Ankle Spec. 2018;11(5):467–70.
37. Yu EC, Garfin SR. Closed dorsal dislocation of the metatarsophalangeal joint of the great toe. A surgical approach and case report. Clin Orthop Relat Res. 1984;185:237–40.
38. Parekh T, Parekh SG. The outcome of turf toe injuries in NFL players. American Orthopaedic Foot and Ankle Society 2019 Annual Meeting, 2019 Sept 12–15; Chicago, IL.

39. Drakos MC, Fiore R, Murphy C, DiGiovanni CW. Plantar-plate disruptions: "the severe turf-toe injury" three cases in contact athletes. J Athl Train. 2015;50(5):553–60.
40. Faltus J, Mullenix K, Moorman CT 3rd, Beatty K, Easley ME. Case series of first metatarsophalangeal joint injuries in division 1 college athletes. Sports Health. 2014;6(6):519–26.
41. Lee S, James WC, Cohen BE, Davis WH, Anderson RB. Evaluation of hallux alignment and functional outcome after isolated tibial sesamoidectomy. Foot Ankle Int. 2005;26(10):803–9.
42. Ford SE, Adair CR, Cohen BE, Davis WH, Ellington JK, Jones CP, et al. Efficacy, outcomes, and alignment following isolated fibular sesamoidectomy via a plantar approach. Foot Ankle Int. 2019;40(12):1375–81.
43. Donley BG. Acquired hallux varus. Foot Ankle Int. 1997;18(9):586–92.
44. Barp EA, Temple EW, Hall JL, Smith HL. Treatment of hallux Varus after traumatic adductor Hallucis tendon rupture. J Foot Ankle Surg. 2018;57(2):418–20.
45. Cheung CN, Lui TH. Traumatic hallux Varus treated by minimally invasive extensor Hallucis Brevis Tenodesis. Case Rep Orthop. 2015;2015:179642.
46. Rodeo SA, Warren RF, O'Brien SJ, Pavlov H, Barnes R, Hanks GA. Diastasis of bipartite sesamoids of the first metatarsophalangeal joint. Foot Ankle. 1993;14(8):425–34.

Plantar Plate Injuries

3

Adam E. Fleischer, Rachel H. Albright, Erin E. Klein, and Lowell Weil Jr

Introduction

Plantar plate injury and subluxation of the lesser metatarsophalangeal (MTP) joint are a relatively common phenomenon [1–3], and growing attention has been given to this problem in recent years as evidenced by the fivefold increase in the number of publications with "plantar plate" in their title in just the past 5 years. Injuries to the plantar plate can allow for advancement of hammertoe deformities and have become increasingly recognized also for their role as pain generators [3–6]. As a result, primary repair of the tissue and restoration of the anatomy, as opposed to indirect repair (e.g., flexor to extensor tendon transfer), have become an increasingly more common practice among foot and ankle surgeons around the world [2].

The vast majority of patients who present with this problem are women between 45 and 60 years of age [7, 8]. The previous and/or current use of high heeled shoes is common, but not always described [8]. Patients may have had a previous first ray surgery without complete restoration of motion at the first MTP joint [9], limiting the patient's ability to fully load the first MTP joint, leading to lateralization of pressure while walking. History of cortisone injection in the lesser MTP joints is also believed to exacerbate and accelerate plantar plate pathology [9]. The pathogenesis and progression of plantar plate injuries are closely linked to the magnitude and duration of weight-bearing stress encountered at the lesser MTP joint. Although conceivably anything that contributes to overloading of the lesser MTP joints will contribute to the development of plantar plate injuries (e.g., high heels, limited ankle joint dorsiflexion, first ray insufficiency, etc.), the role of the long second

A. E. Fleischer (✉) · E. E. Klein · L. Weil Jr
Weil Foot and Ankle Institute, Mount Prospect, IL, USA
e-mail: aef@weil4feet.com; eek@weil4feet.com; lwj@weil4feet.com

R. H. Albright
Stamford Health, Stamford, CT, USA

© Springer Nature Switzerland AG 2022
J. D. Cain, M. V. Hogan (eds.), *Tendon and Ligament Injuries of the Foot and Ankle*,
https://doi.org/10.1007/978-3-031-10490-9_3

53

metatarsal cannot be overstated and should be addressed intraoperatively whenever possible [10–14].

Advanced imaging has evolved over the years within the forefoot. Magnetic resonance imaging (MRI) and ultrasound are important for localizing and confirming the presence of plantar plate injuries, especially when faced with an equivocal clinical exam. Similarly, operative treatment has been refined over the years and now includes a multitude of techniques and approaches; however, the most widely reported and studied method (and our preferred method) involves direct repair of the plantar plate through a single dorsal incision and lesser metatarsal shortening (Weil) osteotomy.

The majority of plantar plate injuries are chronic (i.e., progressive) in nature, although acute injuries do occasionally occur. This chapter is written with a focus more on chronic injuries particularly of the second MTP joint (the most common location) in mind. But most of the same principles apply to the diagnosis and management of acute injuries (and those involving other lesser MTP joints) as well. Knowing when and how to repair plantar plate injuries can be an excellent addition to the foot and ankle surgeon's armamentarium. This chapter will review the basic anatomy, clinical and diagnostic pearls, and surgical approaches supported in the literature.

Anatomy

The plantar plate is a primary stabilizing structure of the lesser MTP joints. It measures approximately 20 mm long, 9 mm wide, and 2 mm thick and is situated plantar to the metatarsal head [15–17]. Distally, the attachment to the proximal phalanx is stout, thick, and can have one or two bundles of fibers [16]. The proximal aspect of the plantar plate contains tissue that is thinner and more mobile and blends with the periosteum of the second metatarsal [16].

The dorsal surface of the plantar plate has an articular-like structure composed primarily of type 1 collagen (which resembles fibrocartilage) [15–17]. The fibers on the dorsal surface of the plantar plate are orientated in a longitudinal fashion, which run parallel to its overall anatomic course. The plantar third of the plantar plate has fibers that are organized in a transverse fashion to facilitate the attachments of the plantar plate to the deep transverse metatarsal ligament and is adjacent to the long flexor tendon and its tendon sheath [15–18] (Fig. 3.1).

The plantar plate receives several attachments (directly and indirectly) from surrounding soft tissue structures which assist with stabilizing the MTP joint. For example, the medial and lateral aspects of the plantar plate are continuous with both the deep transverse metatarsal ligament (DTML) and the collateral and suspensory ligaments. The DTML runs medial to lateral across the foot and provides a strong ligamentous structure that prevents undue splaying of the forefoot [19] and is a critical component of the stability of the lesser MTP joints [18, 20, 21]. Cadaveric dissection has identified that sectioning of the DTML may decrease the force needed to dislocate the lesser MTP joint [18, 20].

Additionally, the metatarsoglenoid (suspensory) ligament attaches to the inferior posterior portion of the metatarsal head tubercle and widens as it courses inferiorly to attach to the plantar plate [22]. The lesser MTP joint also has two collateral

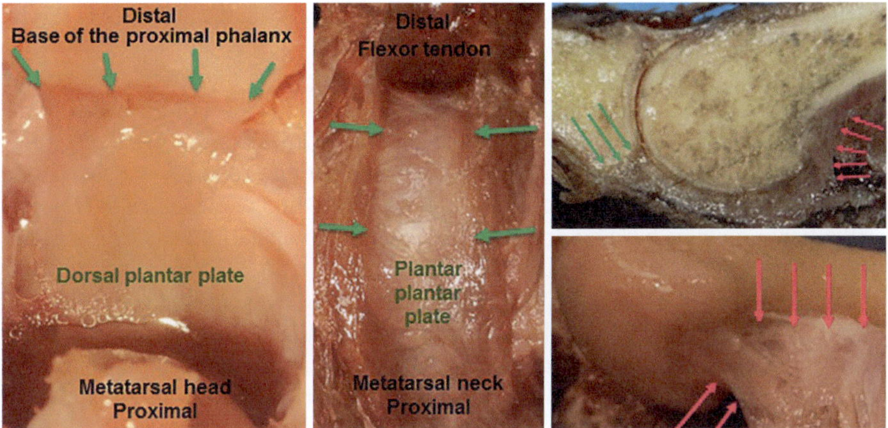

Fig. 3.1 Dorsal and plantar appearance of the plantar plate along with its distal (green arrows) and proximal attachments (pink arrows)

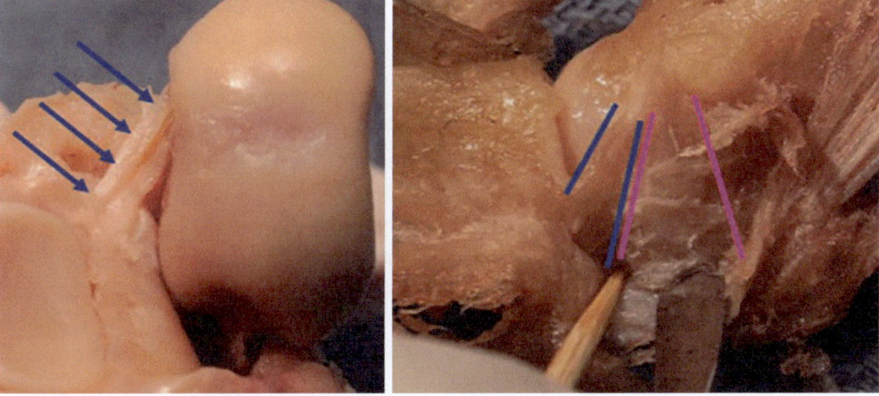

Fig. 3.2 The suspensory (pink lines) and collateral (blue arrows/lines) ligaments of the lesser MTP joint

ligaments on each side of the metatarsal head (medially and laterally) which course anteriorly and inferiorly to attach to the plantar medial or plantar lateral portion of the base of the proximal phalanx. The collateral MTP ligament attaches to the anterior superior portion of the tubercle located immediately proximal to the medial or lateral expansion of the articular cartilage on the metatarsal head. The collateral MTP ligament courses anteriorly and inferiorly to attach to the plantar medial or plantar lateral portion of the base of the proximal phalanx in close proximity to the plantar plate [22] (Fig. 3.2). The collateral ligaments also play an important role in stabilizing the lesser MTP joints in the sagittal plane [20]. Ruptured collateral ligaments are a common finding in cadaveric specimens with crossover toes [4, 23]. Furthermore, cadaveric studies have found that sectioning of (1) only the plantar plate, (2) only the collateral ligaments, and (3) both the plantar plate and collateral ligaments decreases the amount of force needed to dislocate the second MTP joint by 30%, 46%, and 80%, respectively [20].

The plantar plate also has an important relationship with the plantar fascia. The plantar fascia divides into superficial and deep layers at the level of the necks of the metatarsals [19, 24]. Distally, the deep and superficial layers of the five digital slips encompass the flexor tendons [22, 24]. The combination of the plantar fascia, the plantar plate, and the flexor tendons enables plantarflexion at the lesser MTP joints as the flexor tendons have no direct attachment to the metatarsal head or the proximal phalanx in this region.

Finally, the main blood supply to the metatarsal head enters the neck of the metatarsal slightly proximal to the tubercle and the attachment of the collateral ligaments [25]. Care should be taken to avoid serious disruption in this anatomic region during metatarsal osteotomies (Fig. 3.3). It is important also to recognize the proximity of the interdigital nerve to the joint capsule in this area of the forefoot. If there is capsular distension or alteration in joint anatomy, the nerve too can become compressed, resulting in neuroma-like symptoms in the absence of a true neuroma formation.

Diagnosis/Clinical Evaluation

Patients present with sharp and sometimes dull pain beneath one or more of the lesser metatarsal heads, the associated sulcus, and/or base of the proximal phalanges [8, 9]. Pain generally increases in severity as the magnitude of the joint/toe deformity progresses but can be minimal once the toe dislocates fully [8]. Also, burning neuritic symptoms are not uncommon and can be attributed to plantar plate subluxation and localized capsular edema and irritation of the adjacent digital nerve [17, 21].

As the injury to the plantar plate progresses, patients will exhibit weakness with plantar flexion strength at the MTP joint [8, 9]. This can be evaluated using a plantar grip test [8]. This test is performed by asking patients to grip and hold a piece of

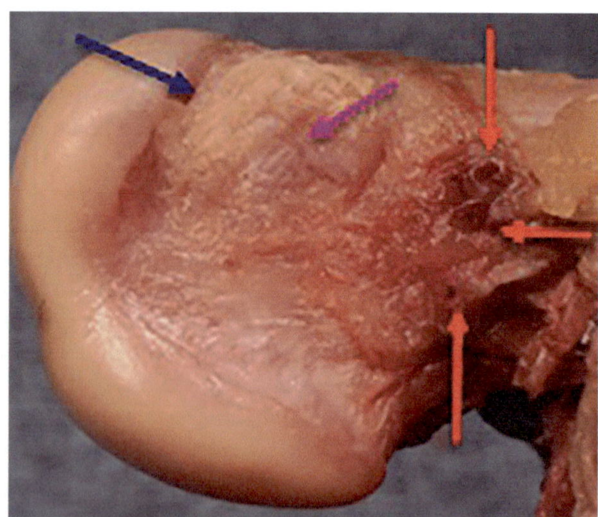

Fig. 3.3 The blood supply to the metatarsal head (red arrows) and its relationship to the suspensory (pink arrow) and collateral (blue arrow) ligament attachments on the metatarsal head

paper to the ground with the injured toe while the examiner tries to pull it away. Additionally, lack of toe purchase during weight-bearing stance may become apparent as the deformity advances [8, 9]. Finally, splaying or separation of the affected toe and adjacent toes upon weight-bearing can also be found in advanced plantar plate injuries [18, 19, 26]. This is due to the disruption of the plantar plate and destabilization of the transverse tie bar (described by Stainsby) [19] and DTML apparatus which allows the affected toe and its adjacent toe to drift apart (Fig. 3.4).

Lesser MTP joint stability should also be assessed using a drawer maneuver (Fig. 3.5). This is a vertical stress test [27]. When the test is performed, the nondominant hand should hold the forefoot stable with the ankle at 90°. The dominant hand should firmly grasp the proximal phalanx and displace the proximal phalanx vertically on the metatarsal head. In equivocal cases, displacement can be compared to the contralateral MTP joint (if unaffected) or an adjacent lesser MTP joint. A positive drawer test is highly suggestive of underlying plantar pate injury with a reported specificity of 99.8%, while a negative drawer, by itself, is not enough to rule pathology out [9].

In cases of progressive plantar plate injury, anterior-posterior (AP) foot X-rays will many times demonstrate a long second metatarsal relative to the first metatarsal. This is important as a long the second metatarsal significantly increases the load beneath the second metatarsal head during ambulation [14] (Fig. 3.6). Using the method of Nilsonne [28] to quantify second metatarsal length (in relation to the first), we previously found that a difference greater than 4 mm was associated with a 2.5× greater risk (multivariate odds ratio 2.5 [95% CI: 1.8–3.3]) of developing

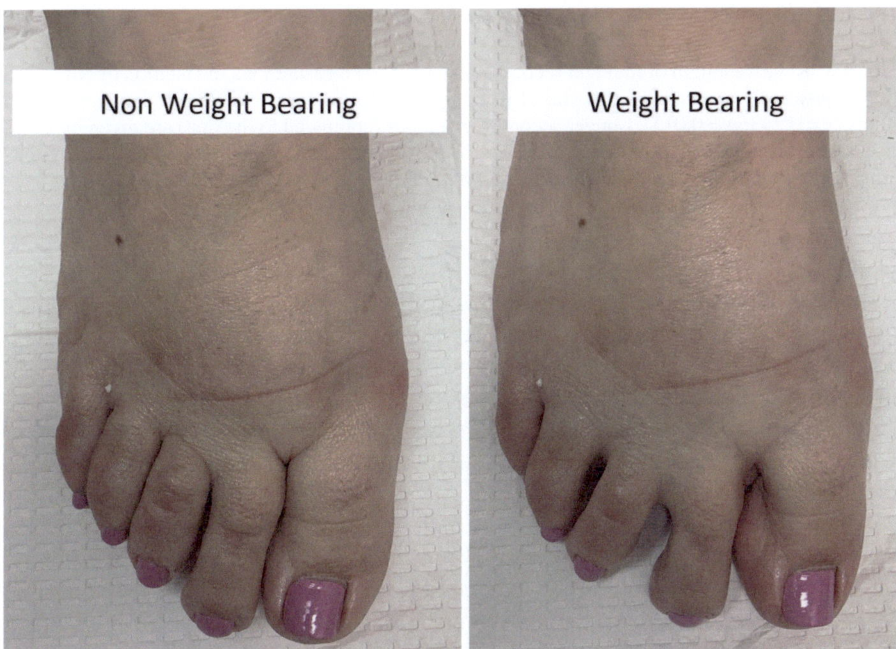

Fig. 3.4 Digital splaying and lateral deviation of the third toe is seen with weight-bearing, suggesting high-grade injury to the second MTP joint plantar plate [26]

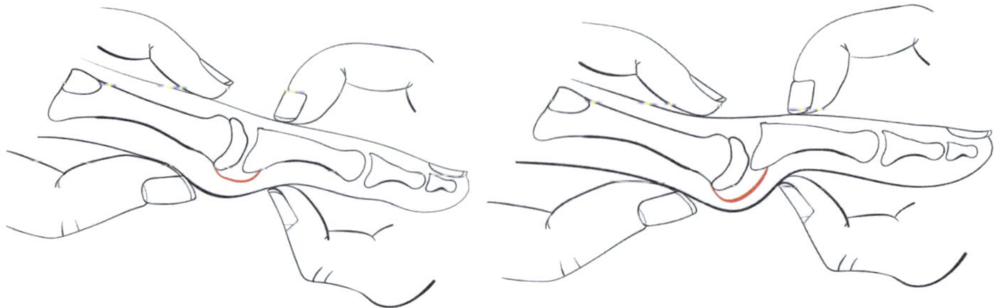

Fig. 3.5 Dorsal drawer test is a straight vertical stress of the lesser MTP joint

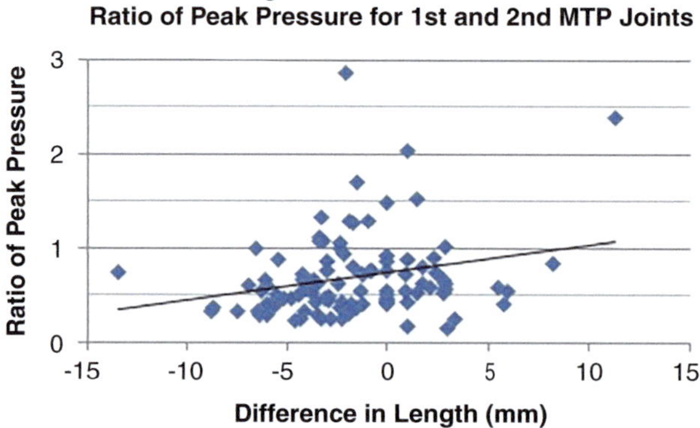

Fig. 3.6 Relative length of first and second metatarsals (as measured via the method of Nilsonne) [28] is positively associated with ratio of peak pressure for first and second metatarsophalangeal joints ($r = 0.243$, $p = 0.015$). Longer second metatarsals (compared to the first) are given by negative values on the x-axis. Relatively higher pressures beneath the second MTP joint on the y-axis are given by smaller values for the ratio of first MTP joint peak pressure/second MTP joint peak pressure [14]

plantar plate pathology [13] (Fig. 3.7). Metatarsal length also exhibited a dose-response relationship in this study, meaning that the risk for plantar plate pathology grew larger as the length discrepancy grew larger. Similarly, using the same method of measurement, Nakagawa and colleagues [12] recently explored how Nilsonne's measurement correlated with rates of postoperative metatarsalgia after bunion surgery. They looked at 51 patients (102 feet) with a mean follow-up of 16 months after hallux valgus surgery and found that the optimal cutoff for avoiding postoperative (sub-second) metatarsalgia was −3 mm, which corresponded to an area under the curve of 0.88 and a sensitivity and specificity of 85% and 88%, respectively. This was a very similar threshold to ours (−4 mm) using the same radiographic method of measurement. Although other methods of assessing relative second metatarsal length have been described, we feel the method of Nilsonne [28] is the single most informative for operative planning.

Advancing imaging in the form of magnetic resonance imaging (MRI) and dynamic ultrasound can be particularly useful in the diagnosis and staging of

Fig. 3.7 Nilsonne's method of metatarsal protrusion distance [28]. Standing AP X-rays are used. The measurement describes the distance in millimeters between a perpendicular line to the longitudinal axis of the second metatarsal at the most distal point of the second metatarsal head to a parallel line that passes through the distal most point of the first metatarsal head. Negative values are reported if the distal end of the first metatarsal is more proximal than the distal end of the second metatarsal. Positive values are reported if the distal end of the first metatarsal is more distal than the distal end of the second metatarsal

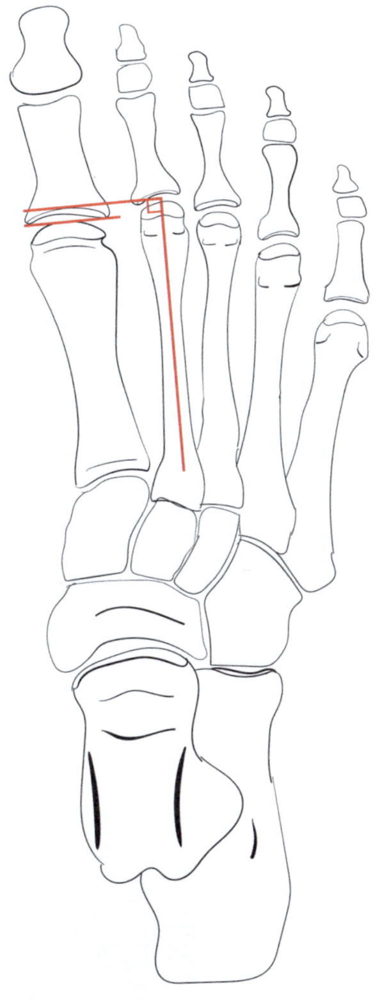

plantar plate pathology (Figs. 3.8 and 3.9). The clear advantage to ultrasound is that it can be performed at the point of care, and it allows the examiner (many times the surgeon him or herself) to perform drawer testing with direct visualization of the plantar plate itself during provocation [29]. In contrast, MRI appears to be a slightly more accurate method of diagnosing plantar plate pathology and can provide added insight into the integrity of the joint's additional supporting structures (e.g., collateral and suspensory ligaments).

Several classification systems have been described for plantar plate injuries; however, the most widely used is the anatomic grading system described by Nery and colleagues [8]:

- Grade 0
- Attenuation and/or capsular dislocation of the plantar plate
- Grade 1

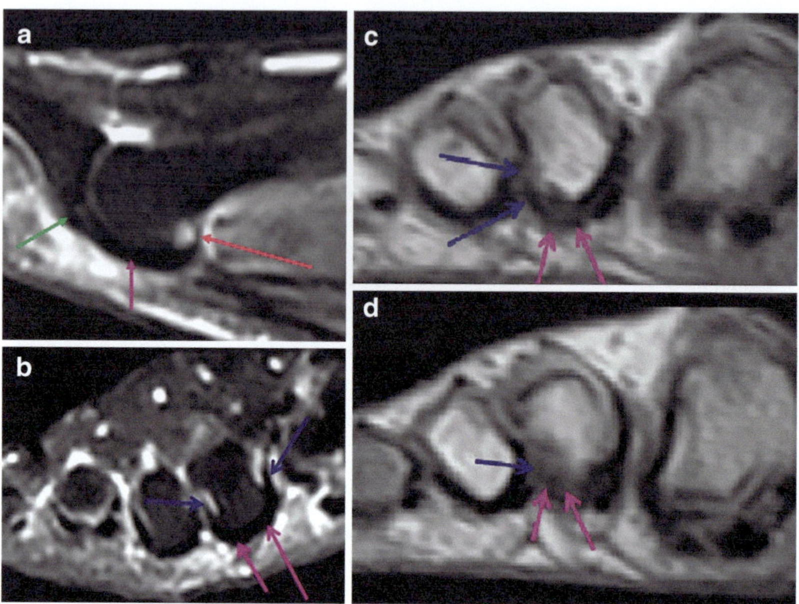

Fig. 3.8 (**a**) The plantar plate (pink arrow) appears hypointense on MRI and has a stout distal attachment (green arrow) with a proximal attachment that blends with the periosteum of the metatarsal (red arrow). (**b**) Collateral ligaments (blue arrows) should appear black and taught on the coronal images. (**c, d**) Coronal MR images depicting a lateral collateral ligament tear (blue arrows) with disruption of the lateral plantar plate (pink arrows)

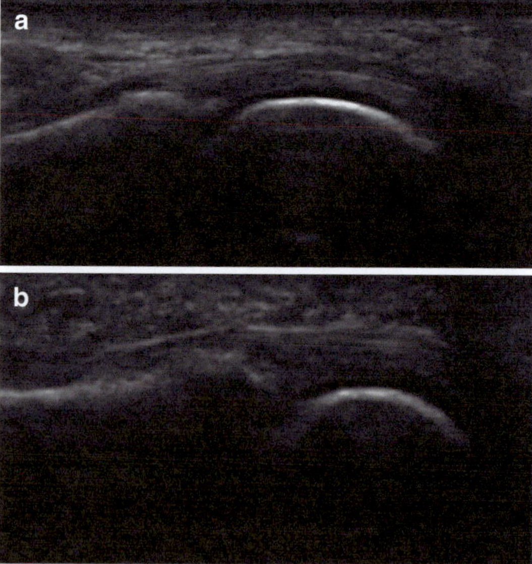

Fig. 3.9 (**a**) The plantar plate normally appears taught and echogenic on diagnostic ultrasound longitudinal scans. (**b**) When injured, it can appear thickened and hypoechoic with distortion of the overlying long flexor tendon as seen here

- Distal transverse lesion (adjacent to the insertion) at the proximal phalanx (<50%); medial/lateral/central area and/or intra-substantial lesion (<50%)
- Grade 2
- Distal transverse lesion (>50%); medial/lateral/central area and/or intra-substantial lesion (>50%)
- Grade 3
- Transverse lesion and/or extensive longitudinal lesion (may involve collateral ligament structures)
- Grade 4
- Extensive lesion in "buttonhole" shape (displacement); combination of transverse and longitudinal plate injuries

The integrity of the plantar plate and lesion configuration is determined at the time of surgery but can also be assessed fairly accurately on dedicated MR imaging preoperatively [30].

Treatment

Nonoperative treatment should be attempted initially, and this centers around supportive measures including over-the-counter and custom foot orthoses, accommodative padding to off-load the symptomatic metatarsal head, NSAIDs, and bracing of the toe via use of commercial splints or spicca dressings [31]. It is still unclear what role regenerative medicine (e.g., platelet rich plasma, amniotic injections, extracorporeal shockwave, etc.) has in this area, but it is unlikely these modalities will help much in the treatment of severe injuries or in patients with unstable joints (i.e., positive drawer test). Surgical treatment includes indirect repair (e.g., flexor to extensor transfers, extensor brevis transfers, and MTP joint arthrodesis) or direct repair of the plantar plate via a dorsal incisional approach or plantar approach. Direct repair through a dorsal incisional approach can be performed either with [6, 12, 32–36] or without [37] a lesser metatarsal osteotomy, and there are several methods of repairing the plantar plate from this approach which include the use of commercially available suture passing systems, Keith needles, and angiocatheter needles [38]. The plantar plate is typically advanced/imbricated to complete the repair and may be fixated a variety of ways (e.g., suture ties, suture button [39], suture anchor [5], and interference screw [40]). Finally, arthroscopic management of plantar plate injuries [41] and radiofrequency shrinkage of the injured tissue [33, 42] has also been described.

Evidence-Based/Critical Appraisal of the Literature

We performed a systematic review and meta-analysis of Medline and CINAHL databases to examine the *diagnostic performance of advanced imaging modalities and exam findings* for plantar plate injuries. We followed standard methodology for performing a meta-analysis using the Preferred Reporting Items for Systematic Reviews and Meta-Analyses (PRISMA) guidelines. Inclusion criteria included any original study that was published in a peer-reviewed journal that tested the diagnostic accuracy for detecting a plantar plate tear using MRI, ultrasound, or dorsal drawer test/Lachman's test. Studies were included if they reported on the sensitivity and specificity of one or more of the above tests. Additionally, unpublished work was included if raw data were available. Visual inspection of the plantar plate (during open surgery or arthroscopically) was used as the reference/gold standard. MeSH search criterion was performed using a PubMed database of words deemed appropriate and in relationship to plantar plate tears and the tools used to diagnose them (see appendix for search strategy). Sensitivity and specificity were obtained and, when possible, pooled from included studies. Summary receiver operating characteristic curves were formed also for diagnostic tests to compare accuracy. Study quality was assessed using the QUADAS scoring system.

The PRISMA flow diagram is depicted in the chapter appendix (Chart 3.1). A total of 1715 unique articles were initially identified, and 10 studies [7, 30, 43–50] met our inclusion criteria, representing 227 plantar plates for MRI and 194 plantar plates for ultrasound (Table 3.1). The overall study quality was good, with generally low ($n = 6$) or medium ($n = 3$) risk for bias across the included studies. MRI displayed a pooled sensitivity of 89% (95% CI: 0.84, 0.93) and pooled specificity of 83% (95% CI: 0.64, 0.94). Ultrasound displayed a pooled sensitivity and pooled specificity of 94% (95% CI:0.89, 0.97) and 55% (95% CI: 0.38, 0.71), respectively (Fig. 3.10). Overall, the diagnostic accuracy of MRI was slightly better than that of ultrasound (Fig. 3.11).

We found only one study that reported formally on the diagnostic performance of a dorsal drawer test [9]. In this study, a positive drawer test was highly suggestive of underlying injury to the plantar plate (specificity 99.8%), but a negative drawer was less able to rule out injury (sensitivity 80.6%).

In order to provide evidence-based recommendations regarding *direct operative repair of plantar plate injuries*, we similarly conducted a systematic review of studies published in Medline and CINAHL databases. We followed standard methodology for performing a systematic review using PRISMA guidelines. The inclusion criteria included any original study published in a peer-reviewed journal that evaluated patients who were treated for lesser metatarsophalangeal joint plantar plate injuries with direct repair and a follow-up time of 6 months or greater. Included studies had to provide a clear description of the technique used and needed to confirm the diagnosis of a plantar plate injury by either ultrasound, MRI, or intraoperative inspection. Prospective and retrospective studies were included. Non-English articles were included. Studies that used cadaver or animal models, focused on indirect repair or radiofrequency shrinkage, and case studies (where $n \leq 2$) were excluded. Summary estimates for mean visual analog scale (VAS) for pain and mean AOFAS scores were generated from included studies. Study quality was assessed using the CARE case report guidelines.

The PRISMA flow diagram is provided in the chapter appendix (Chart 3.2). A total of 2686 unique articles or conference papers were initially identified, and 11 studies met our inclusion criteria, representing 521 plantar plates (Table 3.2). Most studies were clinical level of evidence 4 (i.e., case series, $n = 9$), while two studies

Table 3.1 Diagnostic studies included in the qualitative and quantitative synthesis

Author (year)	Country, setting	Diagnostic test used	Who is reading result of test?	US strength/ frequency of unit used	MRI strength/ frequency of unit used	# of PP	# of subjects	Age (mean ± SD)	Gender (%M, %F)	Risk of bias (QUADAS 2)
Gregg (2006)	Australia	Ultrasound and MRI	MSK Sonographer and MSK Radiologist	Antares scanner (Siemens Medical Systems, Germany) with a high-frequency linear array probe (13-5VF; 11.4 MHz; dynamic range 60 dB; one focal zone)	1.5-T MRI scanner (Signa Hi Speed Plus, General Electric Medical Systems, Milwaukee, WI) with a Medical Advances Quadrature wrist coil	25 PP (10 feet)	10 feet (52 participants with 40 symptomatic and 40 asymptomatic feet)	Symptomatic: 57 y/o Asymptomatic: 31 y/o	Symptomatic: 10% M, 90% F Asymptomatic: 25% M, 75% F	Medium

(continued)

Table 3.1 (continued)

Author (year)	Country, setting	Diagnostic test used	Who is reading result of test?	US strength/ frequency of unit used	MRI strength/ frequency of unit used	# of PP	# of subjects	Age (mean ± SD)	Gender (%M, %F)	Risk of bias (QUADAS 2)
Gregg (2006)_ Cadaver	Australia	Ultrasound and MRI	MSK Sonographer and MSK Radiologist	13–5-MHz linear probe (Antares, Siemens Medical Solutions) + superficial MSK settings (11.4 MHz; 2 cm depth; dynamic range, 60 dB; 1 focal zone)	1.5-T unit (Signa HighSpeed Plus, GE Healthcare) + surface coil, the Med Advances Quadrature wrist coil	24 PP	3 cadavers, 6 feet	74–92 years old	66.6% M, 33.4% F	Low
Klein (2012)	Weil Foot and Ankle Institute – Illinois, USA	Ultrasound and MRI	Fellowship Trained MSK Radiologist and reconstructive foot and ankle fellow	Sonosite M-turbo US (Sonosite, Inc) and a linear 15-6 MHz transducer	0.3 T extremity coil without contrast	51 PP	42 patients	-	-	Low

| Sung (2012) | Weil Foot and Ankle Institute – Illinois, USA | MRI | Radiologist | – | Low-field extremity MRI unit with a field strength of 0.31 Tesla (O-Scan Extremity MRI, Biosound Esaote, Indianapolis, IN) without contrast material | 45 PP | 45 feet in 41 patients | 52.1 years old | 7.3% M, 92.7% F | Low |
| Mazzuca (2013) | Department of Orthopaedic Surgery, University of Minnesota, Minneapolis, MN, USA | MR Arthrography | 2 Radiologists | – | 1.5 Tesla MR scanner, using dedicated extremity coils | 25 PP | 25 patients | 53 years old | 20% M, 80% F | Medium |

(continued)

Table 3.1 (continued)

Author (year)	Country, setting	Diagnostic test used	Who is reading result of test?	US strength/ frequency of unit used	MRI strength/ frequency of unit used	# of PP	# of subjects	Age (mean ± SD)	Gender (%M, %F)	Risk of bias (QUADAS 2)
Carlson (2013)	Loyola University Health Systems Outpatient Clinics – Illinois, USA	Ultrasound	An attending physician in the Department of Radiology	Acuson Sequoia 512 Ultrasound Scanner (Siemens Medical Solutions USA, Inc., Malvern, PA)	–	8 PP	8 patients	51.9 years old	100% F	High
Klein (2013)	Weil Foot and Ankle Institute – Illinois, USA	Longitudinal Ultrasound	Reconstructive foot and ankle fellow	Sonosite M-turbo ultrasound (Sonosite, Inc, Bothell, WA) and a linear 15-6 MHz transducer	–	45 PP	50 patients	–	–	Low

| Donegan (2017) | California, USA | Ultrasound and MRI | Radiologist | Linear array 8- to 18-MHz hockey stick and linear array 6- to 15-MHz wand | 1.5T and 3.0T, dedicated foot and ankle phased-array, 8-channel, high-field open MRI machine | 12 PP | 12 patients | – | | 33% M, 67% F | Low |
| Stone (2017) | Henry Ford Hospital – Detriot, Michicgan, USA | Ultrasound | Fellowship-trained MSK radiologist | LOGIQ E9 ultrasound machine (GE Healthcare, Milwaukee, WI) using an L8-18i probe (GE Healthcare) | – | 24 PP | 6 cadaver feet from 4 cadavers | 69 years old | | 50% M, 50% F | Low |

(continued)

Table 3.1 (continued)

Author (year)	Country, setting	Diagnostic test used	Who is reading result of test?	US strength/ frequency of unit used	MRI strength/ frequency of unit used	# of PP	# of subjects	Age (mean ± SD)	Gender (%M, %F)	Risk of bias (QUADAS 2)
Yamada (2017)	Brazil – Federal University of São Paulo	MRI	2 Radiologists	–	1.5-T units (Signa Excite HD, GE Healthcare; Achieva, Philips Healthcare; or Aera, Siemens Healthcare) w/ dedicated standard extremity coil	45 PP	23 patients	60.5 ± 8.1 years old	43.5% M, 56.5% F	Medium

MRI

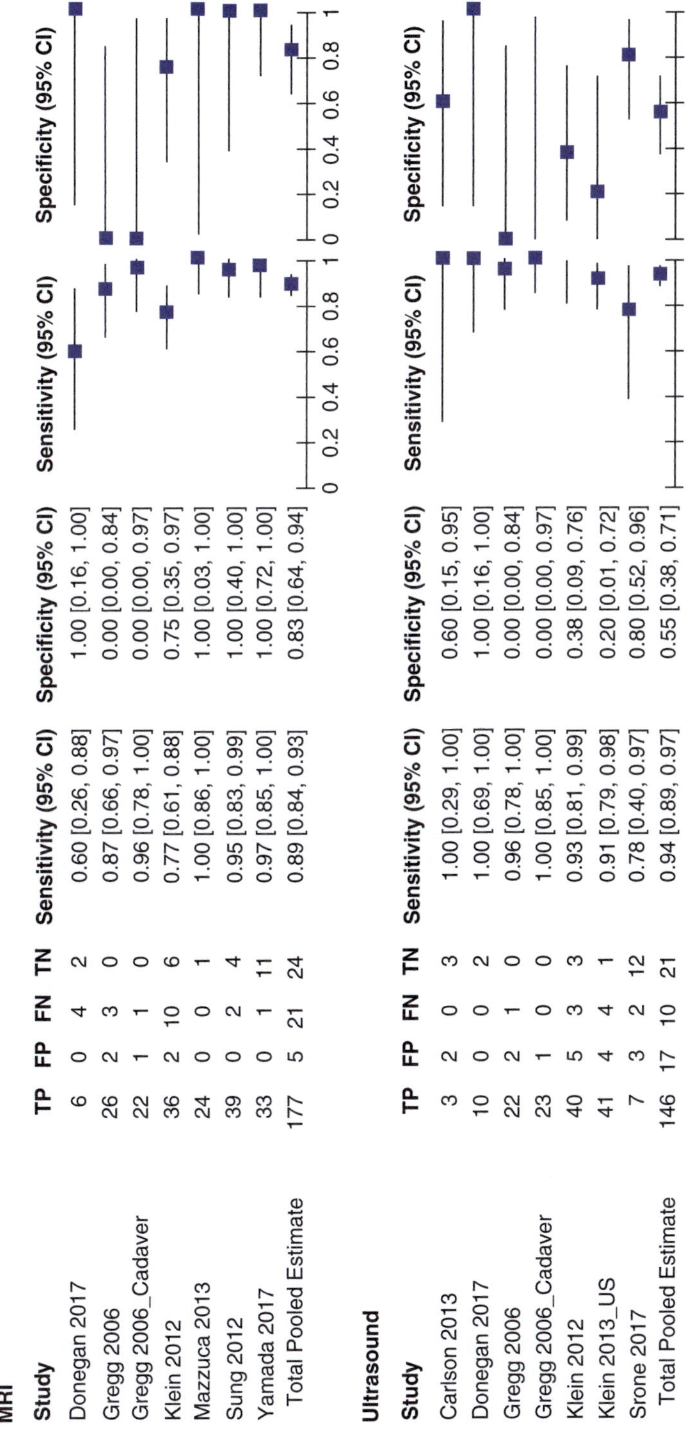

Study	TP	FP	FN	TN	Sensitivity (95% CI)	Specificity (95% CI)
Donegan 2017	6	0	4	2	0.60 [0.26, 0.88]	1.00 [0.16, 1.00]
Gregg 2006	26	2	3	0	0.87 [0.66, 0.97]	0.00 [0.00, 0.84]
Gregg 2006_Cadaver	22	1	1	0	0.96 [0.78, 1.00]	0.00 [0.00, 0.97]
Klein 2012	36	2	10	6	0.77 [0.61, 0.88]	0.75 [0.35, 0.97]
Mazzuca 2013	24	0	0	1	1.00 [0.86, 1.00]	1.00 [0.03, 1.00]
Sung 2012	39	0	2	4	0.95 [0.83, 0.99]	1.00 [0.40, 1.00]
Yamada 2017	33	0	1	11	0.97 [0.85, 1.00]	1.00 [0.72, 1.00]
Total Pooled Estimate	177	5	21	24	0.89 [0.84, 0.93]	0.83 [0.64, 0.94]

Ultrasound

Study	TP	FP	FN	TN	Sensitivity (95% CI)	Specificity (95% CI)
Carlson 2013	3	2	0	3	1.00 [0.29, 1.00]	0.60 [0.15, 0.95]
Donegan 2017	10	0	0	2	1.00 [0.69, 1.00]	1.00 [0.16, 1.00]
Gregg 2006	22	2	1	0	0.96 [0.78, 1.00]	0.00 [0.00, 0.84]
Gregg 2006_Cadaver	23	1	0	0	1.00 [0.85, 1.00]	0.00 [0.00, 0.97]
Klein 2012	40	5	3	3	0.93 [0.81, 0.99]	0.38 [0.09, 0.76]
Klein 2013_US	41	4	4	1	0.91 [0.79, 0.98]	0.20 [0.01, 0.72]
Srone 2017	7	3	2	12	0.78 [0.40, 0.97]	0.80 [0.52, 0.96]
Total Pooled Estimate	146	17	10	21	0.94 [0.89, 0.97]	0.55 [0.38, 0.71]

Fig. 3.10 MRI versus US in the diagnosis of plantar plate tears. Forest plots demonstrating the summary estimates for sensitivity and specificity for each modality. *TP* true positive, *FP* false positive, *FN* false negative, *TN* true negative

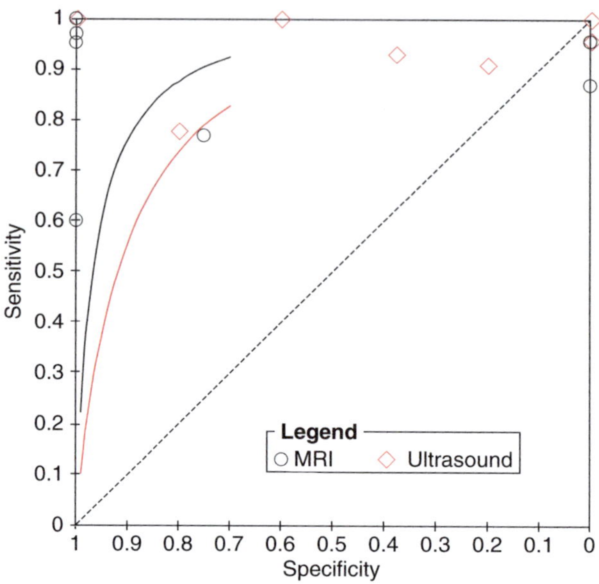

Fig. 3.11 Summary receiver operating characteristic (ROC) curves for diagnosing plantar plate tears. MRI performs slightly better than ultrasound (US) in overall accuracy

had a comparison group (i.e., level 3 evidence). That said, the included studies were generally well conducted with transparent reporting and only low or medium risk of bias. Most studies (9/11, 82%) examined direct repair of the plantar plate from a dorsal incisional approach. Our own unpublished data on 53 patients (53 second MTP joints) with 2 years of postoperative follow-up previously presented at the American Academy of Orthopaedic Surgeons (AAOS) 2016 annual meeting was also included [36]. Overall, patients generally did well following direct repair of the plantar plate, with few reported complications. The pooled mean change in VAS pain from pre- to postoperatively was −5.16 (95% CI: −3.96, −6.35) among articles that examined plantar plate repair from a dorsal approach ($n = 270$ joints) (Fig. 3.12). Patients undergoing direct repair of the plantar plate can also expect significant improvements in function that is maintained at 1–2 years out (pooled postoperative mean AOFAS score 87.4 [95% CI: 84.3–90.5], 6 studies [$n = 228$ patients, 332 joints]). Lack of toe purchase (~20% of the time) and persistent drawer (~5%) were among the most common reported complications.

Many surgeons question, "When is it appropriate to repair an injured plantar plate, and when should it just be left alone?" Some authors have suggested following operative protocols based on the grade of plantar plate injury [33], yet others feel there is value in directly repairing and imbricating the plantar plate in nearly all instances when a shortening osteotomy is performed [6, 51] or when joint instability is suggested [37]. Our recent comparative study from 2020 (86 patients, 65 direct repair from a dorsal approach) found that patients of ours who underwent concomitant plantar plate repair in addition to a shortening osteotomy

Table 3.2 Studies that examined direct operative repair of plantar plate injuries included for qualitative synthesis

Title	Country, setting	Procedure type	# of PP	# of subjects	Age (mean ± SD)	Gender (M, F)	Risk of bias (modified CARE statement)
Weil (2011) [6]	Weil Foot and Ankle Institute, Des Plaines, IL, USA	WMO w/ PPR – dorsal approach	15 feet (second MTPJ)	13	57 ± 7.0 (50–69)	3, 10	Medium
Cook (2018) [37]	Department of Surgery, Mount Auburn Hospital, Cambridge, MA, USA	Anatomic plantar plate and collateral ligament reconstruction – dorsal approach	18 {second, third)	18	58.16 ± 12.1	4, 14	Medium
Bouche (2008) [5]	Seattle, WA, USA	Combined PP and hammertoe repair w/ FDL tendon transfer – plantar approach	17 feet (second, third, fourth MTPJ)	15	53.7 (44–63) (from original 18)	4, 14 (from original 18)	Low
Fleischer (2020) [32]	Weil Foot and Ankle Institute, Mount Prospect, IL, USA	WMO w/ PPR – dorsal approach	65 feet (second MTPJ)	65	60.0 ± 10.2	13, 52	Low
Nery (2014) [33]	Sao Paulo, Brazil	WMO w/ PPR – dorsal approach + lateral soft tissue reefing	40 (second, third, fourth)	22	61	8, 20 (from original 28)	Medium
Kindred (2020) [38]	Podiatric Surgical Residency, Community Health Network, Indianapolis, IN, USA	WMO w/ PPR using low cost materials – dorsal approach	9 (second, third, fourth)	6	63 (44–74)	0, 6	Low

(continued)

Table 3.2 (continued)

Title	Country, setting	Procedure type	# of PP	# of subjects	Age (mean ± SD)	Gender (M, F)	Risk of bias (modified CARE statement)
Flint (2017) [51]	St. Alphonsus Medical Group, Boise, ID, USA	WMO w/ PPR – dorsal approach	97 feet, 138 PP repairs (second, third, fourth)	91	59 (32–82)	10, 81	Low
Prissel (2017) [52]	Orthopedic Foot and Ankle Center, Westerville, OH, USA	PPR – plantar approach w/ or w/o concomitant WMO	144 (second or third MTPJ)	131	58.6 ± 10.2	24, 107	Medium
Yu (2013) [35]	Department of Orthopaedics, Tongji Hospital of Tongji University, Shanghai, China	WMO w/ PPR – dorsal approach	14 (second MTPJ)	14	65.9 (51–82)	4, 10	Medium
Zhou (2015) [53]	Department of Orthopaedics, the First Hospital affiliated to Wen-Hou Medical University, Zhenjiang, China	WMO – dorsal approach	8 (second MTPJ)	5	52	0, 5	Medium
Klein (2016) [36]	Weil Foot and Ankle Institute, Des Plaines, IL, USA	WMO w/ PPR – dorsal approach	53 (second MTPJ)	53	54.5 + 11.2 (20–77)	3, 50	Medium

Study	Preop VAS			Postop VAS				Mean Diff. with 95% CI	Weight (%)
	N	Mean	SD	N	Mean	SD			
Cook 2018	18	5.2	2.5	18	4.8	2.2		2.50 [0.96, 4.04]	12.70
Flint 2017	91	5.4	1.5	91	1.5	1.5		3.90 [3.46, 4.34]	15.77
Hai-bo 2015	5	5.4	1.5	5	.75	1.5		4.65 [2.79, 6.51]	11.57
Klein 2018	53	6.5	1.5	53	1.5	1.5		5.00 [4.57, 5.43]	15.78
Nery 2012	22	8	1.5	22	1	1.5		7.00 [6.11, 7.89]	14.79
Nery 2014	68	7.9	1	68	.95	1		6.95 [6.61, 7.29]	15.90
Weil 2011	13	7.3	1.6	13	1.7	1.8		5.60 [4.29, 6.91]	13.49
Overall								5.16 [3.96, 6.35]	

Heterogeneity: $T^2 = 2.30$, $I^2 = 95.91\%$, $H^2 = 24.46$

Test of $\theta_i = \theta_j$: Q(6) = 154.22, p = 0.00

Test of $\theta = \theta$: z = 8.48, p = 0.00

Random-effects REML model

Fig. 3.12 Forest plots demonstrating the mean change in VAS pain pre- to postoperatively with direct repair of the plantar plate form a dorsal incisional approach

for metatarsalgia reported significantly better foot-specific quality of life scores and less pain at 1 year compared to those undergoing a shortening osteotomy alone for metatarsalgia [32]. This was true despite having generally more severe injuries to their plantar plates to start. We concluded that directly repairing and advancing the plantar plate when a Weil osteotomy is performed may be valuable regardless of the severity of injury in the plate [32]. As a result, we now repair and advance nearly every plantar plate/joint that requires surgery, with the notable exception being those joints with a negative drawer and pristine appearing plantar plate on gross inspection.

Despite the generally favorable outcomes reported in the short and intermediate term with direct repair of the plantar plate, there is still little long-term data with follow-up greater than 2 years in the current literature. It is therefore important to recognize that there is uncertainty at this time as to what kind of longevity can be expected with direct repair.

Final Treatment Algorithm/Author's Preferred Method

Preoperatively, we perform diagnostic ultrasound exams in the office and confirm suspected pathology within the plantar plate and the collateral ligaments with formal MRI. Plantar plate injuries that are unresponsive to nonoperative management are surgically repaired, in nearly all instances, from a dorsal incisional approach. The only exception being an acute rupture in a patient with an already short metatarsal, where a plantar approach might be more desirable.

In this section we illustrate the surgical technique which we originally described in 2011 and have modified very little over the years [6]. The technique is ideal for plantar plate pathology as it addresses an important risk factor in the causal pathway (i.e., a long metatarsal) and avoids a plantar incision in the foot.

First, an incision is made over the dorsal aspect of the lesser metatarsophalangeal joint. This can be either linear (longitudinal) or transverse as pictured in Fig. 3.13a. The extensor tendons and periosteum are then incised and retracted. The collateral ligaments are dissected from the base of the proximal phalanx (Fig. 3.13b), but care must be taken to *avoid* disrupting their proximal attachment on the metatarsal head. A McGlamry-type elevator is utilized centrally over the metatarsal head to mobilize the proximal aspect of the plantar plate. This must be freed up sufficiently to allow for advancement of the plate during the final portion of the procedure (Fig. 3.13c). A Weil osteotomy is created in the metatarsal parallel to the weight-bearing surface. The angle of this cut is depicted in Figs. 3.13d and 3.14. The cut is initiated 2 mm inferior to the dorsal most articular cartilage on the metatarsal head and is therefore intra-articular. If your plan is to shorten the metatarsal length $\geq$ 3 mm, then a small wedge of bone (via parallel cuts) must be removed also at this point to prevent plantarflexion of the metatarsal head upon its translation proximally. The capital fragment is retrograded and provisionally fixated with a k-wire (Fig. 3.13e). A second k-wire is placed in the base of the proximal phalanx. A small joint distractor is now utilized to open up the joint (Fig. 3.13f). The plantar plate can then be inspected and classified according to Nery et al.'s anatomic grading [8]. The plantar plate is then dissected away from the base of the proximal phalanx with a #64 blade (leaving the flexor tendon complex intact), and one flap of tissue is created (Fig. 3.13g). This is similar to what is done during rotator cuff surgery, where a partial tear (when encountered at the phalangeal base) is converted into a complete tear for the purposes of advancing and imbricating the plantar plate.

Nonabsorbable suture (#2 or larger) is then passed through the plantar plate. We typically use a commercially available suture passing system for this (Fig. 3.13h,i). The configuration of suture is dependent upon the extent and orientation of the tear(s) encountered. The final construct should allow the plantar plate to lie flat during mobilization with a suture bridge as wide as possible. K-wires are then utilized to create crossed osseous tunnels through the proximal metaphysis of the proximal phalanx (Fig. 3.13j,k). Suture passers are then placed

Fig. 3.13 Direct repair of the plantar plate from a dorsal incisional approach. (**a**) Dorsal incisional appraoch, (**b**) Perosteal and capslar dissection preserving the collateral attachments on the metatarsal head, (**c**) McGlamry elevator used to free up the plantar plate from the metatarsal head, (**d**) Saw blade depicting the proper angle of the osteotomy through the 2nd metatarsal head, (**e**) Provisional fixation of the metatarsal head, out of the way proximally, (**f**) A second pin is placed in the base of the proximal phalanx allow for distraction of the joint and visualization of the plantar plate, (**g**) The plantar plate is sharply dissected from the base of the proximal phalanx to allow for imbrication and advancement later, (**h**) and (**i**) Nonabsorbable suture is passed through the plate repairing any deficits. The final configuration must allow for a wide suture bridge so that the plate advances evenly. (**j**, **k**) Crossing bone tunnels are created in the base of the proximal phalanx, (**l**, **m**) The nonabsorbable suture is passed from the plantar to dorsal through the tunnels, advancing the plnatar plate onto the undersurface of the proximl phalanx to be tied later, (**n**) The 2nd metatarsal head is "kicked" back into position now ensuring a harmonious forefoot metatarsal parabola has been achieved and permanent fixation applied

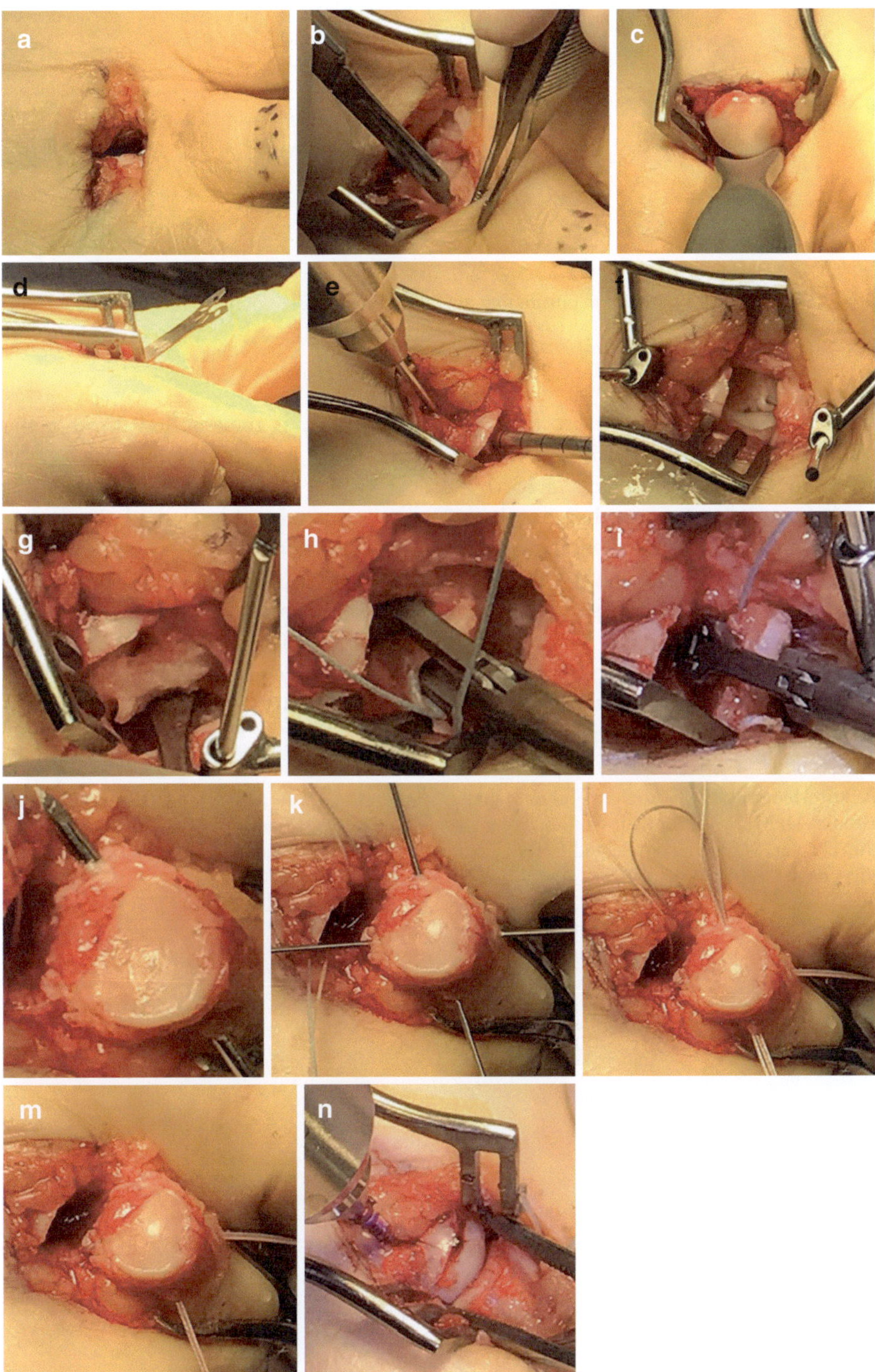

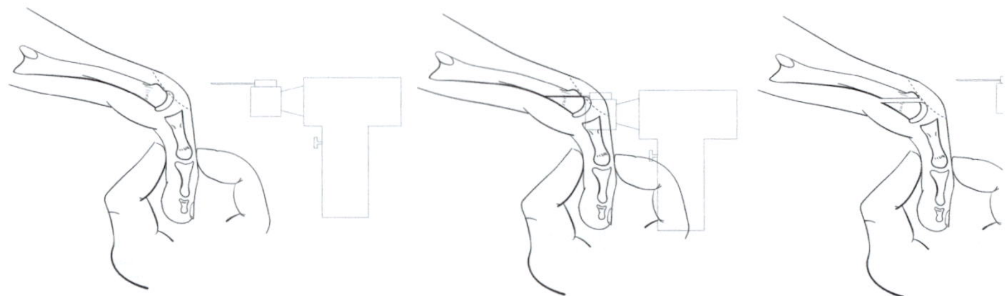

Fig. 3.14 Care must be taken to ensure that angle of the Weil osteotomy is parallel to the weight-bearing surface

through these tunnels. Suture from the plantar plate is then pulled through the osseous tunnels (Fig. 3.13l,m). The Weil osteotomy is then permanently fixated with one or two screws (Fig. 3.13n).

Any prominent or overhanging bone is now resected and smoothed. The toe is held in maximal plantarflexion, and the suture is tied with the toe in plantarflexion. After the suture is tied, the foot is loaded to assure that the toe is in the appropriate position. Postoperatively, patients are partially weight-bearing in a dressing and a surgical shoe for 10 days. The patient then starts to brace at night with the toe in maximal plantarflexion, and physical therapy is commenced. At 1 year postoperatively, the patient should have a stable drawer sign, range of motion adequate for ambulation, and a toe that purchases the floor.

Acknowledgments We are grateful to Manali Chingre, BA, BS, Ryan Jameson, BS, and Brandon Brooks, DPM, MPH, for their work on the systematic reviews and meta-analyses contained within this chapter. We are also indebted to Ryan Jameson for the line art and illustrations contained in this chapter.

Appendix

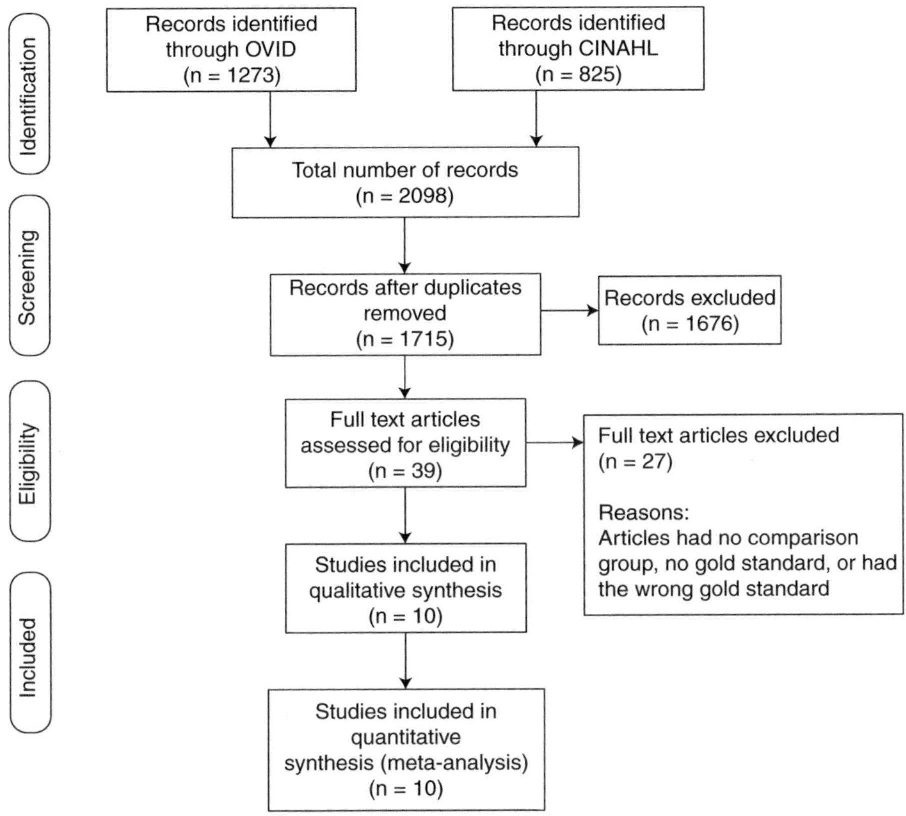

Chart 3.1   PRISMA flow diagram: diagnosis of plantar plate injuries

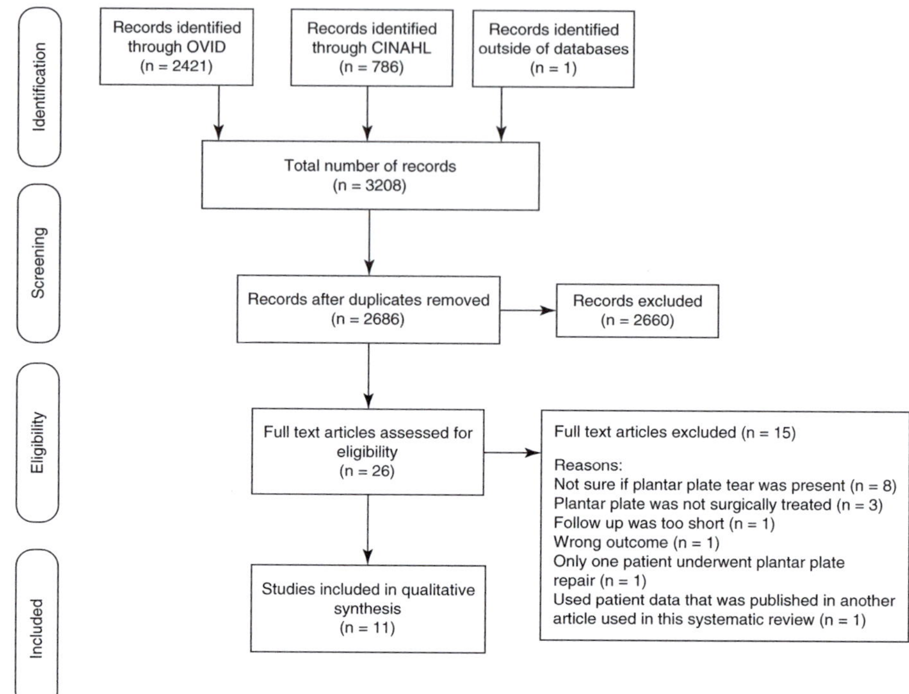

Chart 3.2 PRISMA flow diagram: surgical treatment of plantar plate injuries via direct repair

References

1. Coughlin MJ. Crossover second toe deformity. Foot Ankle. 1987;8(1):29–39.
2. Doty JF, Coughlin MJ. Metatarsophalangeal joint instability of the lesser toes and plantar plate deficiency. J Am Acad Orthop Surg. 2014;22(4):235–45.
3. Doty JF, Coughlin MJ, Weil L Jr, Nery C. Etiology and management of lesser toe metatarsophalangeal joint instability. Foot Ankle Clin. 2014;19(3):385–405.
4. Coughlin MJ, Schutt SA, Hirose CB, Kennedy MJ, Grebing BR, Smith BW, et al. Metatarsophalangeal joint pathology in crossover second toe deformity: a cadaveric study. Foot Ankle Int. 2012;33(2):133–40.
5. Bouché RT, Heit EJ. Combined plantar plate and hammertoe repair with flexor digitorum longus tendon transfer for chronic, severe sagittal plane instability of the lesser metatarsophalangeal joints: preliminary observations. J Foot Ankle Surg. 2008;47(2):125–37.
6. Weil L Jr, Sung W, Weil LS Sr, Malinoski K. Anatomic plantar plate repair using the Weil metatarsal osteotomy approach. Foot Ankle Spec. 2011;4(3):145–50.
7. Klein EE, Weil L Jr, Weil LS Sr, Knight J. Musculoskeletal ultrasound for preoperative imaging of the plantar plate: a prospective analysis. Foot Ankle Spec. 2013;6(3):196–200.
8. Nery C, Coughlin M, Baumfeld D, Raduan F, Mann TS, Catena F. How to classify plantar plate injuries: parameters from history and physical examination. Rev Bras Ortop. 2015;50(6):720–8.
9. Klein EE, Weil L Jr, Weil LS Sr, Coughlin MJ, Knight J. Clinical examination of plantar plate abnormality: a diagnostic perspective. Foot Ankle Int. 2013;34(6):800–4.
10. Klein EE, Weil L Jr, Weil LS Sr, Knight J. The underlying osseous deformity in plantar plate tears: a radiographic analysis. Foot Ankle Spec. 2013;6(2):108–18.

11. Bhutta MA, Chauhan D, Zubairy AI, Barrie J. Second metatarsophalangeal joint instability and second metatarsal length association depends on the method of measurement. Foot Ankle Int. 2010;31(6):486–91.
12. Nakagawa S, Fukushi J, Nakagawa T, Mizu-Uchi H, Iwamoto Y. Association of metatarsalgia after hallux valgus correction with relative first metatarsal length. Foot Ankle Int. 2016;37(6):582–8.
13. Fleischer AE, Klein EE, Ahmad M, Shah S, Catena F, Weil LS Sr, et al. Association of abnormal metatarsal parabola with second metatarsophalangeal joint plantar plate pathology. Foot Ankle Int. 2017;38(3):289–97.
14. Fleischer AE, Hshieh S, Crews RT, Waverly BJ, Jones JM, Klein EE, et al. Association between second metatarsal length and forefoot loading under the second metatarsophalangeal joint. Foot Ankle Int. 2018;39(5):560–7.
15. Deland JT, Lee KT, Sobel M, DiCarlo EF. Anatomy of the plantar plate and its attachments in the lesser metatarsal phalangeal joint. Foot Ankle Int. 1995;16(8):480–6.
16. Johnston RB 3rd, Smith J, Daniels T. The plantar plate of the lesser toes: an anatomical study in human cadavers. Foot Ankle Int. 1994;15(5):276–82.
17. Umans HR, Elsinger E. The plantar plate of the lesser metatarsophalangeal joints: potential for injury and role of MR imaging. Magn Reson Imaging Clin N Am. 2001;9(3):659–69. xii
18. Wang B, Guss A, Chalayon O, Bachus KN, Barg A, Saltzman CL. Deep transverse metatarsal ligament and static stability of lesser metatarsophalangeal joints: a cadaveric study. Foot Ankle Int. 2015;36(5):573–8.
19. Stainsby GD. Pathological anatomy and dynamic effect of the displaced plantar plate and the importance of the integrity of the plantar plate-deep transverse metatarsal ligament tie-bar. Ann R Coll Surg Engl. 1997;79(1):58–68.
20. Bhatia D, Myerson MS, Curtis MJ, Cunningham BW, Jinnah RH. Anatomical restraints to dislocation of the second metatarsophalangeal joint and assessment of a repair technique. J Bone Joint Surg Am. 1994;76(9):1371–5.
21. Chalayon O, Chertman C, Guss AD, Saltzman CL, Nickisch F, Bachus KN. Role of plantar plate and surgical reconstruction techniques on static stability of lesser metatarsophalangeal joints: a biomechanical study. Foot Ankle Int. 2013;34(10):1436–42.
22. Sarrafian SK, Topouzian LK. Anatomy and physiology of the extensor apparatus of the toes. J Bone Joint Surg Am. 1969;51(4):669–79.
23. Deland JT, Sung IH. The medial crosssover toe: a cadaveric dissection. Foot Ankle Int. 2000;21(5):375–8.
24. Bojsen-Moller F, Flagstad KE. Plantar aponeurosis and internal architecture of the ball of the foot. J Anat. 1976;121(Pt 3):599–611.
25. Petersen WJ, Lankes JM, Paulsen F, Hassenpflug J. The arterial supply of the lesser metatarsal heads: a vascular injection study in human cadavers. Foot Ankle Int. 2002;23(6):491–5.
26. Klein EE, Weil L Jr, Weil LS Sr, Bowen M, Fleischer AE. Positive drawer test combined with radiographic deviation of the third metatarsophalangeal joint suggests high grade tear of the second metatarsophalangeal joint plantar plate. Foot Ankle Spec. 2014;7(6):466–70.
27. Thompson FM, Hamilton WG. Problems of the second metatarsophalangeal joint. Orthopedics. 1987;10(1):83–9.
28. Nilsonne H. Hallux rigidus and its treatment. Acta Orthop. 1930;1(1–4):295–303.
29. Feuerstein CA, Weil L Jr, Weil LS Sr, Klein EE, Fleischer A, Argerakis NG. Static versus dynamic musculoskeletal ultrasound for detection of plantar plate pathology. Foot Ankle Spec. 2014;7(4):259–65.
30. Sung W, Weil L Jr, Weil LS Sr, Rolfes RJ. Diagnosis of plantar plate injury by magnetic resonance imaging with reference to intraoperative findings. J Foot Ankle Surg. 2012;51(5):570–4.
31. Yu GV, Judge MS, Hudson JR, Seidelmann FE. Predislocation syndrome. Progressive subluxation/dislocation of the lesser metatarsophalangeal joint. J Am Podiatr Med Assoc. 2002;92(4):182–99.
32. Fleischer AE, Klein EE, Bowen M, McConn TP, Sorensen MD, Weil L Jr. Comparison of combination Weil metatarsal osteotomy and direct plantar plate repair versus Weil metatarsal osteotomy alone for forefoot metatarsalgia. J Foot Ankle Surg. 2020;59(2):303–6.

33. Nery C, Coughlin MJ, Baumfeld D, Raduan FC, Mann TS, Catena F. Prospective evaluation of protocol for surgical treatment of lesser MTP joint plantar plate tears. Foot Ankle Int. 2014;35(9):876–85.
34. Nery C, Coughlin MJ, Baumfeld D, Mann TS. Lesser metatarsophalangeal joint instability: prospective evaluation and repair of plantar plate and capsular insufficiency. Foot Ankle Int. 2012;33(4):301–11.
35. Yu G, Yu Y, Zhang P, Yang Y, Li B, Zhang M. Surgical repair of chronic tears of the second plantar plate. Zhongguo Xiu Fu Chong Jian Wai Ke Za Zhi. 2013;27(12):1446–9.
36. Klein E WJL, Baker J, Sheinkop M, Fleischer A. Intermediate term clinical and patient perceived outcomes of the dorsal approach plantar plate repair. American Academy of Orthopaedic Surgeons (AAOS) Annual Meeting, March 2, 2016; Orlando, FL.
37. Cook JJ, Johnson LJ, Cook EA. Anatomic reconstruction versus traditional rebalancing in lesser metatarsophalangeal joint reconstruction. J Foot Ankle Surg. 2018;57(3):509–13.
38. Kindred KB, Rusher A, Baker A, Groh CN, Fink BR. Outcomes study of an innovative method of direct repair of metatarsophalangeal joint instability with an angiocatheter needle. J Foot Ankle Surg. 2020;59(1):178–83.
39. Judge MS, Hild G. A suture-button technique for stabilization of the plantar plate and lesser metatarsophalangeal joint. J Foot Ankle Surg. 2018;57(4):645–53.
40. Sung W. Technique using interference fixation repair for plantar plate ligament disruption of lesser metatarsophalangeal joints. J Foot Ankle Surg. 2015;54(3):508–12.
41. Lui TH. Correction of crossover toe deformity by arthroscopically assisted plantar plate tenodesis. Arthrosc Tech. 2016;5(6):e1273–9.
42. Nery C, Raduan FC, Catena F, Mann TS, de Andrade MA, Baumfeld D. Plantar plate radiofrequency and Weil osteotomy for subtle metatarsophalangeal joint instablity. J Orthop Surg Res. 2015;10:180.
43. Donegan RJ, Stauffer A, Heaslet M, Poliskie M. Comparing magnetic resonance imaging and high-resolution dynamic ultrasonography for diagnosis of plantar plate pathology: a case series. J Foot Ankle Surg. 2017;56(2):371–4.
44. Gregg J, Silberstein M, Schneider T, Marks P. Sonographic and MRI evaluation of the plantar plate: a prospective study. Eur Radiol. 2006;16(12):2661–9.
45. Gregg JM, Silberstein M, Schneider T, Kerr JB, Marks P. Sonography of plantar plates in cadavers: correlation with MRI and histology. AJR Am J Roentgenol. 2006;186(4):948–55.
46. Stone M, Eyler W, Rhodenizer J, van Holsbeeck M. Accuracy of sonography in plantar plate tears in cadavers. J Ultrasound Med. 2017;36(7):1355–61.
47. Klein EE, Weil L Jr, Weil LS Sr, Knight J. Magnetic resonance imaging versus musculoskeletal ultrasound for identification and localization of plantar plate tears. Foot Ankle Spec. 2012;5(6):359–65.
48. Carlson RM, Dux K, Stuck RM. Ultrasound imaging for diagnosis of plantar plate ruptures of the lesser metatarsophalangeal joints: a retrospective case series. J Foot Ankle Surg. 2013;52(6):786–8.
49. Mazzuca JW, Yonke B, Downes JM, Miner M. Flouroscopic arthrography versus MR arthrography of the lesser metatarsophalangeal joints for the detection of tears of the plantar plate and joint capsule: a prospective comparative study. Foot Ankle Int. 2013;34(2):200–9.
50. Yamada AF, Crema MD, Nery C, Baumfeld D, Mann TS, Skaf AY, et al. Second and third metatarsophalangeal plantar plate tears: diagnostic performance of direct and indirect MRI features using surgical findings as the reference standard. AJR Am J Roentgenol. 2017;209(2):W100–8.
51. Flint WW, Macias DM, Jastifer JR, Doty JF, Hirose CB, Coughlin MJ. Plantar plate repair for lesser metatarsophalangeal joint instability. Foot Ankle Int. 2017;38(3):234–42.
52. Prissel MA, Hyer CF, Donovan JK, Quisno AL. Plantar plate repair using a direct plantar approach: an outcomes analysis. J Foot Ankle Surg. 2017;56(3):434–9.
53. Zhou HB, Chen L, Liu CL. Treatment of the injury of the plantar plate on the second metatarsophalangeal joint with dorsal approach and Weil osteotomy. Zhongguo Gu Shang. 2015;28(11):1059–63.

Lisfranc Injuries

4

Alan Y. Yan, Stephen P. Canton, Xin Ma, Zhongmin Shi, Lorraine Boakye, and MaCalus V. Hogan

Introduction

Lisfranc injury contains a wide spectrum of injuries from frank high energy fracture dislocation to subtle, low-energy midfoot sprain or ligamentous injuries only revealed by stress tests [1, 2]. Missed injuries are noteworthy given the implications on the management of future foot and ankle complications. Previous studies have stated that Lisfranc injuries account for 0.2% of all fractures and a reported incidence of 1 per 55,000 persons per year [3]. However, that number may be an underrepresent. There is an estimated rate of up to 20% for missed diagnosis of Lisfranc injury on plain radiograph due to the unique anatomy of the midfoot which make interpretation of injury difficult [4, 5]. Missed or delayed diagnoses can lead to severe midfoot instability, arch collapse, forefoot abduction deformity, and development of posttraumatic osteoarthritis (PTOA) resulting in stiffness and chronic pain with dysfunction of the foot and ankle complex [6].

A. Y. Yan (✉) · M. V. Hogan
Department of Orthopaedic Surgery, University of Pittsburgh Medical Center, Pittsburgh, PA, USA

Foot and Ankle Injury Research [F.A.I.R.] Group, University of Pittsburgh, Pittsburgh, PA, USA
e-mail: hoganmv@upmc.edu

S. P. Canton · L. Boakye
Department of Orthopaedic Surgery, University of Pittsburgh Medical Center, Pittsburgh, PA, USA

X. Ma
Department of Orthopedics, Huashan Hospital, Fudan University, Shanghai, China

Z. Shi
Department of Orthopedics, Shanghai Jiao Tong University Affiliated Sixth People's Hospital, Shanghai, China

© Springer Nature Switzerland AG 2022
J. D. Cain, M. V. Hogan (eds.), *Tendon and Ligament Injuries of the Foot and Ankle*,
https://doi.org/10.1007/978-3-031-10490-9_4

The Lisfranc joint complex of the midfoot was named after Jacques Lisfranc de St. Martin (1790–1847), a French surgeon and gynecologist, who observed midfoot injury in the cavalry soldiers and did foot amputation at the level of the tarsometatarsal joints [7]. Lisfranc injury is commonly referred as injury of the midfoot, which refers to the various injury combinations of the TMT (tarsometatarsal) joints 1–5 and from single joint to multiple joints or from Lisfranc joints (tarsometatarsal joints) to the concomitantly involved structures including the entire midfoot with extension to the proximal levels of the inter-cuneiform joints, cuneiform-navicular joint, navicular, and cuboid. The preferred term for this injury is Lisfranc joint complex injury as it may even have combined injury to peritalar structures, ankle, and distal tibia [8].

The hallmark of the injury is any combination of bony and/or ligamentous disruption at the base of the metatarsals, articulating tarsals, and any associated concomitant proximal and distal bony or ligamentous injuries. The Lisfranc ligament is one of the strongest ligamentous supports in the complex. Lisfranc complex injuries are most commonly results of either high-energy motor vehicle accidents or falls from height; however, low-energy injuries may occur in daily activities. The mechanism of the Lisfranc injury has been proposed as direct injury of midfoot crush or indirect injuries with forefoot twisting and axial loading mechanism of the plantar flexed foot [8].

In low-energy and sports-related Lisfranc injury, the clinical findings of the injury may be subtle. Faciszewski and colleagues reported subtle injury patterns of the Lisfranc joint in 15 patients in 1990. The lesion from injury was defined as a diastasis of 2–5 mm between the bases of the first and second metatarsals on plain X-ray [9].

Anatomy

The Lisfranc joint itself is comprised of the articulation of nine bones including metatarsals M1 to M5, cuneiform C1 to C3, and cuboid (Cu) arranged in a fashion of inherent stability (Fig. 4.1). There is an inherent stable osseous arrangement of the midfoot. The keystone arrangement is the trapezoidal metatarsal bases forming a Roman arch structure in the axial section (Fig. 4.2). The mortise of the second metatarsal base is formed with the recessed second metatarsal base wedging proximally in between the C1 and C3 about 8 mm and 4 mm, respectively (Fig. 4.3). The entire midfoot is also kept in a stable configuration with keystone pegging of the navicular and cuboid at the medial and middle column and lateral column [10].

Transversely, there are intermetatarsal ligaments which are arranged as dorsal, interosseous, and plantar components connecting the bases of the second to the fifth metatarsal but missing the link of the first and second base of metatarsal or with only very weak fibers [10]. Thomas L. described in 1926 from 50 adult feet dissection that there are three sets of interosseous ligaments corresponding to the first, second, and third tarsometatarsal joints [11]. Solan et al. in their biomechanical measurement objectively demonstrated that the Lisfranc ligament and distinctive plantar ligament combined are stronger than the dorsal ligament – with the interosseous Lisfranc ligament demonstrating the most relative superior strength [12]. A recent anatomical study by Panchobhavi et al. in 2013 revealed in their findings that

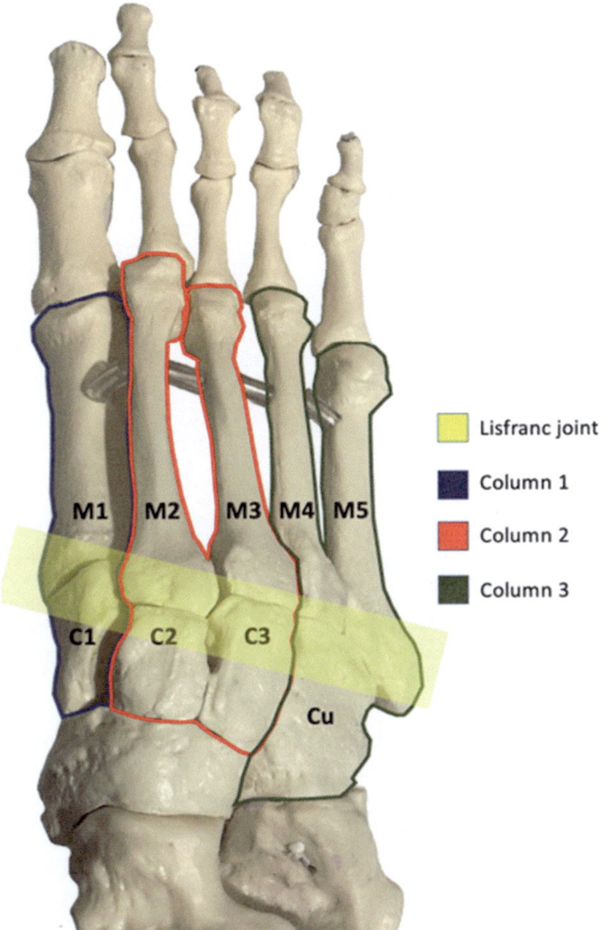

Fig. 4.1 Lisfranc complex – Lisfranc joint and three-column model Courtesy of Stephen Chen, MD

Fig. 4.2 Keystone Roman arch structure of the Lisfranc joint complex

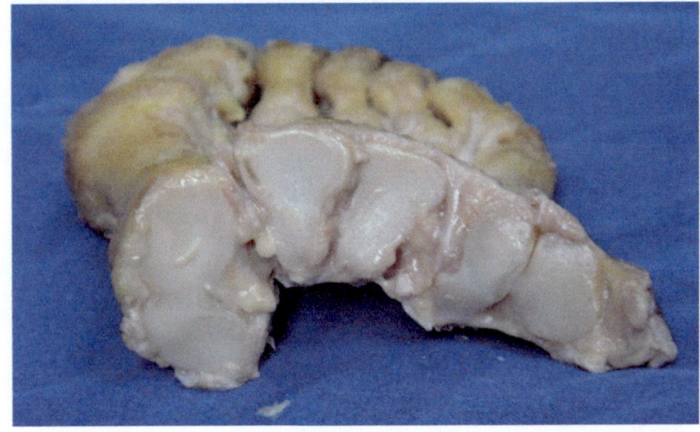

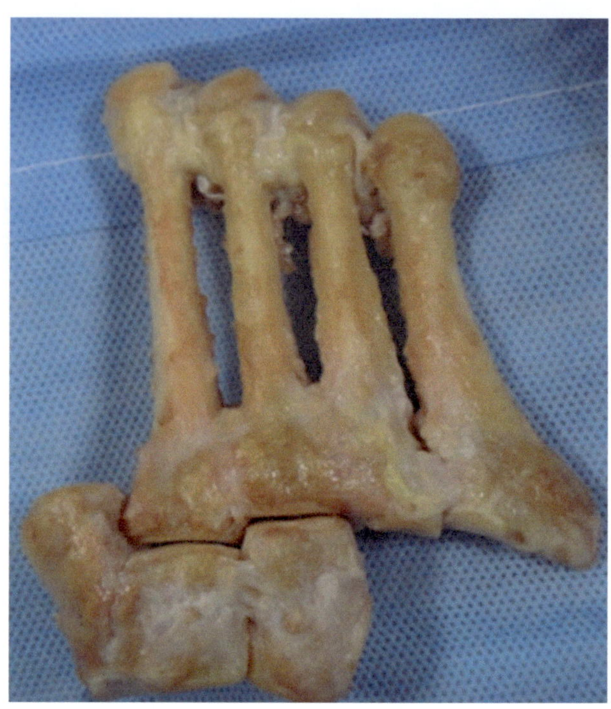

Fig. 4.3 Second TMTJ (tarsometatarsal joint) recess keystone arrangement

there are either one or two bundle Lisfranc interosseous components from C1 to M2 and a plantar ligament of the complex from C1 to M2 and M3 [13]. The dorsal and plantar portion are referred as dorsal ligament and plantar ligament here. There are three distinct synovial joint system of the tarsometatarsal joints correlated to the three columns of the foot. C1M1, C2,3 and M2,3, and CU and M4,5 are the three synovial compartments [14] and corresponding to the medial, middle, and lateral column of the foot.

An in vitro study on midfoot motion showed that the three columns of the midfoot vary at each joint in dorsiflexion-plantar flexion/supination-pronation with the lateral column having considerably more motion than the medial and middle columns. In the sagittal plane and supination-pronation, the cuboid-metatarsal joints have approximately 10° of motion, whereas cuneiform-metatarsal joint motion ranges of the three from medial to lateral are 3.5°, 0.6°, and 1.6° [15]. Lakin's group showed [16] the second and third tarsal metatarsal joints bearing most of the forces in the midfoot and comprising the rigid middle column construct. For the aforementioned reasons, there is a consensus to keep the lateral column mobile in the management of this injury.

Diagnosis and Clinical Evaluation

Diagnosis of the low impact subtle Lisfranc complex disruption can be difficult. The injury occurs more often in males and common in athletes which may cause significant morbidity and huge time loss before RTP (return to play). One of the most

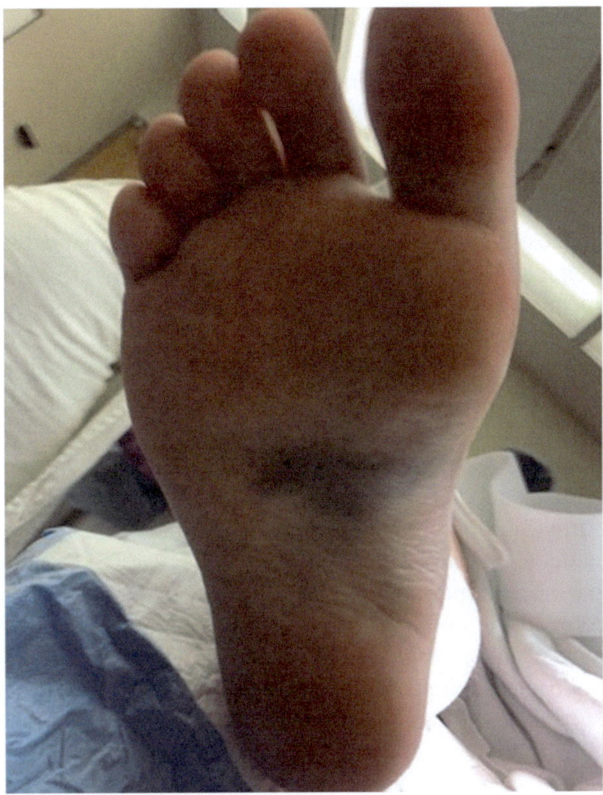

Fig. 4.4 Plantar ecchymosis sign in Lisfranc complex injury

often quoted numbers of missed Lisfranc injuries from initial physical exam and imaging study is about 20–24% [9, 17–22].

A high index of suspicion is needed for all foot injuries with persistent swelling and pain with walking [23]. Aronow describes clinical presentation for missed Lisfranc injuries in patients who may be in pain with limitations of athletic activity or reduced walking tolerance [24]. Glen and colleagues described the plantar ecchymosis sign as a very helpful aid in the diagnosis of Lisfranc injury (Fig. 4.4). Although it is an unspecific finding, it often raises suspicion and necessitates further aggressive evaluation of the injury with stress exam using x-ray or fluoroscopy under anesthesia [23].

Palpation of point of tenderness at the TMT joint region is important for the patient with swelling, pain on activity and with a history of a suspected Lisfranc injury mechanism. Careful examination of the patients may also require a provocative maneuver by compressing midfoot dorsally, plantar deviation of the first metatarsal, passive pronation abduction of the forefoot, and squeezing the first and second metatarsal interspace in the coronal plane. Weight-bearing pain with single limb stance can be used as a way of stress also [25, 26]. Initial imaging should consist of AP, lateral, and 30 degree internally rotated oblique views of the foot. Weight-bearing film should be obtained unless not tolerable by the patients. Bilateral comparison with AP view of both feet can be helpful [27]. Many studies showed a high rate of missed Lisfranc injuries on regular and especially non-weightbearing X-rays with missing rates being reported to be as high as 20% to 50% [21]. Robert Stein summarized radiological findings of the constant anatomical relationships of the intermetatarsal space on AP view medial border of the second metatarsal, which forms a continuous straight line with the medial border of the middle cuneiform [28].

Coss and colleagues described a line tangential to the medial aspect of the navicular and medial cuneiform (medial column line) that intersected the base of the first metatarsal. Any lateral displacement of the forefoot to this line, which is referred to as the "Mills line," indicates disruption of Lisfranc ligaments complex. Fraciszewski, Burks, and Manaster in 1990 also described the flattening of the arch with medial cuneiform plantar to the fifth metatarsal in Lisfranc injury [9]. Particular signs indicating Lisfranc injury are coined the "fleck sign" as a symbol of Lisfranc complex injury for a small bone fragment, which represents an avulsion fracture from the medial base of the second metatarsal or the lateral side of the medial cuneiform [8]. Stress X-ray is helpful in the diagnosis of such injury and is recommended under anesthesia with fluoroscopy [25]. Passive pronation and abduction maneuver have been reported as stress maneuver under anesthesia looking for instability patterns in the midfoot [18, 29]. Diastasis of more than 2 mm between the first and second tarsometatarsal articulations is usually considered unstable. Fraciszewki and colleagues defines instability of Lisfranc injury as 2–5 mm diastasis of the first and second base of metatarsal versus a normal of 1.3 mm [9].

Multiplanar CT is ideal for detecting subtle osseous fractures and subluxation which are not evident on plain radiograph [30]. Siddiqui and colleagues [27] proposed measuring the narrowest transverse gap between the main articular surfaces of the C1 and M2 for pathologic widening. For the inconclusive midfoot sprains, MRI imaging is superior to other modalities for evaluation of soft tissue ligamentous conditions. As per Siddiqui and colleagues [27], most common signs of Lisfranc injury include frank ligament disruption, ligament elongation, and periligamentous edema. Bone scintigraphy is not a routine exam; however, it has been shown its usefulness in low-grade injuries.

For a better understanding of the injury and guiding of the management, there are a series of efforts in the classification of the injury. Earliest classification by Quenu and Kuss divided Lisfranc fracture dislocation into homolateral, isolated, and divergent types [31]. Several modifications based on mechanisms of injury were then described with the most notable classifications proposed by Hardcastle et al. on the basis of their experiences on 119 TMT (tarsometatarsal) injuries [32]. Hardcastle classification is described on the incongruity of the tarsometatarsal joints and divided into (A) complete incongruity, (B) partial incongruity, and (C) with a divergent variation. Myerson et al. modified this system into more detailed classification with type A of total incongruity, type B1 of partial medial incongruity and B2 of partial lateral incongruity, and type C1 of divergent partial and C2 of divergent total displacement [8]. Chiodo and Myerson in 2001 devised a columnar classification of TMT (tarsometatarsal) joint based on three columns of foot in guiding the treatment of the Lisfranc complex injury due to a differential mobility of the columns [33].

Nunley and Vertullo proposed a classification suitable for the low-energy midfoot sprain injury with a combined factor in clinical findings, weight-bearing radiograph, and bone scintigraphy [21]. Stage 1 injury represents dorsal capsule injury with normal weight-bearing X-ray but increased uptake in bone scintigraphy. Stage II injury would have a 2–5 mm diastasis between C1 and M2 but no loss of height. Lisfranc ligament complex would be elongated or disrupted with maintenance of plantar capsular or ligamentous structures. Stage III has more than 5 mm diastasis and loss in height and thus a disrupted plantar ligamentous structure. While it is useful for low-energy low impact injury in sports injuries, bone scintigraphy has been rarely used in the clinic by many practitioners.

Treatment

The goal of foot injury management is to achieve a stable painless plantigrade foot. The role of nonoperative management is reasonable; however, it is limited only to the Lisfranc injuries that have no evidence of instability [21]. Stage I injuries of Nunley and Vertullo classification can be managed conservatively and treated with non-weight-bearing cast for 6 weeks followed by custom orthosis [21]. Also, extra-articular fractures without signs of instability of the Lisfranc complex from stress views can be treated nonoperatively usually with temporary boot immobilization. Patients are allowed to weight-bear as tolerated, perform gentle range of motion and transition to regular shoes in 4–6 weeks. Repeat weight-bearing films in 2–3 weeks are followed to prevent late displacement [34].

Myerson and Cerrato [25] advocated nonoperative management (boot immobilization) for midfoot injuries with no instability noted on weight-bearing or stress radiographs. Weight-bearing is permitted as tolerated as long as the foot remains stable on repeat weight bearing films made 2 weeks later. Patients are recommended to transit out of the boot once there is no pain at midfoot on stress test. Stiff sole shoes with a rigid orthotics must be worn for 6 months. Return to full play for athletes may take up to 8–9 months.

Surgical management is indicated for the rest of the patients with instability in the setting of displaced fracture, dislocation, and consistent or progressive subluxation with or without stress (indicating unstable soft tissue especially ligamentous injuries) and those with proximal midfoot involvement. However, the detailed parameter of diastasis is not commonly agreed with sufficient evidences.

With the goal of achieving a painless plantigrade foot, the means of surgical management is preferably with joint preserving means if possible or joint sacrificing if it is the most feasible option. In injuries with obvious joint surface destruction, the choice for management is rather straightforward with primary fusion for the joints which are considered nonessential or less mobile and not to interfere with a functional foot. However, for many situations with instability, there is still an ongoing debate with the management options of fusion versus fixation.

Regardless of the surgical interventions, the most important aspect of surgical management of the Lisfranc injury is to obtain and maintain a stable anatomical reduction and congruent joint surfaces in the midfoot. The aforementioned goals can be achieved either via closed reduction with percutaneous fixation or open reduction internal fixation (ORIF) or fusion. Quality of reduction is most crucial for optimal outcomes [8]; therefore, the logical way to achieve anatomical reduction will be open reduction with directly visualizing of the instability pattern.

Closed reduction can be difficult to achieve and undesirable in the setting of fracture, soft tissue interposition entrapment, or delayed presentation [8]. Open reduction, on the other hand, has been the golden rule for reduction and fixation of the Lisfranc fracture dislocation [35]. Different approaches of open reduction exposures have been mentioned and used. Typically, multiple longitudinal incisions are used. Single transverse or longitudinal incision has been reported also [36] (Fig. 4.5a). Complications for the exposures have been reported, including wound dehiscence, skin necrosis, soft tissue infection, neuroma formation, or CRPS [37].

Commonly used incisions include the dorsal double incision which would be separated by skin bridge of at least 4–5 cm [38, 39] (Fig. 4.5b). With the concerns of skin necrosis and struggle between the ideal exposure and ideal skin bridge width, the exposures are likely unsatisfactory. Transverse incision avoids this issue; however, the incision crosses over longitudinal neurovascular structures and it is harder to place the incision right in the level of interests with accuracy. The approach is largely surgeon dependent.

Optimal exposure facilitates good reduction of the injury and further procedures to maintain the achieved reduction. There are many ways of fixation used and reported including wires, trans-articular screws, bridging or compression plates, suture buttons, and staples. Each has been reported throughout the history with lessons of failure, success, and debates.

ORIF has been adopted primarily for lower-energy acute injuries in athletes and younger population. Arntz and Hansen established in 1988 [38] the principles of ORIF with rigid fixation with 3.5 cortical screws at medial and middle column and K wires fixation for the lateral column with later removal, which became the most followed standard of care for most of the Lisfranc complex injury. Full weight-bearing in boot is allowed at around 3 months [40]. Since then, many other implants with different modalities of fixation have been used.

K-wires have been traditionally used for intraoperative provisional fixation and maintenance for reduction. K-wire percutaneously placed for the lateral column fixation is usually buried subcutaneously to decrease infection risk and removed in 6 weeks. Use of screws has been questioned in regard to the potential damage of the otherwise intact joint surfaces and risk of creating arthritis. Also, fracture comminution and fractures with intra-articular extension may not be good indications for screw fixation given the concern for instability. Broken screws in joints also increase difficulty in removal. Therefore, bridge plating may offer a viable alternative [34].

Alberta et al. reported in their study of biomechanical comparison of dorsal plate and trans-articular screw fixation [41] and indicated that there was no significant difference between plates and screws with respect to ability to realign and maintain

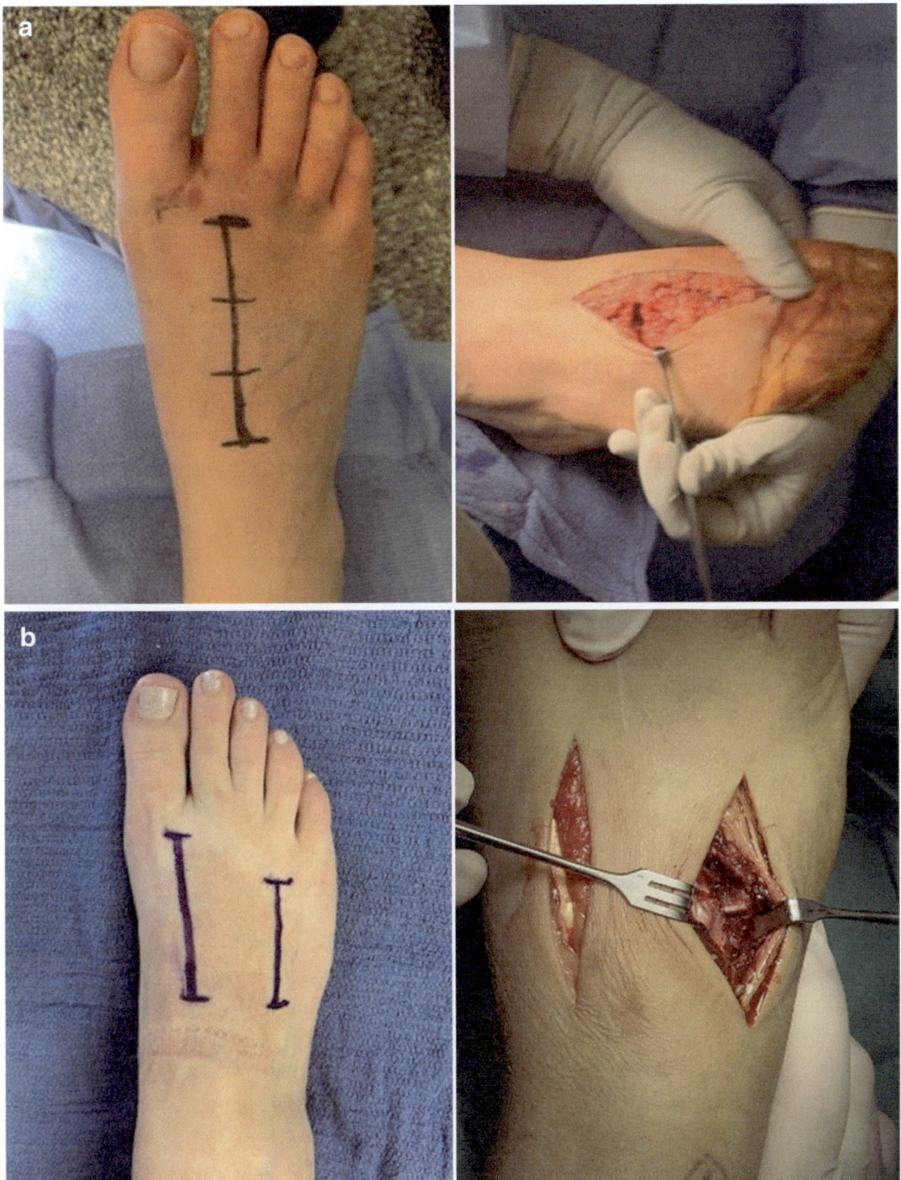

Fig. 4.5 (**a**) Dorsal single incision versus (**b**) dorsal dual incisions

the TMT (tarsometatarsal) joints. They also quantify the articular surface destruction in that study as the area of the visible articular surface damaged at the TMTJ (tarsometatarsal joint) caused by a single 3.5 mm screw varied from 2.0% to 4.6%. Gaines et al. showed injury to the TMTJ (tarsometatarsal joint) during fixation of

Lisfranc dislocations by changing the placement of the guidewire across the mid-foot [42]. Ardoin and Anderson advocated locking screws for use in the distal and proximal holes and nonlocking at the holes close to the joint so the surgeon can direct screws away from the joint if needed [43].

In addition to dorsal spanning extra-articular bridge plating, Anderson also popularized open approach to subtle sports Lisfranc injury and fixation with "home run" Lisfranc screw and inter-cuneiform screws [44]. In the athletic population, Anderson's group advocates ORIF and avoids primary fusion for the concerns of malunion, nonunion, and secondary transfer metatarsalgia. Primary fusion is reserved for patients with subacute or late presentations or with severe articular damages. The "home run screw" or the "Lisfranc screw" was first described in 1990 by Sangeorzan, Veith, and Hansen [45] using 3.5 or 4.0 mm cortical lag screw from medial cuneiform to the base of second metatarsal. Home run Lisfranc screw follows the course of the Lisfranc ligament and essentially extra-articular [44]. The home run screw reduces the medial column to the middle column together with the inter-cuneiform screw.

Panchbhavi proposed an alternative and preferred way for inserting the Lisfranc screw. Instead of medial to lateral orientation, Panchbhavi advocates cannulated partial threaded 4.0–5.0 mm screw directed from the base of second metatarsal into the medical cuneiform. The advantages for this orientation are easier targeting, better purchasing, and easier removal if broken [46, 47].

A similar principle of extra-articular fixation with the same orientation while using endo-button was described by Panchbhavi [48]. As there is likely no one-size-fits-all solution for different Lisfranc complex injuries, there are certain subsets of the population in which specific concerns and strategies should be employed. Panchbhavi and colleagues also found suture button fixation provided stability similar to that provided by screw fixation in cadaver specimens after isolated transection of the Lisfranc ligament [49].

The most debated topics on the management of the Lisfranc complex injury are likely the choice of primary arthrodesis versus open reduction internal fixation. Most of the historical studies indicate favorable outcomes in ORIF with an anatomical reduction achieved. However, there is still a high rate of PTOA (post traumatic osteoarthritis) regardless of the quality of reduction. Kuo and colleagues found a 25% rate of posttraumatic arthritis [50] in 48 patients following ORIF of TMT (tarsometatarsal) injuries at a mean follow-up of 52 months. Increased arthritis were observed in patients with pure ligamentous injuries (presence of arthritis in 40%) despite anatomic reduction from surgeries performed. Of note, pure ligamentous injury pattern was diagnosed based on the plain film diagnosis and also includes those with "fleck sign." No CT scan was used in diagnosis in their study. The degree of posttraumatic arthritis was directly proportional to the degree of gross damage to the articular surface. The authors commented that it may be more of the injury rather than the treatment that determines the outcome. In addition, primary fusion is likely better for the pure ligamentous injury. It is reasonable to deduce that joint damage from injury will dictate a poor outcome later for a secondary PTOA (post traumatic osteoarthritis). However, ligamentous damage may cause a worse outcome regardless of reduction due to poor fixation and inherent poor healing capacity of the soft tissue as compared to bone; Also, the small, flat bony anatomy may be predisposed to perpetuated instability.

One of the most quoted studies that adds to the controversy of the topic is the level 1 study by Ly and Coetzee (2006) on primary ligamentous Lisfranc injuries [51]. Forty-one patients with isolated or subacute primarily ligamentous Lisfranc injury were enrolled in a prospective randomized trial comparing primary fusion of the medial 2 or 3 rays (21 patients) with ORIF (20 patients). Total follow-up time is 42.5 months. Two years postoperatively, mean AOFAS midfoot score was 68.6 points in ORIF versus 88 points in fusion group. Five of the ORIF were ultimately fused due to persistent pain with deformity or arthrosis. Postoperative activity level of fusion was 92% versus 65% in ORIF group. A total of 16/20 in the ORIF group underwent secondary surgery to remove prominent and painful hardware. Only 4/21 patients in the fusion group underwent secondary surgery for removal of hardware. It should be noted that most patients (16/20 in the ORIF group and 17/21 in the fusion group) sustained high-energy injury. The authors speculate that pure ligamentous injury treated with fixation generates insufficient stability by only the healing of the soft tissue, i.e., ligaments and capsules.

Ly and Coetzee adopted partial medial two- or three-ray fusion. A similar approach and results were also noted by Sangeorzan et al. and Komenda et al. [45, 52] who advocated keeping unlimited motion of the lateral two rays. Besides major ligamentous injury with multidirectional instability, initially missed and delayed presentation of the Lisfranc injuries over 6 weeks usually does poorly [2]. Primary arthrodesis of Lisfranc produces acceptable results, and quality of reduction is the major predictor of good outcome. Henning and colleagues [53] investigated whether performing a primary arthrodesis resulted in improved functional outcome and fewer subsequent surgeries as compared to primary open reduction and internal fixation in another prospective randomized study in 40 patients in intervals of 3, 6, 12, and 24 months. There is a significant difference in secondary surgeries needed including removal of hardware and salvage fusion for 78.6% in the ORIF versus 16.7% in the fusion group. Primary arthrodesis however has not been supported in young athletic populations with low-energy injuries. No high-level evidences support the decision.

Lewis and Anderson [44] expressed their preference to perform ORIF for all unstable midfoot segments in low-energy athletic-type injuries and also for higher-energy mechanisms with significant bony involvement concerning potential nonunion or malunion and secondary transfer metatarsalgia with possible end results of not able to perform in higher level of function needed for the sports. Primary fusion is reserved for patients with subacute or late presentations or in case of severe articular damage. Due to the paucity of evidence, the authors feel that there is little data to define a clear guideline. Unfavorable sequelae does occur in participation of sports requires high-level function after midfoot fusion, including periarticular arthrosis, nonunion, malunion, and stress fracture [21].

Myerson and Cerrato [25] do not recommend primary arthrodesis for athletes. In their opinion, maintenance of motion of medial column is necessary for restoration of full function. Nunley and Vertullo [21] reported their outcomes and classification in 15 athletes with Lisfranc injuries and management accordingly. Nonoperative management was adopted for their stage I (nondisplaced), and anatomic reduction with fixation was done for stages II (diastasis with no arch height loss) and III (diastasis with arch height loss). Their reported outcome was excellent in 93% of the patients in an average of 27 months. However, Cochran et al. [54] in a level III study compared 14 fusion versus 18 ORIF of low-energy Lisfranc injuries in active duty military personnel. Primary fusion patients had an earlier return to full military activity and better fitness test scores after 1 year besides a lower rate for hardware removal. The authors noted that 69% of the patients had a diagnosis of primarily ligamentous injury patterns. However, the ORIF and primary fusion were not randomized. Most of the acute cases were treated with ORIF, and those who presented more than 6 weeks post-injury were treated with fusion except for three of the primarily ligamentous acute injury patients.

In regard to rigid implants for either fusion or fixation, there is emerging interest in a new generation of staples with shape memory and purported benefits of ease of use, low profile, and maximization of joint coaptation. Schipper and colleagues [55] showed a radiographic union of 93.8% (60/64) of patients and 95.1% (98/103) of joints using the nitinol staple construct. Flexible fixation, as we mentioned as suture button for special subset of patients, may be reasonable for maintaining of the foot flexibility. There are also investigational reports for other synthetic and allograft reconstruction.

Caio Nery et al. [56] evaluated physiologic fixation with a novel suture augmented neoligamentplasty of fiber tape on cadaveric models compared with a transarticular screw fixation construct and showed no difference in stability with less variability. Weglein and colleagues [57] reported allograft fixation on cadavers also showing adequate strength and stability and did not differ significantly compared to intact foot or foot with screw fixation.

Optimal timing of the surgery is still not clearly defined. Most follow the general rule the sooner the better and as soon as the swelling decreases. Myerson and Cerrato [25] recommended operating within 6 weeks. However, in their experience, patients with Lisfranc injury of midfoot subluxation were successfully managed 1 year after initial injury. Postoperative management is usually followed by 2–6 weeks of no weight-bearing with splint, cast, or boot immobilization. Then patients are allowed to start transition to removable boot with weight-bearing progression and walk in stiff shoe with supportive orthotics in 3 months.

Hardware usually remains in foot for at least 4 months [25, 58]. There is no evidence-based consensus for whether the hardware removal is necessary beyond indications due to hardware prominence with irritation, broken hardware with irritation, or loosening. Questions remains for removal all of the hardware versus selectively removal of the joint violating hardware while maintaining the home run or inter-cuneiform screws or substitution of flexible fixation to prevent later diastasis. It is up to the surgeon's discretion without consensus. Interestingly, Coetzee raised the question that if the surgeon believes the screws should not be removed then how would that be different from performing primary fusion. He referred the surgeons in that category as closet fusers [59].

Return to play are important in athlete patients. McHale and colleagues showed 90% of the 28 NFL players returned to play at professional level at 11.1 months [60]. Nunley and Vertullo [36] reported an average return to play after surgical management at around 14.4 weeks. Myerson and Cerrato [25] however opined their experiences with return to play at 6 months with a gradual systematic rehabilitation program and no running with cutting activities until 6 months postoperatively due to concerns of midfoot torsion stress.

Evidence-Based/Critical Appraisal of the Literature

Over the years, we have realized that the best outcomes of the management of Lisfranc complex injuries are related to the quality of anatomical reduction. In 1963, Cassebaum recognized that anatomic reduction was associated with greater satisfaction [1]. Myerson and colleagues in 1986 evaluated 76 fracture dislocations of the Lisfranc tarsometatarsal joint complex patients. Of which, 52 patients with 55 Lisfranc injuries were analyzed with an average follow-up of 4.2 years. 22/26 feet (85%) had acceptable anatomic reductions by closed or open methods achieved good or excellent clinical results. Quality of the initial reduction was identified as a major determinant of clinical results with a linear direct relationship of the PFCS score and quality of reduction [8]. However, trauma to the joint complex is also important. 4/26 (15%) patients with good or excellent initial reductions developed painful arthritis.

Arntz, Veith, and Hansen reported a consecutive series of 40 adults of 41 TMT fracture dislocations treated with open reduction internal fixation. For 34 patients with 35 Lisfranc complex injuries who had been followed up for 3.4 years, a good or excellent functional result was obtained in all but 2 of the 30 injuries in whom an anatomical reduction had been achieved. The development of PTOA (post traumatic osteoarthritis) was directly related to damage to the articular surfaces or related to inadequate reduction or both [35].

Richter and colleagues from Germany again demonstrated [61] highest functional scores of AOFAS-ET, AOFAS-Midfoot, Hannover Scoring System (HSS), and Hannover Questionnaire (Q) in patients treated with early open reduction and operative fixation of all 155 patients with midfoot fractures. Correct length of the medial and lateral column and shape of the longitudinal arch correlated with good results in all scoring systems. As empirical experiences and many evidences showed us, a prompt early achievement of anatomical reduction is a key to the long-term good outcome. However, evidence also shows that even with anatomic reduction, a good result may not be guaranteed [8, 45, 50, 62].

Teng and colleagues looked into the functional outcome following anatomic restoration of tarsal metatarsal fracture dislocation [62]. Eleven patients with excellent radiographic results following surgical treatment of unilateral closed Lisfranc injury were evaluated at an average of 41.2 months. 10 of 11 cases had anatomic reduction. Yet 8 of 11 patients had evidence of TMTJ (tarsometatarsal joint) arthritis. In spite of excellent clinical objective results measured by restoration of normal alignment and walking patterns, the subjective function outcome was not good with an average AOFAS midfoot score of 71. The patients perceived a definite loss of joint motion. However, the authors were not able to define key elements with vertical ground reaction force loading patterns.

Kuo and colleagues studied a group of 92 adults in a 7-year period retrospectively at the outcome measured with AOFAS-midfoot and long form Musculoskeletal Function Assessment score (MFA) after ORIF of Lisfranc joint injuries [50]. Forty-eight of the injured patients were followed for an average of 52 months. PTOA (post traumatic osteoarthritis) was a complication associated with Lisfranc injury in about 25% of the patients.

Many studies showed the amount of arthritis directly proportional to the area of damage on the articular surface [8, 45, 50]. Besides the joint destruction, perpetuated instability is likely another key factor dictating the long-term outcomes. Kuo and colleague's works showed again that anatomical reduction is the major determinant of a good result; however, the subgroup of patients with pure ligamentous showed poorer outcomes regardless of anatomical reduction and screw fixation [50].

Repeated evidences from different authors indicate that one of the key factors to achieve a better outcome of the Lisfranc complex injury is anatomical reduction of the injury. Comparing closed reduction and open reduction, the likelihood for getting a better anatomical restoration is achieved via open approach. Schepers and colleagues [63] studied the influence of approach and implant on reduction accuracy and stability in Lisfranc fracture dislocation at TMTJ (tarsometatarsal joint). Only 33% closed reduction were acceptable, while 86% open reduction were anatomic. About 37.5% patients had loss of reduction treated with K-wires and no loss of reduction in those treated with rigid fixation with screws or plates. However, on the other hand, we know that anatomical reduction and even with rigid fixation thereafter does not guarantee a painless fully functional foot PTOA (post traumatic osteoarthritis) can still occur. It is likely related to the joint surface damage from the initial injury and degree of instability the injury caused.

For those injuries with already damaged joint surfaces, grossly unstable joints, and pure ligamentous injuries (predictors of perpetuated instability), primary arthrodesis makes more sense than fixation. The practice of fixation without removal of hardware is just a de facto compromised fusion without a good preparation of the joint surfaces. Due to the existence of a wide spectrum of injury pathology, individualized care plans are necessary for optimal management of the particular Lisfranc complex injury. Despite well-known best practices, there are still reality checks needed to guide and support our reasoning and evaluating the empirical ways of management. We need to take a critical look at evidences, especially high-level evidences.

Traditionally, open reduction and internal fixation are the most accepted standard for acute Lisfranc complex injury and conversion to secondary fusion as a salvage in posttraumatic arthritis [45, 64]. However, more emerging reports have proposed primary fusion as definitive management and shown better outcome of primary arthrodesis in certain type of Lisfranc injury [50]. This has become the most debated topic in Lisfranc injury with discussions on topics of pain level after surgery, anticipated secondary procedure necessity and economy, removal of hardware, and functional outcomes.

One of the most quoted papers in this debate is likely the level I study conducted by Ly and Coetzee [50]. This was a prospective randomized trial comparing primary fusion of the medial 2 or 3 rays (21 patients) with ORIF (20 patients). Forty-one patients with isolated or subacute primarily ligamentous Lisfranc injury were enrolled. Total follow-up time is 42.5 months. Two years postoperatively, the mean AOFAS midfoot score was 68.6 points in the ORIF versus 88 points in the fusion group. Five of the ORIF went on fusion eventually due to persistent pain with deformity or arthrosis. Post-op activity level of fusion was 92% versus 65% in the ORIF group. 16/20 cases in the ORIF group underwent secondary surgery to remove prominent and painful hardware. Only 4/21 patients in the fusion group underwent secondary surgery for removal of hardware. Of note, most of the patients (16/20 in the ORIF group and 17/21 in the fusion group) sustained high-energy injury and very few low-energy sports injuries. Therefore, it is prudent not to extrapolate the result to the low-energy sports injury. The authors speculate that pure ligamentous injury will not achieve lasting stability without the support of hardware and not sufficient support with merely the healing of the soft tissue, i.e., ligaments and capsules.

Sheibani-Rad and colleagues [65] performed a qualitative, systematic review of literature in 2012 to compare two of the most common procedures for Lisfranc fractures: primary arthrodesis and ORIF. A total of 193 patients in six articles were analyzed. At 1-year follow-up, the mean AOFAS score of ORIF was 72.5. The AOFAS score was 88.0 for the fusion patients. Both procedures yield satisfactory and equivalent results with slight advantages showing in primary fusion in terms of clinical outcomes.

Evaluating the mechanism of injury by percentage of occurrence of the six studies showed 57% was motor vehicle accident, 21% was fall from height, 8% was work related, 5% was crush injury, and only 9% was sports-related low-energy injury. Henning et al. conducted another prospective randomized study involving 40 acute TMTJ (tarsometatarsal) fracture or fracture dislocation injuries. 32 injuries were followed at intervals of 3, 6, 12, and 24 months after surgery. Their results showed patients treated with ORIF had a higher rate of additional surgery compared with those treated with primary fusion (78.6% vs. 16.7%) [53]. There was no statistical significance; however, the SMFA scores demonstrated a trended improvement in primary fusion as compared to primary fixation group at 2 years.

In 2016, Smith and colleagues performed a systematic review and meta-analysis looking at Lisfranc trauma outcome between ORIF and primary fusion [66]. Four questions were looked into from the literature on whether ORIF or primary fusion led to (1) fewer reoperation for hardware removal, (2) less frequent revision surgery, (3) higher patient outcome scores, and (4) more frequent anatomic reduction. They observed a higher risk ratio of hardware removal was 0.23 for ORIF than fusion. Except for that, there were no favored ratio toward either modalities in regard to revision surgery, patient-reported outcomes, and risk of nonanatomic alignment. The papers analyzed include studies from Henning et al., Ly and Coetzee study, and Mulier et al. [51, 53, 64]. As authors pointed out, the breadth of injury patterns and relative few direct comparative studies with limited numbers of cases call for future well-designed prospective RCTS to further our knowledge for defining a clearer understanding of the treatment modalities and indications for Lisfranc complex injuries.

Magill and colleagues [67] conducted a systematic review and meta-analysis in 2019 under PRISMA guideline including two RCTs and three nonrandomized observational studies compiling a total of 187 subjects and a mean follow-up of 62.3 months. The overall analysis demonstrated a higher need for revision surgery in ORIF and a significantly higher rate of persistent pain in ORIF group. However, the authors believe the available evidence is limited and not adequately robust to make explicit conclusions and call for a need for a high-quality and adequately powered RCTs.

The most recent systematic review and meta-analysis by Alcelik et al. [68] updated the systematic review and meta-analysis with inclusion of outcomes not assessed in the previous studies. Two RCTs and 6 non-RCT studies with a total of 547 patients were included. The authors found no significant difference between the outcomes of ORIF versus primary fusion in terms of return to work or activity. There is higher risk for further surgery in ORIF group to remove hardware or undergo secondary fusion. Overall complication rates were similar in both. However, low power of most of the studies and heterogeneity of the injuries made the studies inconclusive.

Stodle et al. [69] compared primary arthrodesis of the first TMTJ (tarsometatarsal joint) to temporary bridge plating in unstable Lisfranc injuries in a level I randomized controlled trial. Forty-eight patients were included and followed for 2 years. Twenty-four of which were randomized to primary fusion of the medial third TMTJ (tarsometatarsal joint), and another 24 used temporary bridge plating over the first TMTJ (tarsometatarsal joint) and fusion of the second and third TMTJ (tarsometatarsal joint). Outcomes were measured by AOFAS midfoot scale and also SF-36 and VAS pain. CT scans were obtained pre- and post-surgery. Dorsal plates were removed at 4–5 months after the initial surgery fixation. Overall, both groups had good outcome scores. The first metatarsal was better aligned in the bridge plating group but also had a high incidence of radiographic osteoarthritis. 11/24 cases showed osteoarthritis, but only one needed conversion to fusion due to pain.

Lau et al. reported in a level III study of functional outcomes of patients treated with dorsal bridge plating versus screws or combination of the two [70]. The authors found the best predictor of functional outcomes was the quality of anatomical reduction as opposed to the choice of fixation implant used. Also, high-velocity mechanism is a risk factor of poor outcome regardless of the fixation technique used.

There is also a level III systematic review on percutaneous fixation of Lisfranc joint injuries reported by Starvrakakis and colleagues [71]. Seven studies on closed reduction and percutaneous screw fixation were included in the analysis. A total of 106 patients were separated into five groups according to the Myerson classification. The analysis showed percutaneous fixation is a relatively simple and safe modality that leads to a good functional outcome especially in Type B injury and fracture dislocation provided that anatomical reduction has been achieved. However, this review has some major limitations with limited power and different following-up periods among subjects.

As we have not yet reached a solid conclusion on primary fusion versus ORIF, there is a preference for fixation over fusion in the low-energy Lisfranc injury in the young athletic population [21, 25, 43]. Vertullo and Nunley studied participation in sports of patients after arthrodesis of the foot or ankle. Considering the possible effect of arthrodesis which may limit athlete's capability of performing some fundamental motion, excessive burden on surrounding joints, and risk for stress fracture or pseudo-arthrosis, they reported on the questionnaire responses of AOFAS surgeons on their opinions on return to sports participation after arthrodesis [72]. Less than 75% of surgeons recommended RTP (return to play) for running, football, soccer, and basketball after Lisfranc fusion.

Nunley and Vertullo reported [21] the outcome of treatment in 15 athletes with their own classification: nonoperative for stage I nondisplaced injury, anatomic reduction with fixation for stage II diastasis with no arch height loss, and stage III diastasis with arch height loss injuries. They reported an overall 93% excellent outcome in average of 27 months follow-up. RTP (Return to Play) average in these 15 patients was 14.4 weeks.

Porter et al. studied the injury pattern in ligamentous Lisfranc injuries in competitive athletes [73]. Their data showed that proximal extension of disruption in inter-cuneiform ligament tear occurred in 50% of the 82 patients. Mean time RTP (Return to Play) was 7.5± 2.1 months. The pattern they defined as medical column dislocation required longest time to return to sports. All patients were treated with ORIF according to the injury instability pattern, and all returned to their preinjury sports.

Cochran and colleagues reported outcomes of primary arthrodesis versus ORIF in low-energy sports injury in young athletic population of active duty personnel at a single institution [54]. This is a level III comparative cohort study. Total of 32 patients with Lisfranc complex injury included in the study. 14 patients treated with fusion versus 18 treated with ORIF. The primary fusion group outperformed in return to full duty time at 4.5 months comparing to 6.7 months in ORIF patients. The fusion group had lower implant removal rate and better fitness test scores after 1 year. There was no difference in FAAM score in 3 years. In this study, the ORIF was indicated for most of the cases presented acutely. Primary fusion was selected for any patients presented over 6 weeks and those with primary ligamentous injuries. Due to the unknown long-term impact of the young athletic population, primary fusion still cannot be recommended universally.

Mora and colleague reported return to sports and physical activities after ORIF of Lisfranc injuries in recreational athletes in 2018 [74]. Thirty-three patients aged 55 years or younger presented with Lisfranc injury and underwent ORIF using Lisfranc screw with bridge plating. Approximately 94% of them were able to return to some form of sport, 66% of them returned to play at or above their preinjury level in a mean follow-up of 2.9 years, and 33% had some degree of ongoing pain and limited ability to RTP (return to play) 33% of patients had continued pain and not able to play.

MacMahon et al. studied return to sports and physical activities after primary partial arthrodesis for Lisfranc injuries in young patients [75]. This is a level IV retrospective case series conducted in 2016 in 38 patients with a mean follow up of 5.2 years with a mean age at surgery of 31.8 years. Patients were able to return to most of their previous sports and physical activities at follow-up including high impact activities. However, they experienced increased difficulty and impaired participation levels in a third and a quarter of physical activities.

Dubois Ferriere et al. reported clinical outcomes and development of symptomatic osteoarthritis 2–24 years after surgical treatment with either ORIF or primary fusion of TMT (tarsometatarsal) complex injuries [76]. This was a retrospective study involving 61 patients. AOFAS, FFI, and VAS pain were used for functional outcome assessment. SF 12 PCS was also adopted. Radiographic evidence of arthritis was noted in 72.1% of the patients. Approximately 54.1% of the cases were symptomatic arthritis with worse outcomes. Risk factors for arthritis were nonanatomic reduction, type C Myerson classification, and smoking. However, most patients can return to their previous level of function and employment with little need for secondary surgery. Of note, in this report, most injury mechanisms are related to high-energy trauma. Approximately 82% of patients underwent ORIF, and 18% of patients underwent primary fusion. There was no significant difference in outcome scores of the patients who underwent primary fusion versus ORIF.

There is another report of outcomes after temporary internal fixation for ligamentous and osseous injuries with prolonged recovery protocol. 135 Lisfranc injuries were managed with a different post-operatively protocol of much longer immobilization and restricted weight bearing of 3 months in cast followed by arch support for another 4 to 6 weeks showed outcomes with no significant difference in pure ligamentous versus osseous injury pattern [77]. Contrary to previous reports, inferior outcome in ligamentous injures was not found in patients treated with this particular protocol postoperatively.

Overall, the current evidence shows that Lisfranc complex injury is a difficult clinical issue in foot and ankle pathologies, with a wide spectrum of severities, instability patterns, and concomitant joint conditions. So far, there are no concrete evidences supporting any particular treatment modalities. Anatomical reduction achieved with surgery is a priority for a better outcome. Primary arthrodesis may be a better surgical management in those Lisfranc complex injuries with high energy mechanism causing pure ligamentous disruptions, severe damage of the joint surfaces, fracture dislocation with multi directional instability and those with late presentation of the Lisfranc complex injuries. For the young athletes in competitive sports and/ or those require flexibility in the foot for higher performance of athletic tasks, alternative fixation over primary fusion in surgical management may be favored.

Final Treatment Algorithm

In our institution, we use the following algorithm in the management of the Lisfranc complex injury (Fig. 4.6).

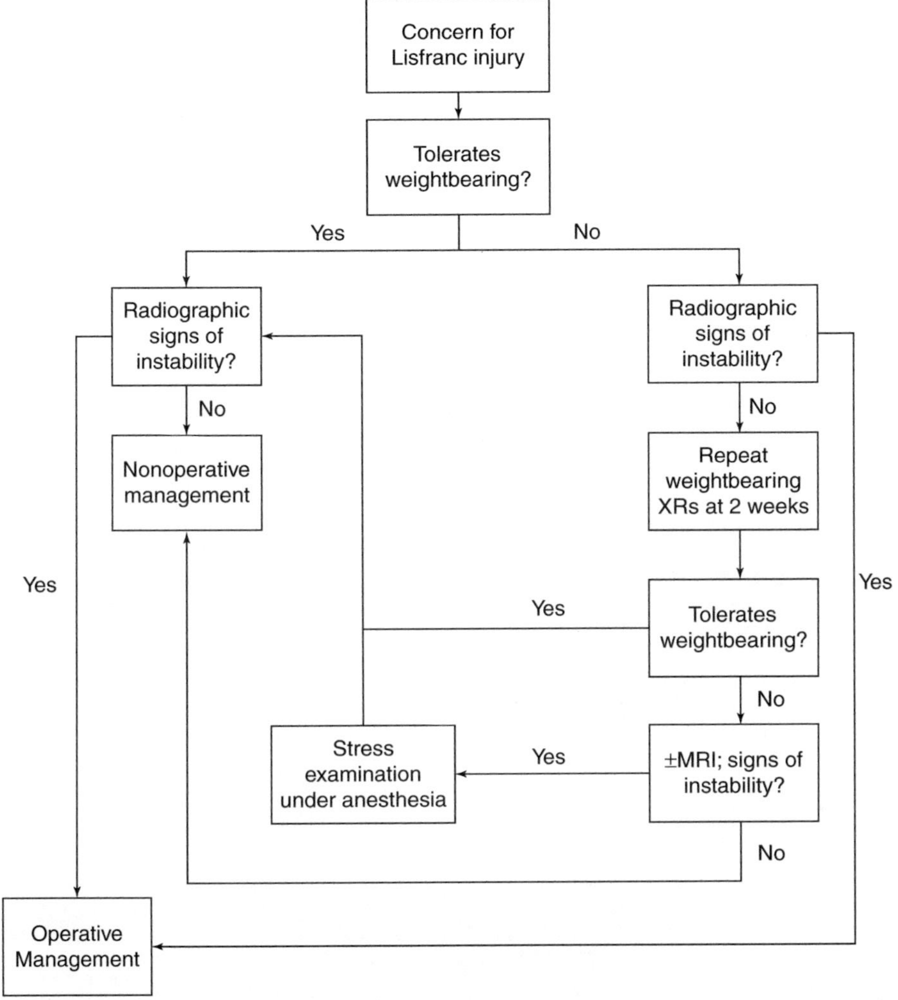

Fig. 4.6 Management algorithm. Courtesy of Stephen Chen, MD

We keep a high index of suspicion for the diagnosis of Lisfranc complex injury in the patients presenting with history of persistent foot swelling and pain on weight-bearing and point tenderness centering around the midfoot region with history of foot injuries with either direct or indirect mechanisms.

Special attention is needed for identifying the clinical signs of plantar ecchymosis on clinical exam and pain at the midfoot with or without provocative maneuvers of rotation with pronating supination, abduction adduction and passive motion of forefoot midfoot in all three columns in sagittal and coronal planes.

All patients with suspected injury of Lisfranc complex will need standard bilateral three-view plain film weight-bearing if they can tolerate. The imaging series include anteroposterior view of both feet on one cassette, 30-degree internal oblique view, and lateral view.

We are looking for the following objective signs of instability on the plain films:

1. If the medial border of the second metatarsal lines up with the medial border of the middle cuneiform on the anteroposterior radiograph (Fig. 4.7a).
2. If the medial border of the fourth metatarsal lines up with the medial border of the cuboid on the oblique radiograph (Fig. 4.7b).
3. If there is a more than 2 mm gap in between the first and second metatarsal base (Fig. 4.7a) or between the medial cuneiform and second metatarsal base on the anteroposterior radiograph (Fig. 4.7a).

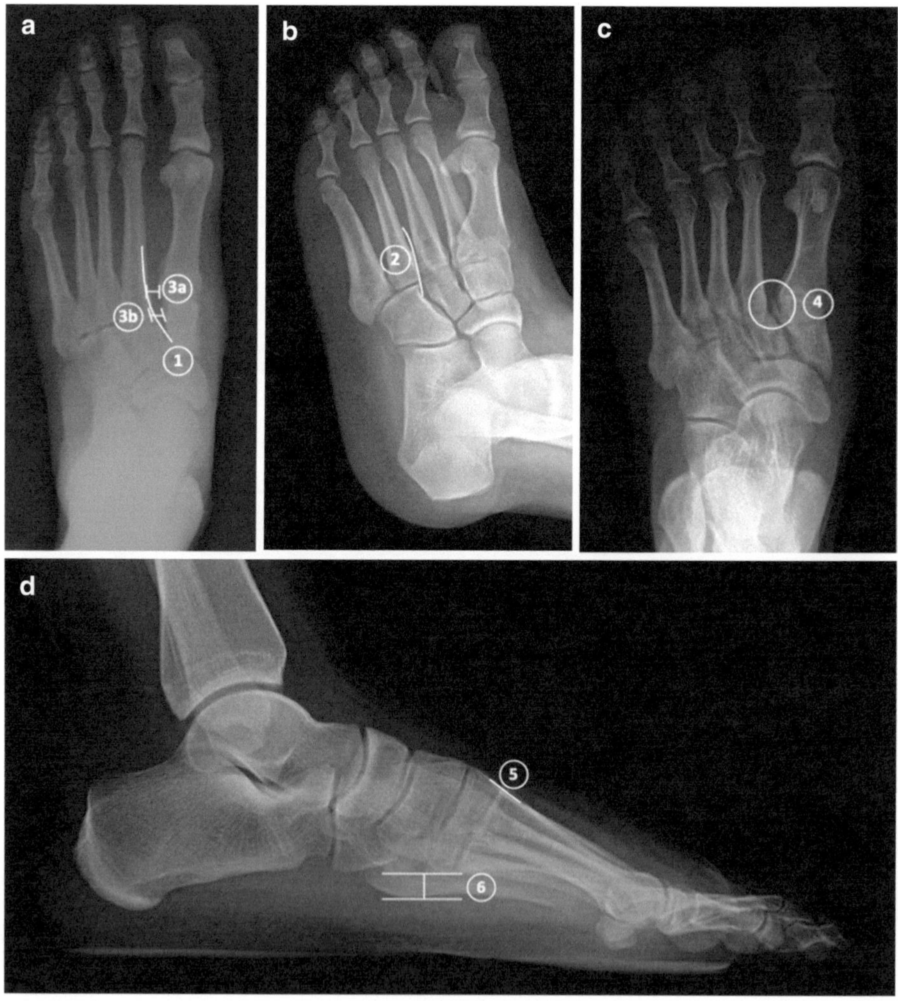

Fig. 4.7 Radiographic signs for diagnostic assessment of Lisfranc injury. Courtesy of Stephen Chen, MD

4. If there is any small avulsion fragment fracture from lateral edge of the medial cuneiform or the medial second metatarsal base as we referred to as "fleck sign" [8] (Figs. 4.7c and 4.8).
5. If the dorsal cortex of the first metatarsal to the medial cuneiform has a normal smooth continuity without any step off on the lateral radiograph (Fig. 4.7d).
6. If the plantar border of the medial cuneiform stays above the plantar border of the fifth metatarsal (Fig. 4.7d).
7. If there are any associate signs suggesting Lisfranc complex injury including compression fracture of cuboid, metatarsal base or neck fractures, and metatarsal phalangeal joint dislocation subluxation [43].

For the patient who has a typical history of injury resulting in Lisfranc complex injury and positive characteristic clinical signs and symptoms, we may still treat the patient with nonoperative management if the patient is able to tolerate weight-bearing and there are no detectable radiographic signs of instability on weight-bearing radiograph. Also if the, diastasis detected on weight bearing Xray in between medial and middle column measures less than 2 mm and there is no arch collapse detected clinically, we follow the recommendation of nonoperative management from expert opinions [25, 36, 44, 59]. The patient will be treated without

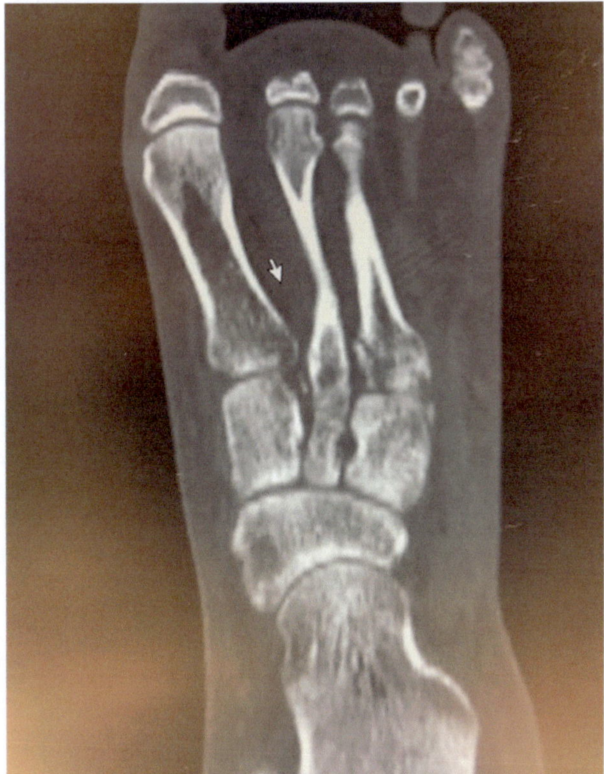

Fig. 4.8 Computed tomography (CT) showing the "fleck" sign

surgery and put in short leg cast for 1–2 weeks. Alternatively, the injured foot of the patient can be immobilized in boot non-weight-bearing at initial visit of acute injury. Progressive protected weight-bearing is permitted if repeat weight-bearing film showing stable foot in 2–3 weeks and patient has progressively reduced pain and swelling in the injured foot. A firm orthotic arch support is prescribed when taking off the boot at 6 weeks. Athlete patient is allowed to train and exercise if there is no pain on stress at 3 months. Return to full sports activities may start at 6–8 months.

If the patient is not able to tolerate weight-bearing but there are no signs of radiographic instability at initial non-weight-bearing exam, a repeat weight-bearing radiograph is required in 2 weeks at follow-up visit. If the patient is still not able to tolerate weight-bearing, then a stress exam under anesthesia is a reasonable option. If the patient at the follow-up visit presents with persistent swelling, pain, and persistent plantar ecchymosis from the initial presentation, even the patient is able to tolerate weight-bearing with pain, we will still plan for stress examination under anesthesia and consent for possible surgical reduction and fixation versus primary arthrodesis pending our findings of the instability patterns during the exam. The stress maneuver under anesthesia includes rotation stress maneuver by pronation supination of the forefoot, sagittal stress maneuver by passive dorsiflexion and plantarflexion of the three columns of the foot, and coronal stress maneuver by passive abduction and adduction of the forefoot midfoot in testing the border columns and squeezing of the forefoot. We look for any radiographic signs of instability and any associated subtle signs with Lisfranc complex fractures of the midfoot forefoot. We pay particular attention to any proximal variant of instability to the Lisfranc joints. On abduction stress, we observe the presence or absence of the lateral displacement of the entire forefoot to the tangential line of the medial navicular and medial cuneiform [29]. Any positive findings of instability will be subjected to surgical management.

If the patient is not able to bear weight and there are characteristic clinical signs and symptoms of Lisfranc complex injury with detectable radiographic instability, we will plan for operative management including stress exam under fluoroscopy under anesthesia to detect and confirm the instability pattern and determine operative modalities accordingly.

We routinely obtain CT scan before planning for surgery for the patient with high-energy injury mechanism and plain radiography showing complex midfoot fracture or dislocation with comminution. Dynamic stress exam is still planned during surgery for detailed instability pattern recognition. MRI will be obtained for the patient with equivocal clinical exam and not willing to undergo stress exam under anesthesia. If only dorsal ligaments of the Lisfranc joint complex are involved, we will manage the patient nonoperatively [78]. Both CT and MRI are static exams and do not give useful information on instability pattern which can mostly be provided by dynamic stress exam.

Any detected instability of the midfoot Lisfranc joint complex from distal TMTJ (tarsometatarsal joint) to the proximal navicular cuneiform and intercuneiform regions will need surgical management in our institution unless the diastasis of the medial and middle column is less than 2 mm without arch collapse and there is no proximal extension beyond Lisfranc joint [59].

In the OR, we routinely perform stress exam to recognize and confirm all possible patterns of instability. We use dorsal joint sparing plate for metatarsal base fracture comminution with instability but preserved joint surfaces. Screws will be used also per surgeon's preference. Open reduction internal fixation is favored over percutaneous fixation except for those cases which we can achieve anatomical reduction in a closed manner (Fig. 4.9a). If there are any destruction of the joint surfaces in the Lisfranc complex, we will proceed with partial fusion of the nonessential joints of the medial and middle column and percutaneous fixation with Kirschner wires at the lateral column of fourth and fifth TMTJ (tarsometatarsal joint) with subsequent removal of the wires at 6 weeks follow-up (Fig. 4.9b). We use 3.5 mm cortical screws in non-compression mode for trans-articular fixation if needed and Lisfranc home run extra-articular screw fixation. We prefer to perform Lisfranc home run screw retrograde from the base of the lateral second metatarsal to the medial cuneiform [46]. The length of the inter-cuneiform screw is determined by the instability pattern of involvement. We will use medial column plating if there is extended instability medially and proximally to the naviculocuneiform joint.

For the high-energy mechanism Lisfranc complex injury with fracture dislocation and or complete ligamentous disruption, we prefer primary arthrodesis of the medial and middle columns due to the destruction of the joint surface or multidirectional instability regardless of sometime intact joint surfaces (Fig. 4.10). If the patient chooses to preserve the joint with fixation over fusion, we will adopt more

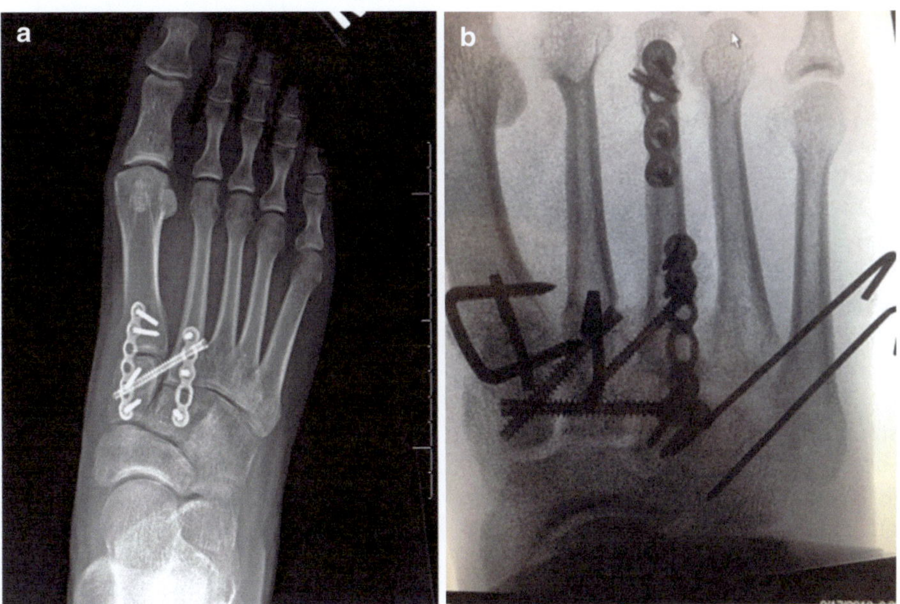

Fig. 4.9 (**a**) Anteroposterior radiograph demonstrating dorsal bridge plating and Lisfranc screw fixation and (**b**) intraoperative fluoroscopy demonstrating primary fusion of the medial and middle columns and temporary fixation of the lateral column

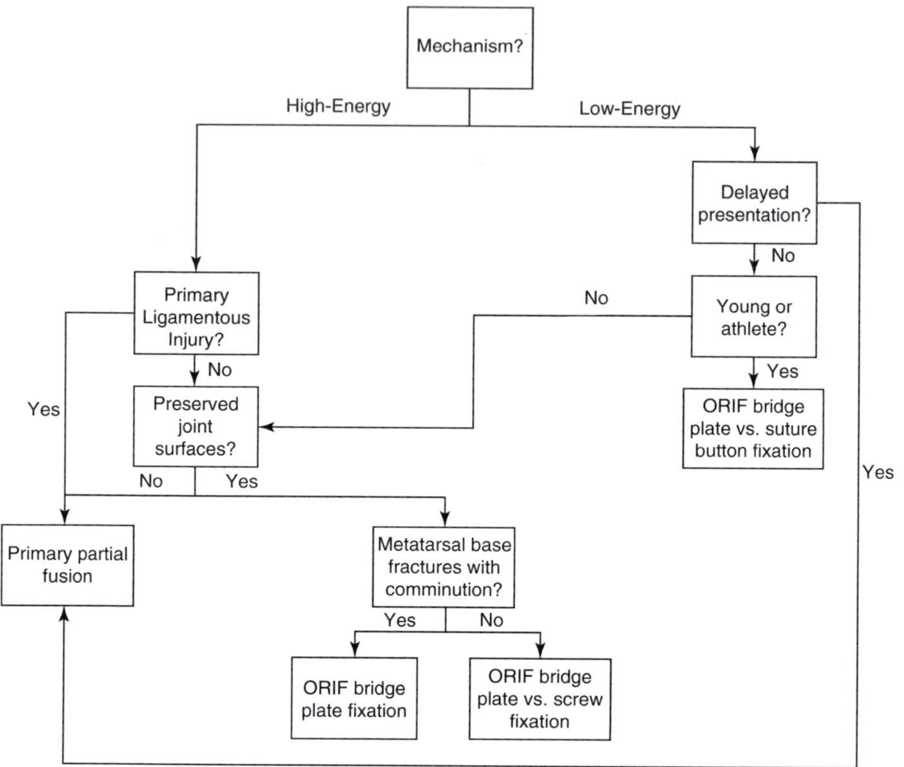

Fig. 4.10 High-energy versus low-energy management algorithm. Courtesy of Stephen Chen, MD

conservative postoperative protocol to keep the patient non-weight-bearing of the injured foot up to 12 weeks.

In regard to young athletes with low-energy injury of the Lisfranc complex, we prefer ORIF over primary fusion unless there is obvious destruction of the joint surfaces detected during the surgery exposure or very late presentation over 6 weeks with pure ligamentous and multidirectional instability patterns.

We will consider flexible fixation with suture button in the isolated Lisfranc ligament injury in young athletes in the sports requiring high performance and flexibility of the foot. Postoperatively, patient is placed in bulky Jones non-weight-bearing splint for 2 weeks. Suture is removed at 2 weeks. Splint is removed and changed to short leg casting till week 6. We typically apply another new short leg cast at week 4. Weight bearing progression will start at week 6 when patient's cast will be taken off and transit to a boot. For elite athlete, we follow the protocol of Ardoin and Anderson [43] for which we take off splint and put the patient in boot at week 2 after surgery and start rehabilitation. Custom mold shoe orthosis will be needed for 6 months post-injury.

We will remove the hardware for the patient who underwent ORIF in between 4 and 6 months. We usually only remove the trans-articular screws of the

TMTJ (tarsometatarsal joint) and leave the Lisfranc screw and inter-cuneiform screws in unless there is clinical irritation or radiological signs of loosening.

With the current available evidences, we adopted our current Lisfranc management algorithm and protocols which are considered safe and prudent. However, many studies so far have limited evidence level. Prospective high-level studies will be needed in many aspects of the Lisfranc complex injury to guide our future treatment modalities and to achieve a better patient long-term outcome.

References

1. Cassebaum WH. Lisfranc fracture-dislocations. Clin Orthop Relat Res. 1963;30:116–29.
2. Hardcastle PH, Reschauer R, Kutscha-Lissberg E, Schoffmann W. Injuries to the tarsometatarsal joint. Incidence, classification and treatment. J Bone Joint Surg Br. 1982;64(3):349–56.
3. Aitken AP, Poulson D. Dislocations of the tarsometatarsal joint. J Bone Joint Surg Am. 1963;45-A:246–60.
4. Goossens M, De NS. Lisfranc's fracture-dislocations: etiology, radiology, and results of treatment. A review of 20 cases. Clin Orthop Relat Res. 1983;176:154–62.
5. Groulier P, Pinaud J. Les luxations tarso-métatarsiennes. Rev Chir Orthop. 1970;56:303–24.
6. Philbin T, Rosenberg G, Sferra JJ. Complications of missed or untreated Lisfranc injuries. Foot Ankle Clin. 2003;8(1):61–71.
7. Fischer L-P. Jacques Lisfranc de Saint-Martin (1787–1847). Hist Sci Med. 2005;39(1):17–34.
8. Myerson MS, Fisher RT, Burgess AR, Kenzora JE. Fracture dislocations of the tarsometatarsal joints: end results correlated with pathology and treatment. Foot Ankle. 1986;6(5):225–42.
9. Faciszewski T, Burks RT, Manaster BJ. Subtle injuries of the Lisfranc joint. J Bone Joint Surg Am. 1990;72(10):1519–22.
10. Kelikian AS, Sarrafian SK. Sarrafian's anatomy of the foot and ankle: descriptive, topographic, functional. Philadelphia: Lippincott Williams & Wilkins; 2011.
11. Thomas L. Research on the interosseous ligaments of the Lisfranc joint: anatomical study and embryo. Arch Anat Histol Embryol. 1926;5:104.
12. Solan MC, Moorman CT 3rd, Miyamoto RG, Jasper LE, Belkoff SM. Ligamentous restraints of the second tarsometatarsal joint: a biomechanical evaluation. Foot Ankle Int. 2001;22(8):637–41.
13. Panchbhavi VK, Molina D, Villarreal J, Curry MC, Andersen CR. Three-dimensional, digital, and gross anatomy of the Lisfranc ligament. Foot Ankle Int. 2013;34(6):876–80.
14. de Palma L, Santucci A, Sabetta SP, Rapali S. Anatomy of the Lisfranc joint complex. Foot Ankle Int. 1997;18(6):356–64.
15. Ouzounian TJ, Shereff MJ. In vitro determination of Midfoot motion. Foot Ankle. 1989;10(3):140–6.
16. Lakin RC, DeGnore LT, Pienkowski D. Contact mechanics of normal tarsometatarsal joints. JBJS. 2001;83(4):520.
17. Meyer SA, Callaghan JJ, Albright JP, Crowley ET, Powell JW. Midfoot sprains in collegiate football players. Am J Sports Med. 1994;22(3):392–401.
18. Curtis MJ, Myerson M, Szura B. Tarsometatarsal joint injuries in the athlete. Am J Sports Med. 1993;21(4):497–502.
19. Englanoff G, Anglin D, Hutson HR. Lisfranc fracture-dislocation: a frequently missed diagnosis in the emergency department. Ann Emerg Med. 1995;26(2):229–33.
20. Haapamaki VV, Kiuru MJ, Koskinen SK. Ankle and foot injuries: analysis of MDCT findings. Am J Roentgenol. 2004;183(3):615–22.
21. Nunley JA, Vertullo CJ. Classification, investigation, and management of midfoot sprains: Lisfranc injuries in the athlete. Am J Sports Med. 2002;30(6):871–8.

22. Chesbrough RM. Strategic approach fends off charges of malpractice program provides tips for avoiding litigation. Diagn Imaging. 2002;24(13):44–51.
23. Ross G, Cronin R, Hauzenblas J, Juliano P. Plantar ecchymosis sign: a clinical aid to diagnosis of occult Lisfranc tarsometatarsal injuries. J Orthop Trauma. 1996;10(2):119–22.
24. Aronow MS. Treatment of the missed Lisfranc injury. Foot Ankle Clin. 2006;11(1):127–42.
25. Myerson MS, Cerrato RA. Current management of tarsometatarsal injuries in the athlete. JBJS. 2008;90(11):2522–33.
26. Shapiro MS, Wascher DC, Finerman GA. Rupture of Lisfranc's ligament in athletes. Am J Sports Med. 1994;22(5):687–91.
27. Siddiqui NA, Galizia MS, Almusa E, Omar IM. Evaluation of the tarsometatarsal joint using conventional radiography, CT, and MR imaging. Radiographics. 2014;34(2):514–31.
28. Stein RE. Radiological aspects of the tarsometatarsal joints. Foot Ankle. 1983;3(5):286–9.
29. Coss LHS, Usnr M, Manos LRE, USNR M, Buoncristiani LA, USNR M, et al. Abduction stress and AP weightbearing radiography of purely ligamentous injury in the tarsometatarsal joint. Foot Ankle Int. 1998;19(8):537–41.
30. Lu J, Ebraheim NA, Skie M, Porshinsky B, Yeasting RA. Radiographic and computed tomographic evaluation of Lisfranc dislocation: a cadaver study. Foot Ankle Int. 1997;18(6):351–5.
31. Quenü E, Küss G. Study on metastarsal dislocation. Rev Chir Paris. 1909;39:281.
32. Hardcastle P, Reschauer R, Kutscha-Lissberg E, Schoffmann W. Injuries to the tarsometatarsal joint. Incidence, classification and treatment. J Bone Joint Surg. 1982;64(3):349–56.
33. Chiodo CP, Myerson MS. Developments and advances in the diagnosis and treatment of injuries to the tarsometatarsal joint. Orthop Clin N Am. 2001;32(1):11–20.
34. Clare MP. Lisfranc injuries. Curr Rev Musculoskelet Med. 2017;10(1):81–5.
35. Arntz C, Hansen S Jr. Dislocations and fracture dislocations of the tarsometatarsal joints. Orthop Clin North Am. 1987;18(1):105–14.
36. Vertullo CJ, Easley ME, Nunley JA. The transverse dorsal approach to the Lisfranc joint. Foot Ankle Int. 2002;23(5):420–6.
37. Philpott A, Lawford C, Lau SC, Chambers S, Bozin M, Oppy A. Modified dorsal approach in the management of Lisfranc injuries. Foot Ankle Int. 2018;39(5):573–84.
38. Arntz CT, Veith RG, Hansen ST Jr. Fractures and fracture-dislocations of the tarsometatarsal joint. J Bone Joint Surg Am. 1988;70(2):173–81.
39. Mann RA, Prieskorn D, Sobel M. Mid-tarsal and tarsometatarsal arthrodesis for primary degenerative osteoarthrosis or osteoarthrosis after trauma. J Bone Joint Surg Am. 1996;78(9):1376–85.
40. Benirschke SK, Meinberg E, Anderson SA, Jones CB, Cole PA. Fractures and dislocations of the midfoot: Lisfranc and Chopart injuries. J Bone Joint Surg Am. 2012;94(14):1325–37.
41. Alberta FG, Aronow MS, Barrero M, Diaz-Doran V, Sullivan RJ, Adams DJ. Ligamentous Lisfranc joint injuries: a biomechanical comparison of dorsal plate and transarticular screw fixation. Foot Ankle Int. 2005;26(6):462–73.
42. Gaines RJ, Wright G, Stewart J. Injury to the tarsometatarsal joint complex during fixation of Lisfranc fracture dislocations: an anatomic study. J Trauma. 2009;66(4):1125–8.
43. Ardoin GT, Anderson RB. Subtle Lisfranc injury. Tech Foot Ankle Surg. 2010;9(3):100–6.
44. Lewis JS Jr, Anderson RB. Lisfranc injuries in the athlete. Foot Ankle Int. 2016;37(12):1374–80.
45. Sangeorzan BJ, Veith RG, Hansen ST Jr. Salvage of Lisfranc's tarsometatarsal joint by arthrodesis. Foot Ankle. 1990;10(4):193–200.
46. Panchbhavi VK. Orientation of the "Lisfranc screw". J Orthop Trauma. 2012;26(11):e221–e4.
47. Panchbhavi VK, Boutris N, Patel K, Molina D, Andersen CR. CT density analysis of the medial cuneiform. Foot Ankle Int. 2013;34(11):1596–9.
48. Panchbhavi VK. Extraarticular stabilization of Lisfranc injury. Tech Foot Ankle Surg. 2012;11(4):175–80.
49. Panchbhavi VK, Vallurupalli S, Yang J, Andersen CR. Screw fixation compared with suture-button fixation of isolated Lisfranc ligament injuries. JBJS. 2009;91(5):1143–8.
50. Kuo R, Tejwani N, Digiovanni C, Holt S, Benirschke S, Hansen S Jr, et al. Outcome after open reduction and internal fixation of Lisfranc joint injuries. JBJS. 2000;82(11):1609.

51. Ly TV, Coetzee JC. Treatment of primarily ligamentous Lisfranc joint injuries: primary arthrodesis compared with open reduction and internal fixation: a prospective, randomized study. JBJS. 2006;88(3):514–20.
52. Komenda GA, Myerson MS, Biddinger KR. Results of arthrodesis of the tarsometatarsal joints after traumatic injury. JBJS. 1996;78(11):1665–76.
53. Henning JA, Jones CB, Sietsema DL, Bohay DR, Anderson JG. Open reduction internal fixation versus primary arthrodesis for Lisfranc injuries: a prospective randomized study. Foot Ankle Int. 2009;30(10):913–22.
54. Cochran G, Renninger C, Tompane T, Bellamy J, Kuhn K. Primary arthrodesis versus open reduction and internal fixation for low-energy Lisfranc injuries in a young athletic population. Foot Ankle Int. 2017;38(9):957–63.
55. Schipper ON, Ford SE, Moody PW, Van Doren B, Ellington JK. Radiographic results of nitinol compression staples for hindfoot and midfoot arthrodeses. Foot Ankle Int. 2018;39(2):172–9.
56. Nery C, Baumfeld D, Baumfeld T, Prado M, Giza E, Wagner P, et al. Comparison of suture-augmented ligamentplasty to transarticular screws in a Lisfranc cadaveric model. Foot Ankle Int. 2020;41(6):735–43.
57. Weglein DG, Andersen CR, Morris RP, Buford WL Jr, Panchbhavi VK. Allograft reconstruction of the Lisfranc ligament. Foot Ankle Spec. 2015;8(4):292–6.
58. Panchbhavi VK. Current operative techniques in Lisfranc injury. Oper Tech Orthop. 2008;18(4):239–46.
59. Coetzee JC. Making sense of Lisfranc injuries. Foot Ankle Clin. 2008;13(4):695–704. ix
60. McHale KJ, Rozell JC, Milby AH, Carey JL, Sennett BJ. Outcomes of Lisfranc injuries in the National Football League. Am J Sports Med. 2016;44(7):1810–7.
61. Richter M, Wippermann B, Krettek C, Schratt HE, Hufner T, Therman H. Fractures and fracture dislocations of the midfoot: occurrence, causes and long-term results. Foot Ankle Int. 2001;22(5):392–8.
62. Teng AL, Pinzur MS, Lomasney L, Mahoney L, Havey R. Functional outcome following anatomic restoration of tarsal-metatarsal fracture dislocation. Foot Ankle Int. 2002;23(10):922–6.
63. Schepers T, Oprel PP, Van Lieshout EM. Influence of approach and implant on reduction accuracy and stability in Lisfranc fracture-dislocation at the tarsometatarsal joint. Foot Ankle Int. 2013;34(5):705–10.
64. Mulier T, Reynders P, Dereymaeker G, Broos P. Severe Lisfrancs injuries: primary arthrodesis or ORIF? Foot Ankle Int. 2002;23(10):902–5.
65. Sheibani-Rad S, Coetzee JC, Giveans MR, DiGiovanni C. Arthrodesis versus ORIF for Lisfranc fractures. Orthopedics. 2012;35(6):e868–e73.
66. Smith N, Stone C, Furey A. Does open reduction and internal fixation versus primary arthrodesis improve patient outcomes for Lisfranc trauma? A systematic review and meta-analysis. Clin Orthop Relat Res. 2016;474(6):1445–52.
67. Magill HH, Hajibandeh S, Bennett J, Campbell N, Mehta J. Open reduction and internal fixation versus primary arthrodesis for the treatment of acute Lisfranc injuries: a systematic review and meta-analysis. J Foot Ankle Surg. 2019;58(2):328–32.
68. Alcelik I, Fenton C, Hannant G, Abdelrahim M, Jowett C, Budgen A, et al. A systematic review and meta-analysis of the treatment of acute Lisfranc injuries: open reduction and internal fixation versus primary arthrodesis. Foot Ankle Surg. 2020;26(3):299–307.
69. Stødle AH, Hvaal KH, Brøgger HM, Madsen JE, Husebye EE. Temporary bridge plating vs primary arthrodesis of the first tarsometatarsal joint in Lisfranc injuries: randomized controlled trial. Foot Ankle Int. 2020;41(8):901–10.
70. Lau S, Guest C, Hall M, Tacey M, Joseph S, Oppy A. Functional outcomes post Lisfranc injury—transarticular screws, dorsal bridge plating or combination treatment? J Orthop Trauma. 2017;31(8):447–52.
71. Stavrakakis IM, Magarakis GE, Christoforakis Z. Percutaneous fixation of Lisfranc joint injuries: a systematic review of the literature. Acta Orthop Traumatol Turc. 2019;53(6):457–62.
72. Vertullo CJ, Nunley JA. Participation in sports after arthrodesis of the foot or ankle. Foot Ankle Int. 2002;23(7):625–8.

73. Porter DA, Barnes AF, Rund A, Walrod MT. Injury pattern in ligamentous Lisfranc injuries in competitive athletes. Foot Ankle Int. 2019;40(2):185–94.
74. Mora AD, Kao M, Alfred T, Shein G, Ling J, Lunz D. Return to sports and physical activities after open reduction and internal fixation of Lisfranc injuries in recreational athletes. Foot Ankle Int. 2018;39(7):801–7.
75. MacMahon A, Kim P, Levine DS, Burket J, Roberts MM, Drakos MC, et al. Return to sports and physical activities after primary partial arthrodesis for Lisfranc injuries in young patients. Foot Ankle Int. 2016;37(4):355–62.
76. Dubois-Ferrière V, Lübbeke A, Chowdhary A, Stern R, Dominguez D, Assal M. Clinical outcomes and development of symptomatic osteoarthritis 2 to 24 years after surgical treatment of tarsometatarsal joint complex injuries. JBJS. 2016;98(9):713–20.
77. Abbasian MR, Paradies F, Weber M, Krause F. Temporary internal fixation for ligamentous and osseous Lisfranc injuries: outcome and technical tip. Foot Ankle Int. 2015;36(8):976–83.
78. Raikin SM, Elias I, Dheer S, Besser MP, Morrison WB, Zoga AC. Prediction of midfoot instability in the subtle Lisfranc injury: comparison of magnetic resonance imaging with intraoperative findings. J Bone Joint Surg Am. 2009;91(4):892–9.

Tibialis Anterior Tendon Injuries

5

Dekarlos M. Dial, Hayden L. Hoffler, and John P. Bonvillian

Introduction

Tibialis anterior injuries are rare to the lower extremity with few cases reported in the literature. An injury to this tendon is defined as a partial or complete disruption in the continuity. Injuries to the tendon can produce destabilization, disability, and loss of functionality to the foot and ankle. Although they can occur at all ages, tibialis anterior injuries are more commonly found in older individuals and can be located from the anterior aspect of the distal tibia to the medial arch of the foot. Risk factors for injury include older age, steroid injections, fluoroquinolone usage, inflammatory arthritis, active individuals, and cavus foot structure [1–5]. The mechanism of action is multifactorial and includes internal and external methods of injury. Internally, tendon injuries occur from excessive intensity producing abnormal tension to the tendon, normal intensity in a high-level activity such as sports, and low intensity on a diseased tendon. External injuries to the tendon are due to direct impact, often with a contusion or laceration present. Different treatment modalities are aimed at the various disorders that can come with injury to this tendon. Following an adequate workup and treatment plan, patients are able to return back to normal function.

D. M. Dial (✉) · H. L. Hoffler · J. P. Bonvillian
Podiatric Medicine and Surgery Residency, Department of Orthopaedic Surgery, Wake Forest Baptist Medical Center, Winston-Salem, NC, USA
e-mail: ddial@wakehealth.edu; jpbonvil@wakehealth.edu

© Springer Nature Switzerland AG 2022
J. D. Cain, M. V. Hogan (eds.), *Tendon and Ligament Injuries of the Foot and Ankle*,
https://doi.org/10.1007/978-3-031-10490-9_5

Anatomy

The muscle belly of the tibialis anterior originates from the lateral condyle and upper and middle portions of the lateral shaft of the tibia, interosseous membrane, and the deep surface of the deep fascia [1, 3]. The tendon courses distally across the ankle in a synovial sheath under the medial portion of the superior and inferior extensor retinaculum and inserts on the medial and plantar surfaces of the first cuneiform and first metatarsal [6–8]. There are a couple of classifications that define the insertion location of the tibialis anterior tendon. They are defined by the amount of the tendon that inserts in each portion of the bone [9, 10]. Further classifications divide the insertion of the tendon based on the size of the insertion [11]. Figure 5.1 demonstrates the wide variety of insertions for the tibialis anterior that have been described in the literature. The majority of the literature states that there is an equal insertion of the tendon into the first cuneiform and first metatarsal base (Fig. 5.2).

The tibialis anterior muscle and tendon are supplied by the anterior tibial artery and its branches. Specifically, the anterior tibial recurrent artery provides blood supply proximally, and the medial tarsal artery supplies blood distally (Fig. 5.3). In the early 1990s, Geppert reported homogenous blood supply throughout the tendon, while other literature states that there is a watershed area 10.1 mm from insertion that predisposes the tendon to be injured in the area [12]. The watershed area spans from 45 to 67 mm located under the superior and inferior retinaculum (Fig. 5.4). It is these gliding regions where the tendon changes direction consisting of fibrocartilage which is avascular producing an area susceptible to injury [13].

Tibialis anterior is innervated by the deep peroneal nerve which branches from the common peroneal nerve as it courses inferior to the neck of the fibula. This tendon has numerous functions to the foot and ankle. The tibialis anterior is the strongest dorsiflexor of the foot, supplying 80% of the dorsiflexion at the ankle [14]. Other functions include inverting and adducting the foot, and a key stabilizer of the longitudinal arch. Tibialis anterior is the second strongest inverter to the foot behind the tibialis posterior tendon. This tendon is the antagonist to the peroneus longus tendon which plantarflexes and everts the foot [1, 9, 13]. In gait, along with the other dorsiflexors, tibialis anterior has the two main functions as described by Scheller [15]. They include deceleration of the ground reactive forces at heel strike to prevent foot slap and ground clearance during the swing phase. Using the anatomy of the tibialis anterior, the clinician can adequately diagnose various disorders and provide adequate treatment options based on the structures involved.

Type	Musial (1963) [n/%]	Arhornhurasook and Gaew lm (1990) [n/%]	Brenner (2002) [n/%]	Willegger et al. (2017) [n/%]	Current study – anatomical part [n/%]	Current study – US part [n/%]
Two equal size bands that inserts to the MCB and FM	46/ 37.7	25/ 56.5	43/ 27.6	3/ 7.3	31/ 31	20/ 20
Wider component inserts to the MCB and narrower component inserts to the FM	69/ 56.5	12/ 27.3	71/ 45.5	20/ 48.8	24/ 24	35/ 35
Wider component inserts to the FM and narrower component inserts to the MCB	2/ 1.7	–	37/ 25.6	1/ 2.4	11/ 11	13/ 13
Wider component inserts to the FM and MCB and accessory slip to the distal part of the FM	5/ 4.1	–	–	–	2/ 2	–
Single band inserts to the MCB	–	7/ 15.9	2/ 1.3	–	32/ 32	20/ 20
Two bands inserts to the MCB	–	–	–	–	–	12/ 12
Single band inserts to the FM	–	–	3/ 1.9	–	–	–
Narrow inserts both MCB and FM	–	–	–	17/ 41.5	–	–

Fig. 5.1   Table from Olewnik et al. [10] study demonstrating the wide variety of insertions seen with the tibialis anterior tendon

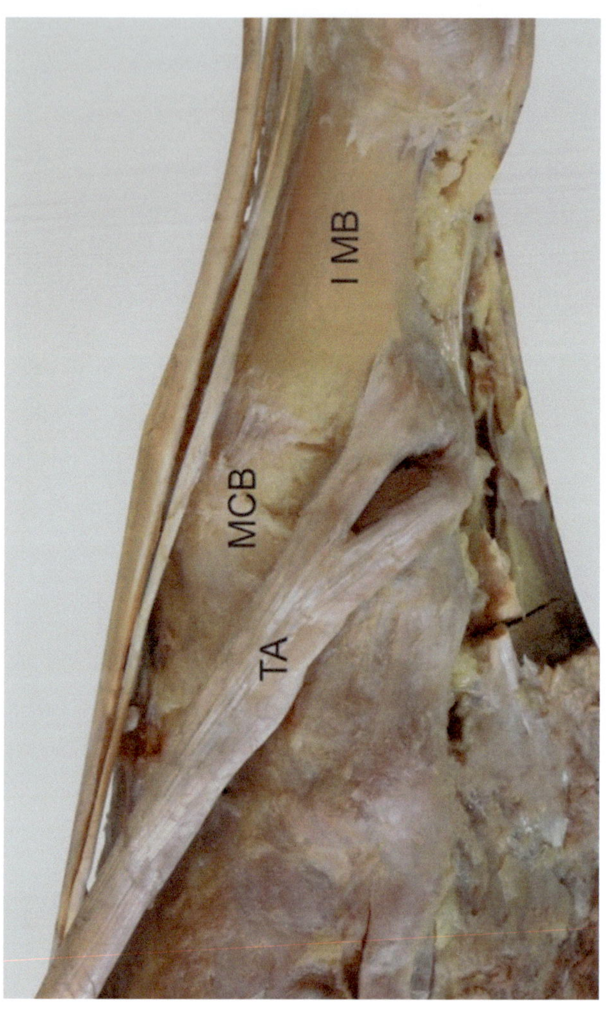

Fig. 5.2 Cadaveric limb demonstrating insertion of the tibialis anterior tendon into the medial cuneiform and first metatarsal base

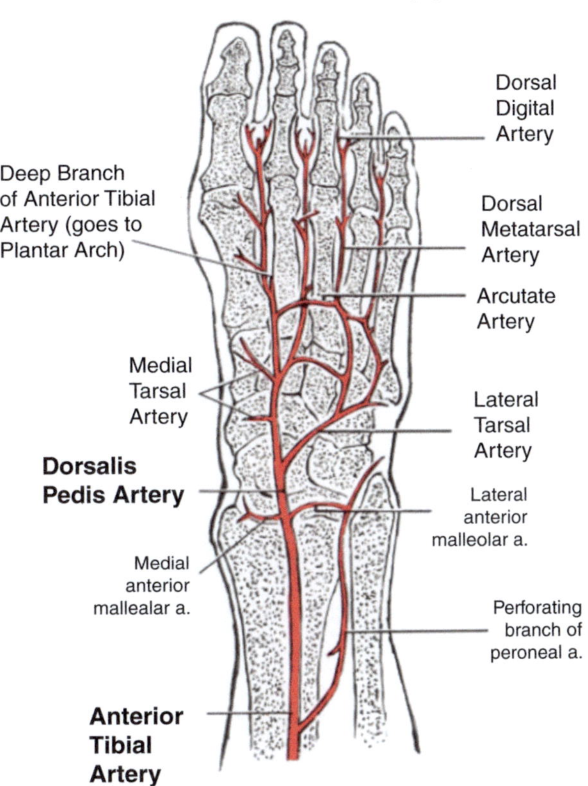

Fig. 5.3 Blood supply of the tibialis anterior supplied distally by the medial tarsal artery which is a branch of the anterior tibial artery

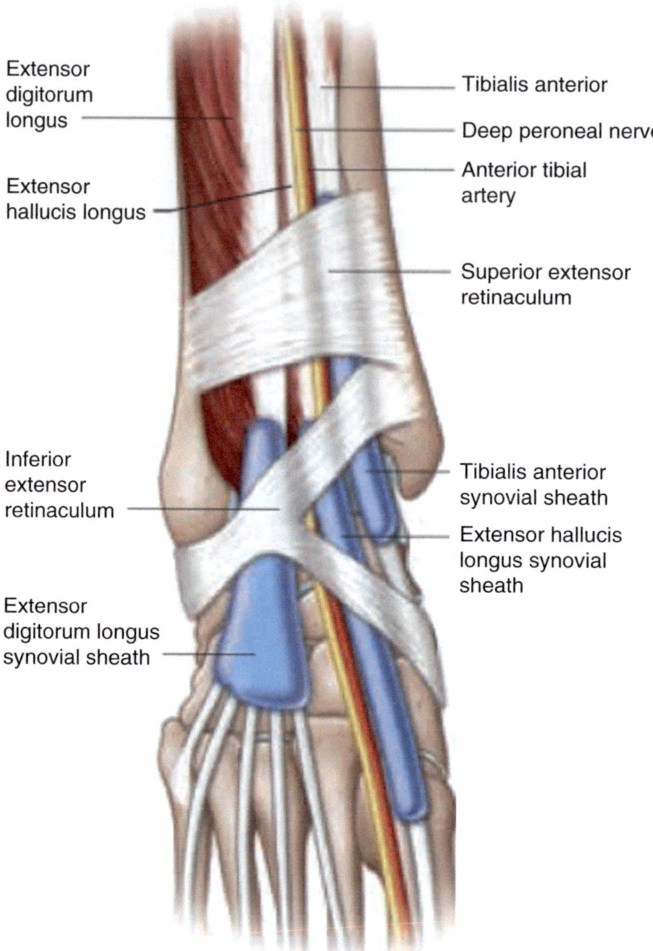

Fig. 5.4 Location of the retinaculum on anterior ankle and foot which is the watershed area of the tibialis anterior tendon

Diagnosis/Clinical Evaluation

Clinical Evaluation

Diagnosing tibialis anterior tendon injuries starts with a proper history and physical examination. Patient's usually recall a specific trauma to the associated foot that caused them immediate pain in discomfort. In other situations, patients describe pain, weakness, and discomfort that has gotten worse over time not remembering a certain incident. Past medical history should be thoroughly examined to look for disorders that put the individual at risk for a tendon injury. These can include diabetes, inflammatory arthritis, history of local corticosteroid injection, or fluoroquinolone use (Fig. 5.5). After a sufficient history, a detailed clinical exam should be performed. Visual inspection is the first indicator of an injury, with pain and weakness often apparent. In acute injuries, there is often pain over the anterior ankle and medial foot with limited dorsiflexion. In chronic injuries, there can be swelling with mass formation over the anterior ankle, drop foot, clawing of the digits, callus formation, and a slapping gait. A unique finding in chronic injuries is that they can be painless due to compensation from adjacent tendons in the anterior compartment of the leg. In 2009, Sammarco described a triad of key indicators of an injury to the tibialis anterior tendon. This included a pseudotumor on the anterior ankle, loss of contour of the tendon, and weak dorsiflexion combined with hyperextension of the toes [16].

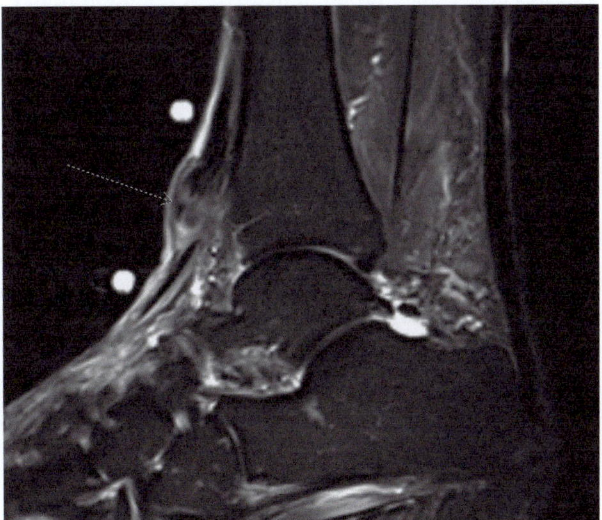

Fig. 5.5 T2 MRI demonstrating a rupture of the tibialis anterior tendon secondary to a local steroid injection

Clinical tests are next initiated to examine the strength and integrity of the tendon. Beginning with palpation, pain, swelling, and discontinuity can sometimes be appreciated as a sign of injury. Palpation should begin from the distal tibial metaphysis and continue to the insertion points of the medial midfoot. Muscle strength is performed by having the patient actively dorsiflex and invert against resistance. In ruptures, strength is decreased but can be normal in tendinopathy, tenosynovitis, and tendonitis. First ray range of motion is another way of assessing injury. In diseased tendons, there is often increased plantarflexion noted of the first ray, due to the lack of dorsiflexion provided by the tendon. The only clinical test with high sensitivity and specificity that has been described for a specific tibialis tendon injury is the Tibialis Anterior Passive Stretch Test (TAPS) for distal tendinopathy [7]. In this maneuver, the ankle is put in plantarflexion, hindfoot eversion, and a midfoot abduction, and pronation force is applied. The test is positive when pain is reproduced or increased [17]. With sufficient clinical testing, adjunctive imaging is performed next to analyze the precise location and extent of the tibialis anterior injury.

Diagnostic Imaging

Radiographs

Plain film radiographs are the initial imaging source commonly used in assessing tibialis anterior tendon injuries because they are the most accessible. They are useful in identifying soft tissue contour and density changes such as a mass on the anterior ankle that can be indicative of a tendon injury [18]. Radiographs also help rule out avulsion fractures at the tendon insertion and other occult fractures associated with the injury (Fig. 5.6). Furthermore, they assist in identifying calcifications that can occur within the tendon.

Ultrasound

Another imaging modality commonly used today is ultrasound. Ultrasound allows a skilled clinician to dynamically evaluate underlying tendon pathology with minimal morbidity to the patient. This modality is useful to assess tendon injuries in patients with underlying hardware which may otherwise obscure the image due to artifact. Fortunately, due to its superficial location in the anterior ankle, the tibialis anterior is easily visualized with a high frequency ultrasound probe (between 12 and 15 Hz). This gives better spatial and contrast resolution. The patient is best positioned with their knee flexed to 45° and their foot flat on a chair. The tendon is examined longitudinally and transversely from the myotendinous junction to the bony insertion. A normal tibialis anterior tendon's appearance is hyperechoic with its diameter twice the size of the other extensor tendons (Fig. 5.7). A diseased tibialis anterior tendon appears hypoechoic with disorganized tendon fibers, interstitial or peritendinous edema, and occasional surrounding fluid present [7, 19].

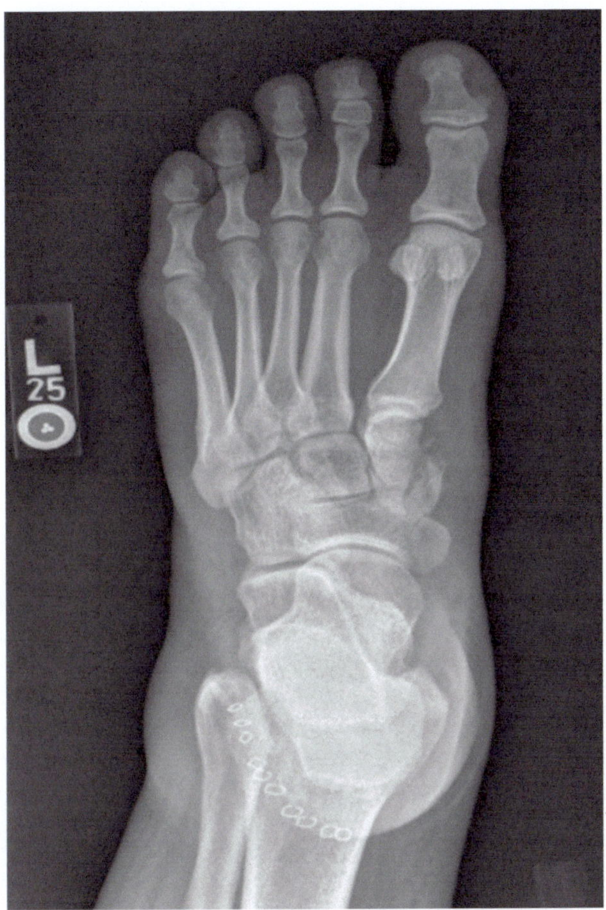

Fig. 5.6 Anterior posterior radiograph demonstrating an avulsion fracture off the medial cuneiform due to tibialis anterior injury

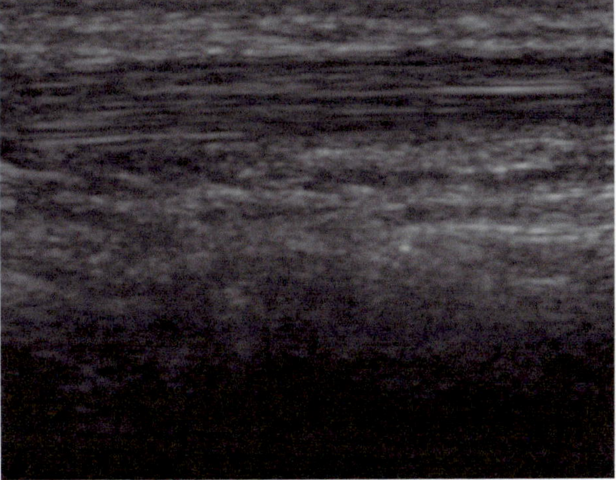

Fig. 5.7 Ultrasound image showing normal hyperechoic signs indicating an intact tibialis anterior tendon

Magnetic Resonance Imaging

The most sought out imaging modality for diagnosis of tibialis anterior injuries is Magnetic Resonance Imaging (MRI) because it can look at all tissues in the foot and ankle [20]. MRI is beneficial in that it is noninvasive and allows for multiplanar imaging. Physicians can look at the TA tendon directly to evaluate for a complete or partial tear, tenosynovitis, and tendinopathy. The normal tibialis anterior appearance is homogenous throughout with thin fibers surrounding the tendon demonstrating the retinaculum. In a diseased tendon, the tibialis anterior can appear heterogenous, with increased signal located around or within the tendon. Partial tear or split longitudinal tears are characterized by increased signal intensity in the intrasubstance of the tendon on a T2 weighted image [19]. A rupture of the tibialis anterior is commonly viewed at the level of the superior extensor retinaculum and is characterized by a complete discontinuity or defect of the tendon [20].

Differential Diagnosis

Anterior Tibial Stress Syndrome

Anterior Tibial Stress Syndrome, also known as "shin splints," is an overuse injury of the distal tibia. It is apparent in 10–15% of all running injuries [21]. It is caused by traction periostitis of the tibialis anterior on the tibia and the interosseous membrane. Risk factors include highly active patients and patients with active overpronation of the subtalar joint. Symptoms of shin splints involve pain along the anterior distal tibia that decreases with activity. Physical exam reveals a tight Achilles, pes planus foot type, and tenderness along the tendon. Upon imaging, X-rays can demonstrate stress fractures of the tibia [22]. More advanced imaging such as an MRI can show periosteal edema along the tibia. Bone scans have even been used to rule out a stress fracture.

Tendinopathy

Distal tendinopathy or tendinosis of the tibialis anterior tendon is not as common as other tendinopathies in the foot and ankle. It is most common in obese females in the fifth to seventh decade. This disorder involves degeneration of the tendon distally, most often occurring at the insertion site. Patients commonly complain of burning, nocturnal pain on the medial side of the midfoot, with pain on palpation at the insertion site [23, 24]. The TAPS test mentioned previously is the most useful test in the diagnosis with sensitivity of 90% and specificity of 95% [17]. Imaging on X-ray is relatively normal, with arthrosis shown in the medial midfoot. Ultrasound is useful, as it demonstrates hypoechoic tendon swelling distally possibly with longitudinal tears that appear fluid filled [7]. More advanced imaging such as an MRI shows tendon thickening, edema within the tendon, and increased signal within the distal aspect of the tendon near the insertion site. Degenerative changes such as osteophytes in the first tarsometatarsal joint, navicular cuneiform joint, and talonavicular joints are often seen [25, 26]. Correlation between the tendinopathy and degenerative changes has not been reported in the literature at this time and is therefore unknown.

Tendonitis

Whenever too much tension is placed on the tibialis anterior tendon, a condition known as tendonitis can form. Tibialis anterior tendonitis is most commonly seen in patients who are involved in active exercises such as running, walking, or kicking. It can also be seen by applying tight shoes or straps over the anterior ankle. Patients complain of pain along the tendon over the anterior ankle that has gradually gotten worse over time. On exam, patients may have pain with resisted dorsiflexion of the foot as well as pain on palpation of the insertion of the tendon at the first metatarsal cuneiform joint. Imaging is not used, as this disorder is a clinical diagnosis.

Tenosynovitis

Tibialis anterior tenosynovitis is another uncommon overuse injury that occurs due to repeated dorsiflexion. It is common in sports such as hiking, cycling, and skiing. Irritation from the upper edge of the shoes can contribute to the inflammation of the tendon. Patients usually complain of pain upon dorsiflexion and palpation to the anterior ankle joint [27]. X-rays are unremarkable for tenosynovitis. Ultrasound reveals hypoechogenic tendon thickening, thickening of the synovial sheath, and fluid collection within the sheath [7]. MRI demonstrates increased signal intensity on a T2 weighted image surrounding the tendon indicative of fluid collection (Fig. 5.8).

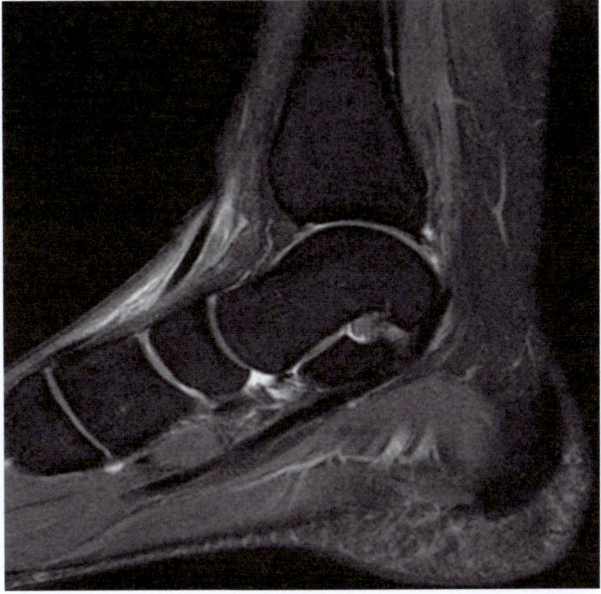

Fig. 5.8 T2 MRI demonstrating increased signal intensity surrounding the tibialis anterior tendon consistent with tenosynovitis

Rupture

First described by Brüning in 1905, tears of the tibialis anterior tendon are rare to the foot and ankle literature, with around only a couple hundred reported [28] They are the third most common tendon rupture in the lower extremity behind the Achilles and patellar tendons. The most common mechanism of rupture is a plantarflexed and everted foot combined with contracted tibialis anterior [29]. Ruptures can occur from the myotendinous junction, which is less common to the insertion site. The most common location is 5–30 mm from the insertion point [12]. Although more common as spontaneous ruptures in older people, ruptures can occur in younger individuals through open or closed blunt trauma [7, 30]. Spontaneous ruptures are a result of repetitive microtrauma on a weakened tendon combined with systemic diseases such as diabetes mellitus, hyperparathyroidism, and gout to name a few. Tears due to trauma can be very painful to younger patients. In older individuals, minimal pain is reported across the anterior ankle. Upon physical exam, the outline of the tibialis anterior tendon is not well appreciated. A firm mass can also be noted to the anterior ankle (Fig. 5.9). When placing the foot through ranges of motion, dorsiflexion can appear normal if the integrity of the extensor hallucis longus and extensor digitorum longus is intact. It is this reason that tibialis anterior ruptures often go undiagnosed during the first visit. Chronic ruptures can reveal not only a mass, but calluses underneath the metatarsal heads, clawing of the digits, and foot slap during gait [16, 31]. Radiographs are the first imaging source obtained to rule out accompanied trauma, especially in high energy impact injuries that occur in younger individuals. Ultrasound reveals irregular, hypoechoic, and enlarged tendon fibers, specifically over the lump that forms (Fig. 5.10). Fluid collection can also be apparent surrounding the tendon [7]. On MRI, a complete rupture is indicated by increased signal intensity in a T2 weighted image with tendon discontinuity and proximal retraction of the tendon commonly at the level of the superior extensor

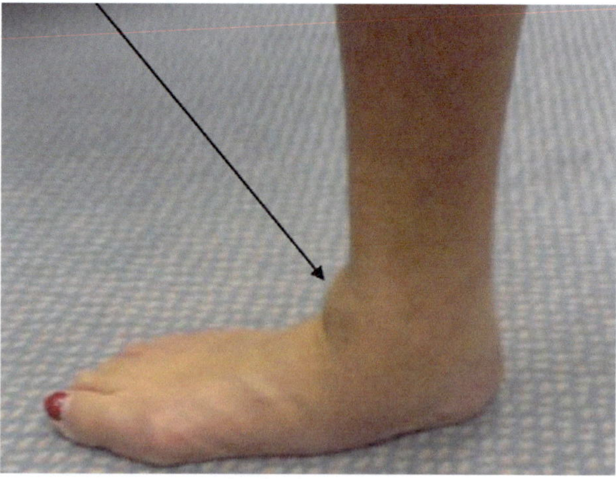

Fig. 5.9 Lateral picture showing a pseudotumor on the anterior ankle indicating a tibialis anterior rupture

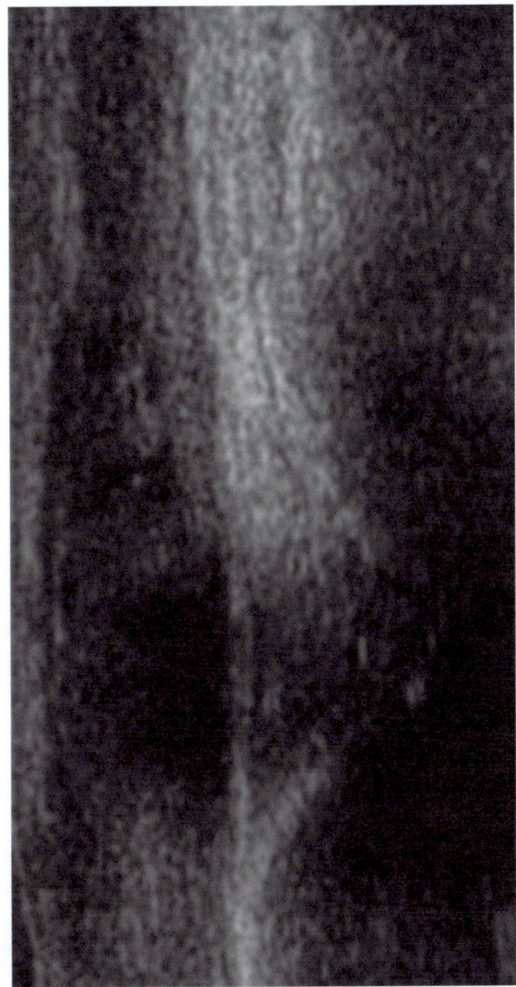

Fig. 5.10 Ultrasound demonstrating hypoechoic changes within the tibialis anterior tendon which are consistent with a rupture

retinaculum. A partial rupture or split longitudinal tear is characterized by increased signal intensity within intrasubstance of the tendon in a T2 weighted image [32, 33]. Overall, an MRI may be useful with preoperative planning.

Other disorders such as lumbar radiculopathy, superficial peroneal nerve entrapment, stress fractures, and compartment syndrome should be included in the differential diagnosis as they present with similar symptoms and exam findings [29, 34–36]. However, these must be ruled out before an appropriate treatment plan can be initiated. With an appropriate neuromuscular exam and imaging, a definitive diagnosis can be obtained, and an adequate treatment plan can be developed to allow the patient to return to normal day to day activities.

Treatment

Conservative

Most injuries of the tibialis anterior tendon can be treated nonoperatively starting with the PRICE protocol. Additionally, nonsteroidal anti-inflammatory medications (NSAIDS), bracing, and physical therapy can be initiated to help with pain, inflammation, and improved function. Steroids are not recommended because they can increase the likelihood of rupture [7, 37, 38]. In ruptures, conservative therapy is indicated in the elderly and less active patients. This involves below the knee cast for 6–8 weeks in a dorsiflexed and inverted position. Due to muscle atrophy from the cast, a decrease in the dorsiflexion can be seen in subsequent follow-up visits. Ankle foot orthotics come into play at this time as they assist in dorsiflexion through the swing phase of gait.

Surgical

Surgical treatment is more often seen in younger patients who would like to maintain a higher level of activity, or ruptures with large gaps that produce obvious functional deficits [39]. For tibialis anterior injuries, there has been surgical treatment that has been described for distal tendinopathy, tenosynovitis, and ruptures.

Tendinopathy

Distal tibialis anterior tendinopathy is usually treated nonoperatively [23, 24]. However, when nonoperative modalities fail, surgical options are considered. Surgical options for DTAT included debridement, augmentation with extensor hallucis longus (EHL) transfer, gastrocnemius recession, and decompressive medial cuneiform exostectomy (DMCE).

A gastrocnemius recession has recently been described in the literature as an adjunct procedure for ruptures but have also been used in DTAT. Contraction of the heel cord, which is an antagonist to the tibialis anterior prevents the ankle from reaching 10° of dorsiflexion which in theory leads to stressing of adjacent structures [24]. Lengthening of the muscle lessens the strain of the antagonist leading to less tension placed on the TA tendon. This decreased the amount of degeneration of tendon fibers seen in tendinopathy.

Another surgical procedure seen in DTAT is the decompressive medial cuneiform exostectomy. This technique involves first debriding the tibialis anterior tendon. While carefully preserving the insertion, the medial prominence of the medial cuneiform is resected in the sagittal plane with an oscillating saw under fluoroscopic guidance (Fig. 5.11). After smoothing the area, the tendon is replaced into the groove, the tenosynovium is excised proximally and a layered closure is performed [25]. Similar to an Achilles tendon procedure, this operation reduces mechanical irritation experienced around the insertion site.

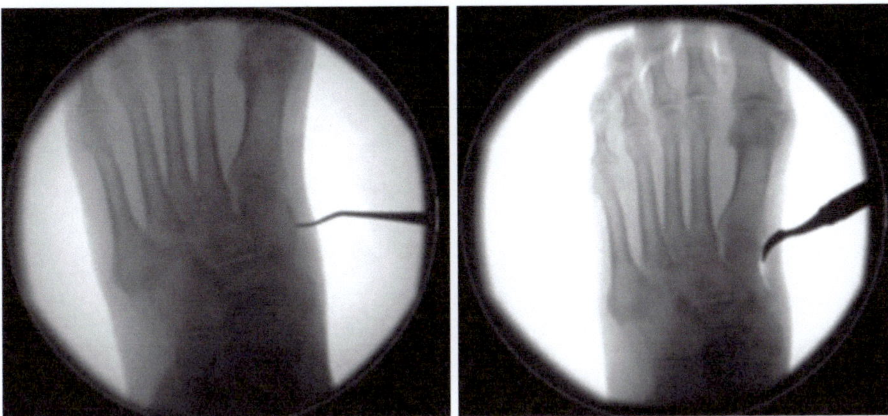

Fig. 5.11 Pre and postoperative anterior posterior fluoroscopic X-rays demonstrating exostectomy of medial cuneiform for tibialis anterior tendinopathy

Tenosynovitis

The only known surgical treatment of the tenosynovitis is excising the synovium. These are commonly done open, however damage to the extensor retinaculum can occur. This produces tendon bowstringing which can precipitate postoperative wound complications. Recently, there has been a push to tendoscopically release the synovium to preserve the integrity of the retinaculum. This is done through three portals: proximal at proximal end of tendon, middle at anterior ankle joint line, and distal at the talonavicular joint. Through these portals, the synovium can be adequately examined, and additionally bone spurs or bursa present can be resected [27].

Ruptures

The repair of tibialis anterior tendon ruptures depends on age, when the rupture occurred, the amount of retraction and how big of a gap there is. For tears that have no retraction, simple end-to-end repair is sufficient [40, 41]. When the tendon is avulsed off the insertion site and minimal retraction is present, reattachment to the bone via tendon anchor or screw is appropriate [18]. If a moderate gap exists between portions of both tendons ends and the tendon is healthy, procedures such as z lengthening and turn down flap are explored [42, 43]. However, this can report in an unusual gait pattern, as the tibialis anterior tendon is only 1/3–1/2 the normal size and the tendon to muscle ratio increases [44, 45].

Several grafts have been explored in the literature that help fill in large rupture gaps. These include semitendinosus, gracilis, Achilles, plantaris, peroneus brevis, extensor digitorum longus, and peroneus longus [29, 46–50] (Fig. 5.12). For example, in a peroneus brevis free graft, the proximal and distal ends are sutured to the peroneus longus while the graft is interposed in the rupture location [48]. Free grafts are advantageous in that they cover large tendon gaps with no functional loss or

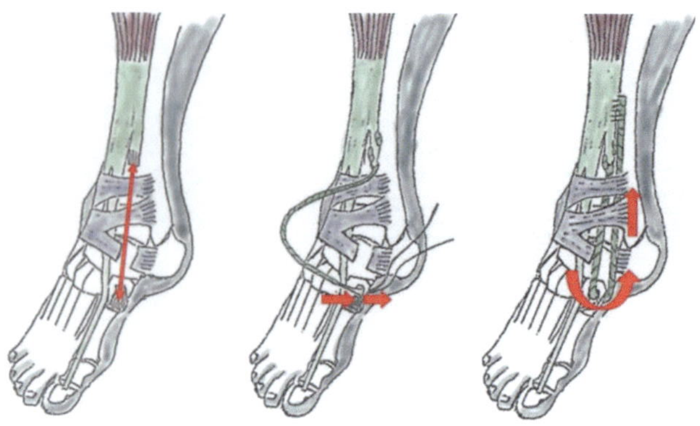

Fig. 5.12 Semitendinosus autograft used to fill in gap after a tibialis anterior rupture

anatomical changes in the foot and ankle (Fig. 5.13). Tendon transfers are also indicated for large gaps. These include the EHL, extensor digitorum longus (EDL), peroneus tertius, and tibialis posterior [5, 23, 39, 51–53]. The EHL and EDL are the most common tendons used in transfers. The EHL transfer, also known as the modified Tohen procedure involves transecting the EHL at the metatarsophalangeal joint and suturing the proximal portion to the medial cuneiform. The tibialis anterior tendon proximally is then sutured to the EHL tendon. The distal aspect of the EHL tendon is sutured to the extensor hallucis brevis (EHB) tendon or sutured to the EDL tendon of the second digit [23, 47]. This transfer is the most common because it's the nearest tendon with a similar function to the tibialis anterior (Fig. 5.14). It also has the additional benefit of eliminating claw toe deformity of the hallux. Using the EDL's second- and third-digit tendon slips, another transfer known as the Kelikian procedure can be performed. This involves the transfer of the second and third EDL tendon slips to the medial cuneiform with the distal aspect of the tendons sutured to the EDB [39, 47]. However, you must be careful of the neurovascular bundle. If a visible contracture of the heel cord is noted, a tendo-Achilles lengthening or gastrocnemius recession should be performed before surgical reconstruction of the tibialis anterior tendon.

Along with all other tendons, tibialis anterior goes through three stages following repair. The first stage is known as the inflammatory phase. This phase lasts about a week and involves the tendon ends being met together and filled in with granulation tissue. Inflammatory cells then move in, producing cytokines and growth factors which lead to the production of fibroblasts. The next stage proliferation lasts several weeks and involves fibroblast proliferation and collagen fibril formation. Lastly, the remodeling phase lasts months and involves collagen fibril alignment and strength [54]. Any disruption in the healing process can delay return to function.

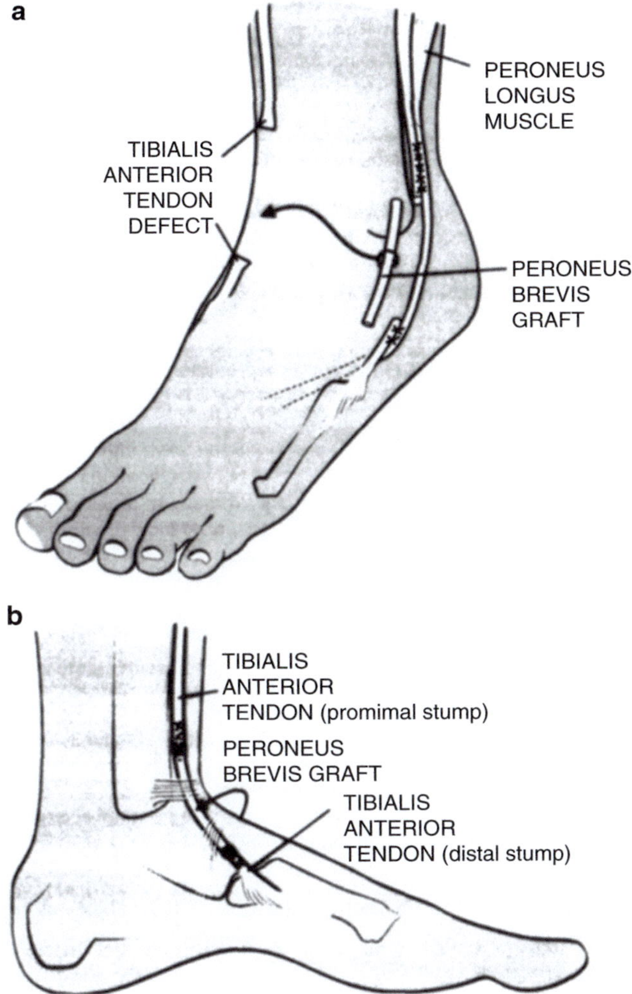

Fig. 5.13 Peroneus brevis free graft used. (**a**) The proximal and distal portions of the tendon are sutured to the peroneus longus. (**b**) The graft is used to fill in the gap of the ruptured tibialis anterior tendon

Post operatively, the patient is non-weight bearing in a cast for 4–6 weeks, with more time spent in patients who received grafts. Then the patient is transitioned to a CAM walker for an additional 6 weeks and physical therapy is initiated to work on range of motion and strengthening exercises. Full weight bearing is initiated at that time. However, patients should not resume full athletic activity until 4–6 months. A full recovery can take up to 1 year. Complications of surgical repair involving

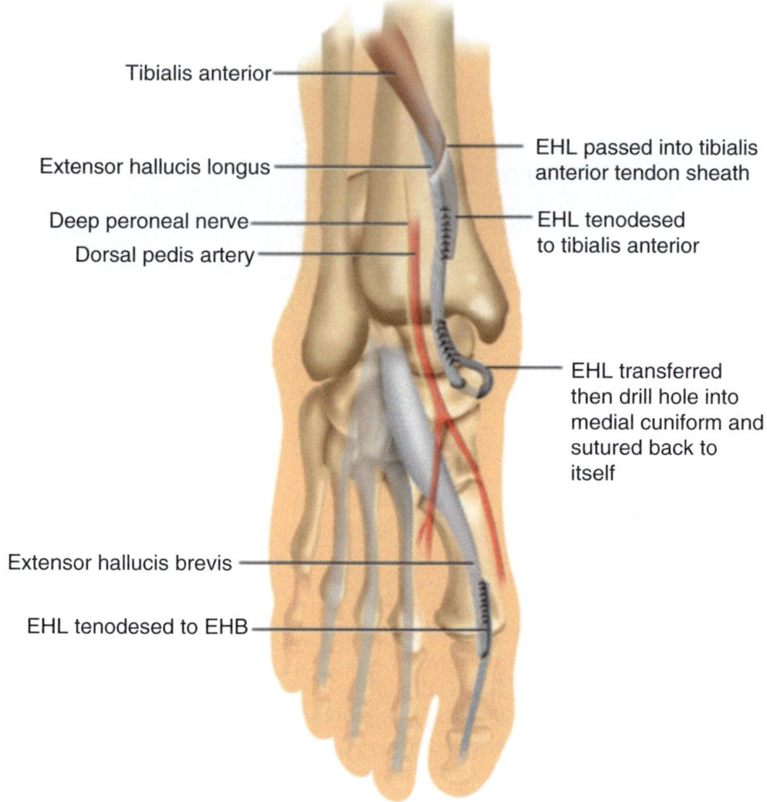

Fig. 5.14 EHL transfer performed to accommodate for tibialis anterior rupture

tibialis anterior injuries include infection, failure of the repair, wound complications, weakness in dorsiflexion, adhesions, and stump neuroma formation. These issues should be addressed on an individual basis to ensure adequate healing, and function is returned in a timely manner.

Evidence Based/Critical Appraisal of the Literature

Comprehensive Literature Search Conforming to PRISMA Statement

A comprehensive literature search was performed, with no time limit to maximize the pool of work available, conforming to the PRISMA statement. The databases used were PubMed, CINAHL, and EMBASE. The terms used for searching were tibialis anterior tendon rupture and repair in human studies. The article abstracts were reviewed, and those that were not involving humans, the management of tibialis anterior tendon injuries, nor had English translation if original articles were not in English were excluded. The search found a literature review of tibialis anterior tendon injuries, which provided further articles that were included, providing 17 studies available for analysis.

Upon review of the literature, injuries to the tibialis anterior are relatively rare [28]. Injuries to the tibialis anterior usually fall into one of several categories including: overuse, degenerative, or traumatic. Overuse injuries usually resolve after a period of conservative treatment, and seldomly require surgical intervention. Although rare, the tibialis anterior is the third most commonly ruptured tendon in the body, following the Achilles and patellar tendons. Ruptures can be either traumatic due to excessive forces acting on the ankle or from direct injury such as a laceration. In older individuals with a past medical history significant for diabetes, local corticosteroid injection, fluoroquinolone use, or gout, degenerative changes to the tibialis anterior may cause a rupture [4]. This rupture may initially be relatively asymptomatic due to the recruitment of the long extensors to aid in dorsiflexion of the foot. A thorough physical exam is of utmost importance to detect any deficiencies in manual muscle testing, any palpable defect along the course of the tendon or subtle findings in the patient's gait. Advanced imaging such as ultrasound (depending on the clinician skill level) or MRI is useful for diagnosis and surgical planning. Intraoperative findings ultimately guide surgical procedure selection based on the percentage of the tendon that is affected for patients with tendinosis and the size of the defect in cases of a complete rupture [40, 41]. Augmentation of the tendon may be necessary for defects larger than 5 cm with tendon allograft or adjacent tendon transfer [29, 46–50]. Post operatively, patients usually are non-weight bearing for 4–6 weeks, followed by a period of protected weight bearing for an additional 6 weeks in a CAM boot.

Author	Year	Study design	N	Level of evidence	Treatment
Forst et al.	1995	Case report	1	V	Use of ipsilateral peroneus brevis tendon grafting in a complicated case of traumatic rupture of TAT
Markarian et al.	1998	Case report	16	IV	No statistically significant difference between the outcomes operative (8) and nonoperative (8) group
Kausch et al.	1998	Case report	1	IV	Acute TAT rupture with transosseous suture repair
Otte et al.	2002	Case report	1	V	Recommend augmented tenoplasty of the TAT in cases of defects up to 4 cm without functional losses
DiDomenico et al.	2008	Case report	1	IV	Treatment of spontaneous TAT rupture in a DM patient with STAT repair
Gundy et al.	2010	Retrospective case series	11	IV	Debridement and repair of DTAT with EHL augmentation for greater than 50% of the tendon

Author	Year	Study design	N	Level of evidence	Treatment
Ellington et al.	2010	Retrospective case series	15	IV	No statistically significant difference between primary tendon repair versus tendon transfer groups when comparing plantarflexion strength or ROM
Aderinto et al.	2011	Case report	1	IV	Delayed repair of TAT rupture with 4 cm deficit with use of Achilles tendon allograft
Goetz et al.	2013	Retrospective study	5	IV	Recommend Z-plasty for ruptures of the TAT with understanding that this technique does not fully restore a physiologic gait pattern
Rajeev et al.	2015	Case report	1	V	Traumatic avulsion of TAT with approximation with a whip stitch and suture anchor
Funk et al.	2015	Case report	7	IV	Repair of TAT rupture using an Endobutton
Huh et al.	2015	Retrospective case series	11	IV	Allograft reconstruction of chronic irreparable TAT ruptures yielded satisfactory strength, pain, and patient reported functional outcomes
Burton et al.	2016	Case report	4	IV	Gracilis allograft reconstruction of TAT with a substantial deficit of greater than 10 cm with favorable results
Patel et al.	2017	Case report	2	IV	Repair of atraumatic TAT rupture with EHL transfer and plantaris autograft
Gossett et al	2019	Case report	1	V	Treatment of DTAT with gastrocnemius recession
Tickner et al.	2019	Systematic review and meta-analysis	134	II	Conservative treatment lead to poorer outcomes when compared to surgical treatment. Use of ipsilateral tibialis split/turn down flap of the TAT, semitendinosus autograft, or direct repair provided the best outcomes compared to EHL autograft
Vosoughi et al.	2020	Retrospective review	81 case reports	IV	For defect <2.5 cm recommend direct repair. Lengthening and rotationplasty procedures for TAT with defects <5 cm. Tendon reconstruction including EHL transfer or tendon allograft for large defects and chronic rupture with significant degeneration. Address any equinus contracture prior to TAT reconstruction

Final Treatment Algorithm

Based on the evidence in the literature and the authors experience, an algorithm can be used to guide treatment for patients with tibialis anterior tendon injuries. As stated above, these injuries can be separated into three broad categories including: overuse injuries, degenerative or chronic tendon injury, or traumatic injury. Patients with overuse type injuries (anterior tibial stress syndrome, insertional tibialis anterior tendonitis, etc.) usually recover with conservative treatment methods alone. These methods include treatments such as PRICE, NSAIDS, appropriate shoe wear, and activity modifications.

In patients with degenerative or chronic tendon injury, the overall patient should be considered. The provider should evaluate things such as the patient's medical comorbidities, activity demand, and functional loss from the injury. In low demand patients with advanced age and multiple comorbidities, conservative management is usually recommended. Treatment options include casting or splinting in dorsiflexion and inversion or an AFO device with or without dorsiflexory assist. In patients with chronic tendon injuries with functional loss that are not of advanced age and are relatively active, surgical intervention may be warranted. The operative procedure depends on the intraoperative findings upon evaluation of the degenerated tendon. When less than 50% of the tendon is involved, operative procedures may include: tendon debridement with tenolysis or tenosynovectomy. If greater than 50% of the tendon is involved or in cases of a neglected tendon rupture, local tendon transfers as well as tendon allograft may be needed to fill large defects [18, 29, 41–50].

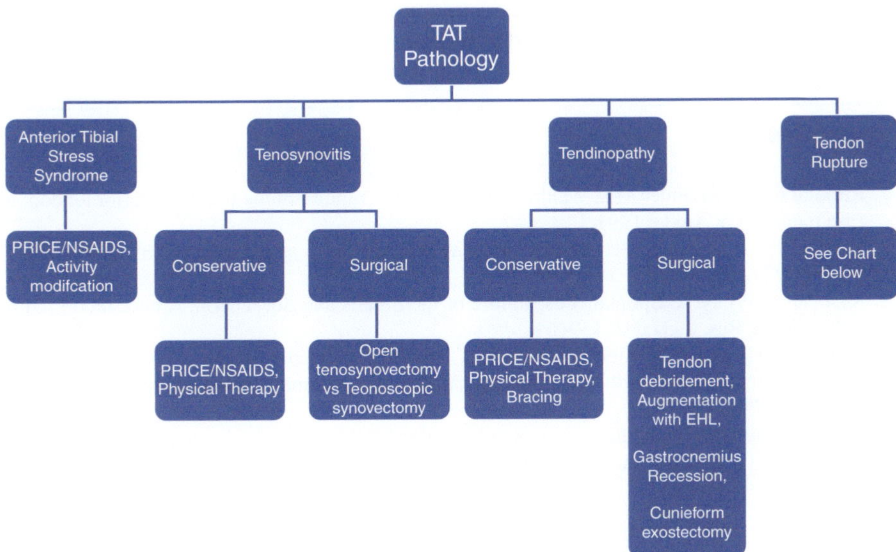

Finally, patients with traumatic injuries to the tibialis anterior, including complete or partial tendon rupture, or tendon laceration with functional deficits will likely benefit from surgical intervention. Again, the procedure of choice is dependent on the surgeon's intraoperative findings, specifically the size of the defect as seen in the flow chart below.

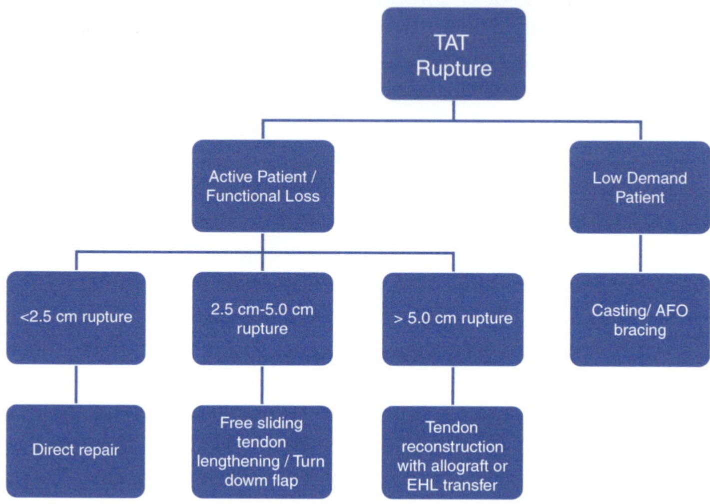

In ruptures with less than 2.5 cm of tendon defect, an end-to-end anastomosis is preferred. In ruptures with a defect of 2.6–5.0 cm, lengthening of the tendon will likely be necessary to achieve tendon apposition. Finally, in defects larger than 5.0 cm tendon allograft or local tendon transfers are recommended.

References

1. Rimoldi RL, Oberlander MA, Waldrop JI, et al. Acute rupture of the tibialis anterior tendon: a case report. Foot Ankle. 1991;12:176–7.
2. Trevino S, Baumhauer JF. Tendon injuries of the foot and ankle. Clin Sports Med. 1992;11:727–39.
3. Kashyap S, Prince R. Spontaneous rupture of the tibialis anterior tendon. A case report. Clin Orthop Relat Res. 1987;216:159–61.
4. Velan GJ, Hendel D. Degenerative tear of the tibialis anterior tendon after corticosteroid injection-augmentation with the extensor hallucis longus tendon, case report. Acta Orthop Scand. 1997;68:308–9.
5. Patten A, Pun WK. Spontaneous rupture of the tibialis anterior tendon: a case report and literature review. Foot Ankle Int. 2000;21:697–700.
6. Sobotta J, Paulsen F. Atlas of human anatomy. Elsevier; 2011.

7. Varghese A, Bianchi S. Ultrasound of tibialis anterior muscle and tendon: anatomy, technique of examination, normal and pathologic appearance. J Ultrasound. 2013;17(2):113–23.
8. Saraffian SK. Retaining systems and compartments. In: Patterson D, editor. Anatomy of the foot and ankle: descriptive, topographic, functional. Philadelphia, PA: Lippincott; 1993. p. 113–8.
9. Willegger M, Seyidova N, Schuh R, et al. Anatomical footprint of the tibialis anterior tendon: surgical implications for foot and ankle reconstructions. Biomed Res Int. 2017;2017:1–5.
10. Olewnik L, Podgorski M, Polguj M, et al. A cadaveric and sonographic study of the morphology of the tibialis anterior tendon—a proposal for a new classification. J Foot Ankle Res. 2019;12(1)
11. Musial WW. Variations in the terminal insertions of the anterior and posterior tibial muscles. Folia Morphol (Warsaw). 1963;22:237–47.
12. Geppert MJ, Sobel M, Hannafin JA. Microvasculature of the tibialis anterior tendon. Foot Ankle. 1993;14(5):261–4.
13. Petersen W, Stein V, Bobka T. Blood supply of the tibialis anterior tendon. Arch Orthop Trauma Surg. 1999;119(7–8):371–5.
14. Lavelle, William F. Foot pain. Current therapy in pain, by Howard S. Smith, Saunders/Elsevier, 2009, pp. 189–194.
15. Scheller AD, Kasser JR, Quigley TB. Tendon injuries about the ankle. Orthop Clin North Am. 1980;11:801–11.
16. Sammarco VJ, Sammarco GJ, Henning C, et al. Surgical repair of acute and chronic tibialis anterior tendon ruptures. J Bone Joint Surg Am. 2009;91(2):325–32.
17. Beischer AD, Beamond BM, Jowett AJL, et al. Distal tendinosis of the tibialis anterior tendon. Foot Ankle Int. 2009;30(11):1053–9.
18. Rajeev A, McDonald M, Newby M, et al. Traumatic avulsion of tibialis anterior following an industrial accident: a case report. Int J Surg Case Rep. 2015;14:125–8.
19. Chang A, Miller MT. Imaging of tendons. Sports Health: A Multidisciplinary Approach. 2009;1(4):293–300.
20. Lee MH, Chung CB, Cho JH, et al. Tibialis anterior tendon and extensor retinaculum: imaging in cadavers and patients with tendon tear. Am J Roentgenol. 2006;187(2)
21. Bates P. Shin splints—a literature review. Br J Sports Med. 1985;19(3):132–7.
22. Devas MB. Stress fractures of the tibia in athletes or "shin soreness". JBone Joint Surg. 1958;40B(2):227–39.
23. Grundy JRB, O'Sullivan RM, Beisher AD. Operative management of distal tibialis anterior tendinopathy. Foot Ankle Int. 2010;31(3):212–9.
24. Gossett L, Gossett PC, Roberts J. Gastrocnemius recession for the treatment of tibialis anterior tendinopathy. Foot Ankle Orthop. 2019;4(3):247301141985294.
25. Laing AJ, Carr C. Decompressive medial cuneiform exostectomy for resistant tibialis anterior insertional tendinopathy. J Foot Ankle Surg. 2018;57(3):531–6.
26. Mengiardi B, Pfirrmann CW, Vienne P, et al. Anterior tibial tendon abnormalities: MR imaging findings. Radiology. 2005;235:977–84.
27. Lee JCY, Lui TH. Tendoscopic synovectomy of tibialis anterior tendon of the ankle. Arthrosc Tech. 2018;7(12)
28. Brüning F. Zwei seltene Fälle von subkutaner Sehnenzerreissung. Münchner Medizinische Wochenschrift. 1905;26(52):1928–9.
29. Tickner A, Thorng S, Martin M, et al. Management of isolated anterior tibial tendon rupture: a systematic review and meta-analysis. J Foot Ankle Surg. 2019;58(2):213–20.

30. Christman-Skieller C, Merz MK, Tansey JP. A systematic review of tibialis anterior tendon rupture treatments and outcomes. Am J Orthop (Belle Mead NJ). 2015;44(4):E94–9.
31. Petersen W, Stein V, Bobka T. Structure of the human tibialis anterior tendon. J Anat. 2000;197(Pt 4):617–25.
32. Khoury NJ, el-Khoury GY, Saltzman CL, et al. Rupture of the anterior tibial tendon: diagnosis by MR imaging. AJR Am J Roentgenol. 1996;167:351–4.
33. Gallo RA, Kolman BH, Daffner RH, et al. MRI of tibialis anterior tendon rupture. Skelet Radiol. 2004;33:102–6.
34. van Acker G, Pingen F, Luitse J, et al. Rupture of the tibialis anterior tendon. Acta Orthop Belg. 2006;72:105–7.
35. Kennelly KD, Shapiro SA, Kumar N, et al. Spontaneous tibialis anterior tendon rupture: a rare cause of foot drop. Neurology. 2007;68:1949–51.
36. Jerome JT, Varghese M, Sankaran B, et al. Tibialis anterior tendon rupture in gout—case report and literature review. Foot Ankle Surg. 2008;14:166–9.
37. Jain K, Asad M, Joshi Y, et al. Tibialis anterior tendon rupture as a complication of first tarsometatarsal joint steroid injection: a case report and review of literature. Foot (Edinb). 2015;25(3):179–81.
38. Gwynne-Jones D, Garneti N, Wyatt M. Closed tibialis anterior tendon rupture: a case series. Foot Ankle Int. 2009;30(8):758–62.
39. Markarian GG, Kelikian AS, Brage M, et al. Anterior tibialis tendon ruptures: an outcome analysis of operative versus nonoperative treatment. Foot Ankle Int. 1998;19:792–802.
40. Neumayer F, Djembi YR, Gerin A, et al. Closed rupture of the tibialis anterior tendon: a report of 2 cases. J Foot Ankle Surg. 2009;48:457–61.
41. Hipp E, Weigert M. Subkutane Ruptur der tibialis-anticus-Sehne. Z Orthop. 1966;101:398–9.
42. Otte S, Klinger HM, Lorenz F, et al. Operative treatment in case of a closed rupture of the anterior tibial tendon. Arch Orthop Trauma Surg. 2002;122:188–90.
43. Trout BM, Hosey G, Wertheimer SJ. Rupture of the tibialis anterior tendon. J Foot Ankle Surg. 2000;39:54–8.
44. Goetz J, Beckmann J, Koeck F, et al. Gait analysis after tibialis anterior tendon rupture repair using Z-plasty. J Foot Ankle Surg. 2013;52:598–601.
45. DiDomenico LA, Williams K, Petrolla AF. Spontaneous rupture of the anterior tibial tendon in a diabetic patient: results of operative treatment. J Foot Ankle Surg. 2008;47:463–7.
46. Burton A, Aydogan U. Repair of chronic tibialis anterior tendon rupture with a major defect using Gracilis allograft. Foot Ankle Spec. 2016;9(4):345–50.
47. Vosoughi AR, Heyes G, Molloy AP, et al. Management of tibialis anterior tendon rupture: recommendations based on the literature review. Foot Ankle Surg. 2019;S1268-7731(19):30099–2. [published online ahead of print, 2019 Jun 21]
48. Forst R, Forst J, Heller KD. Ipsilateral peroneus brevis tendon grafting in a complicated case of traumatic rupture of tibialis anterior tendon. Foot Ankle Int. 1995;16:440–4.
49. Patel R, Fallat L. Surgical techniques for repair of atraumatic tibialis anterior tendon ruptures: a report of two cases. J Foot Ankle Surg. 2017;56:1343–9.
50. Aderinto J, Gross A. Delayed repair of tibialis anterior tendon rupture with Achilles tendon allograft. J Foot Ankle Surg. 2011;50:340–2.
51. Dooley BJ, Kudelka P, Menelaus MB. Subcutaneous rupture of the tendon of tibialis anterior. J Bone Jt Surg Br. 1980;62-B:471–2.

52. Ellington JK, McCormick J, Marion C, et al. Surgical outcome following tibialis anterior tendon repair. Foot Ankle Int. 2010;31:412–7.
53. Gaulrapp H, Heimkes B. Peronaeus-tertius-Plastik nach veralteter traumatischer Ruptur der Tibialis-anterior-Sehne (Kasuistik). Unfallchirurg. 1997;100:979–83.
54. Thomopoulos S, Parks WC, Rifkin DB, et al. Mechanisms of tendon injury and repair. J Orthop Res. 2015;33(6):832–9.

Peroneal Tendons Injuries

6

Francisco Muñoz, Felipe Chaparro, Mario Escudero, Gonzalo F. Bastías, and Manuel J. Pellegrini

Introduction

Pathology of the peroneal tendons is often underdiagnosed when evaluating patients with lateral foot and ankle pain. Likewise, it is sometimes difficult to distinguish the origin of the symptoms at this location [1]. For this reason, a wide knowledge of anatomy, biomechanics, and physiopathology of the peroneal tendons is necessary for diagnosing and treatment. A correct exploration of the patient, and the peroneal tendons, is mandatory to achieve the proper diagnosis. In case conservative treatment fails, a surgical procedure (open or minimally invasive) should be suggested. Current options include the following: (1) peroneal tendoscopy, (2) open debridement and tubularization of the remaining tendon, (3) tenodesis, (4) tendon transfer,

F. Muñoz
Department of Traumatology and Orthopaedic Surgery, Universidad Finis Terrae, Santiago, Chile

F. Chaparro
Department of Foot and Ankle Surgery, Clínica Universidad de los Andes, Santiago, Chile
e-mail: fchaparro@clinicauandes.cl

M. Escudero
Department of Foot and Ankle Surgery, Hospital Clínico Universidad de Chile, Santiago, Chile

G. F. Bastías
Department of Foot and Ankle Surgery, Clínica Las Condes, Santiago, Chile
e-mail: gbastias@clinicalascondes.cl

M. J. Pellegrini (✉)
Department of Foot and Ankle Surgery, Clínica Universidad de los Andes, Santiago, Chile

Department of Foot and Ankle Surgery, Hospital Clínico Universidad de Chile, Santiago, Chile
e-mail: mpellegrini@clinicauandes.cl

© Springer Nature Switzerland AG 2022
J. D. Cain, M. V. Hogan (eds.), *Tendon and Ligament Injuries of the Foot and Ankle*,
https://doi.org/10.1007/978-3-031-10490-9_6

and (5) reconstruction with allograft or autograft. With the goal of reducing comorbidity observed from open surgery, minimally invasive techniques are increasing. In 1998, van Dijk and Kort were the first to describe tendoscopy of the peroneal tendons [2]. Technological advances and instrumentation improvements have increased indications for tendoscopic techniques in the foot and ankle [3–5], including those referred to peroneal tendons tendoscopy.

The objective of this chapter is to offer the orthopedic surgeon complete information related to the peroneal tendons that may help manage patients with lateral pain of the foot and ankle arising from the peroneal tendons.

Anatomy

The peroneal muscles lay in the lateral compartment of the leg and are innervated by the superficial peroneal nerve. The peroneus longus tendon originates proximally from the lateral condyle of the tibia and the head of the fibula, and the peroneus brevis tendon originates from superior 2/3 of the fibula and the interosseous membrane.

Typically, the muscle-tendinous unit of the peroneus brevis tendon is located proximal to the superior peroneal retinaculum; however, it may occasionally present a lower insertion and generates a continent-contained conflict at the retromalleolar groove, increasing pressure in this space and producing pain [6]. Under the same perspective, a quartus peroneus muscle can be located inside this space and produce a similar situation. The prevalence of this muscle oscillates between 10% and 22% and typically originates from the muscle belly of the peroneal brevis and inserts into the peroneal trochlea of the calcaneus [7–10].

Both tendons enter in a common synovial sheath approximately 4 cm proximal to the tip of the lateral malleolus. They run posterior to the lateral malleolus through a fibrous bone tunnel called the retromalleolar groove, with the peroneus longus tendon located posterolateral with respect to the peroneus brevis tendon. Distal to the articulation of the ankle, the synovial sheath separates upon reaching the peroneal trochlea on the lateral face of the calcaneus. The peroneus longus tendon passes underneath the peroneal trochlea, and the peroneus brevis tendon passes over the top. The peroneal tendon transverse inferior retinaculum lays approximately 2–3 cm distal from the tip of the fibula. The peroneus brevis tendon continues directly until its insertion in the tuberosity at the base of the fifth metatarsal. The peroneus longus tendon rotates medially between the groove of the cuboid and the long plantar ligament and inserts in the superficial plantar surface of the first metatarsal and the lateral aspect of the medial cuneiform.

There are two critical zones for the pathology of the peroneal tendons: the retromalleolar groove for both tendons and the cuboid notch for the peroneus longus tendon.

The retromalleolar groove is limited by the superior peroneal retinaculum posterolateral and anterior to the fibula and medially by both talofibular (anterior and posterior) and calcaneofibular ligaments [11, 12]. This groove is lined by fibrocartilage and varies in depth and shape [13], potentially affecting the stability of the peroneal tendons when passing behind the fibula. In a cadaveric study of 178 fibulas, 82% presented a concave retromalleolar groove, 11% flat, and 7% convex [14]. The groove measures between 6 and 7 mm in width and between 2 and 4 mm of depth and is reinforced by a fibrocartilage ridge. The shape of the groove is determined more by its fibrocartilage ridge than by the concavity of the fibula [15, 16]. Although the morphology of the retromalleolar groove can contribute to the subluxation and consequent injury of the peroneal tendons [7, 14, 17], apparently there are no clinical differences considering groove type in patients with and without instability of the peroneal tendons [18]. The superior peroneal retinaculum is the primary restriction to avoid subluxation of the peroneal tendons in the ankle. This structure corresponds to a band of fibrous tissue approximately 1–2 cm of width that originates from the posterolateral and distal fibula, with great variety in its insertion [19].

The passage of the peroneus longus tendon at the level of the cuboid notch represents a zone of direction change and therefore of increased stress for the tendon. The os peroneum, a fibrocartilaginous enlargement, is a structure that increases the resistance of the peroneus longus tendon in this zone of maximum stress, and it is estimated that it ossifies in approximately 20% of the general population [20, 21]. The hypertrophy of the os peroneum is considered a cause of tenosynovitis in the peroneal tendons [9, 21–23], given the mechanical stress trauma and thinning of the sheath that can secondarily alter normal excursion [24].

The peroneal arteries and the perforating branches of the anterior tibial artery irrigate the lateral compartment of the leg. Additionally, they receive irrigation through links that originate from the posterior peroneal artery and from branches of the medial tarsal. These links penetrate the posterolateral aspect of each tendon of its route to the retromalleolar groove. It has been proposed that the peroneal tendons present critical vascular zones that can contribute to tendinopathy [25]. However, the presence of avascular zones has been refuted by many authors [26, 27].

Pathophysiology

Tendinosis and tenosynovitis of the peroneal tendons correspond to an alteration of the normal tendon structure and inflammation of the synovial sheath, respectively [11, 28]. Among its causes are repetitive and prolonged activities, severe inversion ankle sprains, chronic instability of the ankle, peroneal subluxation, and fractures of the ankle or calcaneus [7, 23, 24, 29–33]. Although the etiology of peroneal tendons tears is not completely understood [34], predisposing anatomical factors have been reported to contribute to this pathology. A convex fibula groove, low or abnormal muscle belly, incompetence of the superior peroneal retinaculum, presence of a posterolateral osteophyte, and cavus foot have been associated directly with injury of the peroneal tendons [35, 36].

The primary function of the peroneal muscles is the eversion and plantar flexion of the ankle. Secondarily, the peroneus longus produces plantarflexion of the first metatarsal. Both tendons participate in the dynamic stability of the ankle especially during the partial support and elevation of the heel on the gait [13, 37].

The presence of anatomical variants related both to the retromalleolar trochlea can predispose the presence of pathology of the peroneal tendons. The hypertrophy of the peroneal trochlea also has been implicated in the pathogenesis of this problem increasing the mechanical stress in the peroneal tendons, potentially leading to tendinopathy and restriction of the normal displacement [7, 22, 38–41].

The presence of cavus and/or varus of the foot predisposes to biomechanical alterations of both peroneal tendons, reducing the lever arm and increasing forces of displacement in the lateral malleolus, peroneal trochlea, and in the cuboid notch [42, 43], so the addition of other stress agents can raise the probability of producing disorders at the level of the peroneal tendons.

Tendinopathy and/or tear of the peroneal tendons can cause lateral instability of the ankle and can present acute or chronic. During acute inversion of the ankle, an impingement of the peroneus brevis tendon is produced between the peroneus longus tendon and the posterior aspect of the fibula, which can lead to a longitudinal split tear (Fig. 6.1) or a complete tear of the peroneus brevis tendon [44, 45]. The posterolateral border of the fibula can create a defect in the tendon while it is repeatedly subluxated over the crest. This defect often evolves into a longitudinal tear of approximately 2.5–5 cm in length [46].

Tears of the peroneus longus tendon can occur in an isolated form or in conjunction with tears of the peroneus brevis tendon. Acute tears of the peroneus longus tendon result from sports injuries, lateral instability of the ankle, instability of the peroneal tendons, or traumatic injuries such as tendon avulsion at the level of the os

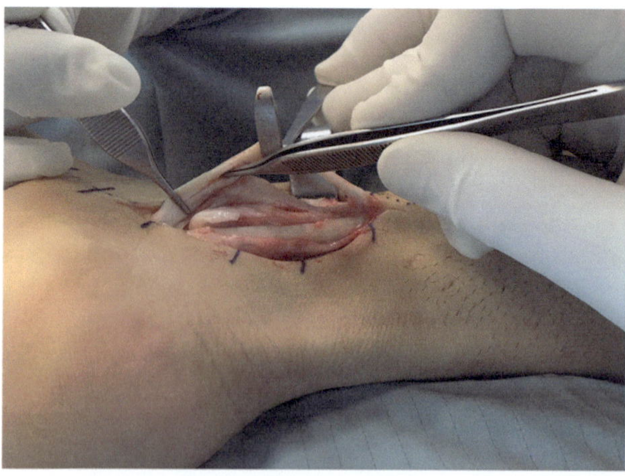

Fig. 6.1 Longitudinal split type tear of the peroneus brevis tendon

peroneum and/or traumatic lacerations of the tendon [17, 23, 30, 47–49]. Classically, these tears occur at the level of the cuboid, in the os peroneum, in the peroneal trochlea, or at the level of the tip of the lateral malleolus [50–54].

Although longitudinal tears are the most frequent, there has also been documented transverse tears of both tendons. These tears occur most frequently in acute injuries and are located distal to the os peroneum but also can occur at the level of the muscle-tendinous unit [55].

Peroneal tendon instability occurs under physiological loads, as the tendons alter their position and/or anatomical location producing symptoms. This condition can be subdivided depending on the competence of the superior peroneal retinaculum and the grade of dislocation (complete or incomplete) of the tendons with respect to the retromalleolar groove. The most frequent form of presentation occurs with a rupture of the retinaculum and producing dislocation of both tendons outside the retromalleolar groove (Fig. 6.2a, b). The most common mechanism is an abrupt contracture of the peroneal tendons during a forced inversion of the ankle or during a forced dorsiflexion of the foot while it is in eversion [15, 56]. This produces disruption of the superior peroneal retinaculum and allows that the peroneal tendons subluxate anteriorly over the lateral malleolus [12, 57]. This condition is frequently associated with lateral instability of the ankle, considering that rupture of the lateral ligamentary complex increases the tension over the superior peroneal retinaculum [58, 59]. A dysplastic retromalleolar groove, hyperlaxity of the superior peroneal retinaculum for a cavovarus hindfoot or congenital absence of the superior peroneal retinaculum, can contribute to the subluxation mechanism of the peroneal tendons [30, 60, 61].

Subluxation of the peroneal tendons can be classified in four grades. In grade 1, the superior peroneal retinaculum is elevated from the fibula at the subperiosteal level. In grade 2, the fibrocartilage crest comes off from the anterior aspect of the fibula. In grade 3, the superior peroneal retinaculum is avulsed from the fibula with a small cortical fragment, and in grade 4, the superior peroneal retinaculum is disinserted at the level of its posterior insertion in the calcaneal and/or the Achilles tendon [16, 62].

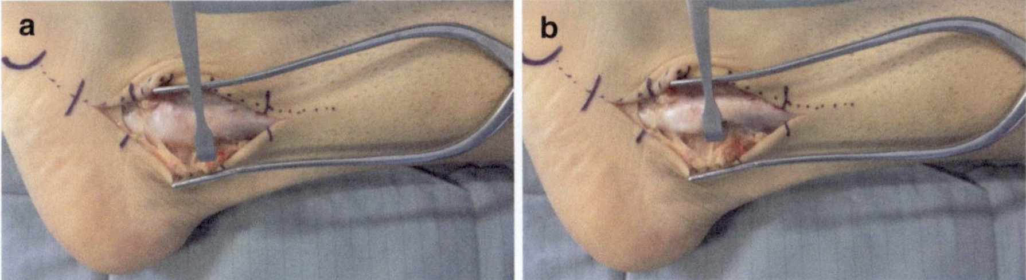

Fig. 6.2 Instability of the peroneal tendons in a left foot. (**a**) Peroneal tendons in anatomical situation and (**b**) dislocated outside the retromalleolar groove

Diagnosis/Clinical Evaluation

A detailed history and a thorough physical exam are essential, in particular, for patients presenting with chronic pain and instability of the ankle. Frequently, patients refer repetitive ankle sprains or malleolar/calcaneal fractures, among other injuries. Associated conditions are rheumatoid arthritis, psoriasis, hyperparathyroidism, diabetic neuropathy, use of fluoroquinolones, and history of infiltration with corticosteroids, which should be investigated [55, 63–65].

Differential diagnosis include lateral instability of the ankle, tarsal sinus syndrome, fifth metatarsal, cuboid and fibula fractures, stress fractures of the calcaneal, cuboid tunnel syndrome, osteochondral injuries of the talus, free bodies (tibiotalar or subtalar), degenerative joint disease, tarsal coalition, sural neuritis, radiculopathy, malign tumor, and accessory muscle or bone [60].

Acute peroneal tendinopathy is defined as symptoms presenting for less than 2 weeks, subacute if the symptoms are present for 2–6 weeks, and chronic if the symptoms persist for more than 6 weeks [11].

Patients with a history of subluxation of the peroneal tendons often describe it as a painful clicking sensation. Tears of the peroneus brevis tendon are often referred to a persistent increase of volume along the trajectory of the tendon, while tears of the peroneus longus tendon pain can flow around the cuboid notch and extend to the plantar aspect of the foot in relation to its distal insertion zone.

The evaluation of the alignment of the hindfoot and forefoot is paramount, due to the coexistence of cavovarus that can predispose it to injuries in the peroneal tendons [37]. Coleman block test can be useful for determining if the cavovarus hindfoot is the primary problem or if it is secondary to a plantar flexed first metatarsal.

Tenderness can be generated while palpation of the peroneal tendons throughout its entire length. The strength of the peroneal tendons should be evaluated for both weakness and pain while performing counter-resistance to eversion of the midfoot, maintaining the ankle in plantar flexion.

Presence of instability can be evaluated with flexion of 90° and requesting the patient to actively perform movements of plantar flexion and dorsiflexion of the ankle while counter resistance is performed. The test is considered positive when you can see or feel the anterior subluxation of the tendons over the lateral malleolus. Sobel et al. [21] described the compression test of the peroneal tendons in the peroneal grove to evaluate the presence of tendinopathy.

Radiological study of patients presenting with lateral pain of the ankle, and in which there is a suspicion of peroneal pathology, should always include X-ray examination. Weight-bearing anteroposterior, lateral, and Saltzman projections of both ankles should be obtained. Abnormal findings indicating pathology of the peroneal tendons include an avulsion at the base of the fifth metatarsal, an avulsion of the distal fibula denominated "fleck sign" (that indicates a grade 3 injury of the superior peroneal retinaculum which is in turn pathognomonic of traumatic subluxation of the peroneal tendons) [66], hypertrophy of the peroneal trochlea, or presence of an os peroneum [37]. X-rays can also reveal fractures of the os peroneum or an os peroneum bi- or multipartite [53, 54].

Ultrasonography (US) is a noninvasive method allowing dynamic evaluations of the tendons [66] which is useful to evaluate competence of the superior peroneal retinaculum.

MRI is the standard method for evaluating disorders in tendons, since it provides a tridimensional evaluation of the peroneal tendons [67]. Axial views with the foot in slight plantar flexion provide the best definition of the contour of the peroneal tendons, the content of the synovial sheath, and the adjacent structures such as the superior peroneal retinaculum or the retromalleolar groove [68, 69]. Both tendons normally present a homogenous intensity in signal T1, T2, and in STIR (short tau inversion recovery). In cases with tenosynovitis, tendinosis or in tears of the tendons, high-intensity signal in T2 or in STIR, decrease in the homogeneity of the signal, or thinning of the tendons can be observed [70, 71] (Fig. 6.3).

Computed tomography is a useful method to define with greater accuracy those bone abnormalities associated with tendinopathy of the peroneal tendons such as hypertrophy of the peroneal trochlea, calcaneum fractures, os peroneum or lateral malleolus avulsion fracture [32].

A tear of the peroneal brevis tendon can be appreciated in the shape of a V ("chevron-shaped"), bisected or with an increased signal in T2 [68]. Common

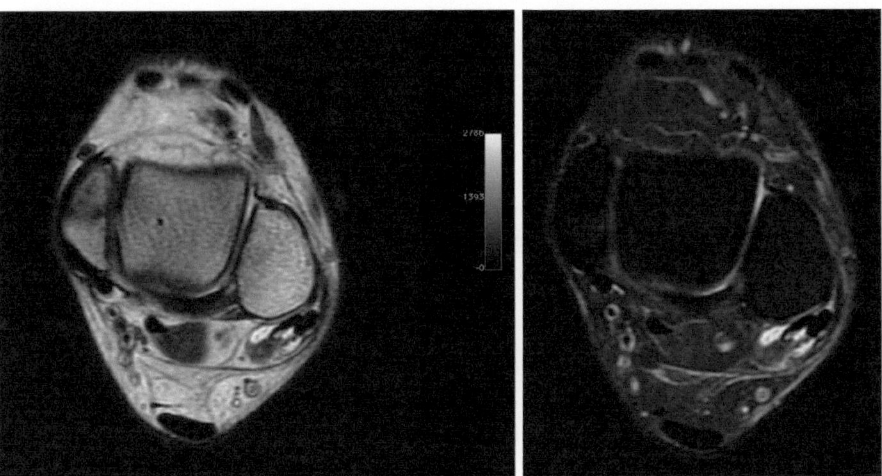

Fig. 6.3 Compatible findings with tear of the peroneus brevis tendon, tenosynovitis, and dissection by synovial liquid of the superior peroneal retinaculum in the fibula, suggesting instability of the peroneal tendons

findings in cases with tears of the peroneal longus tendon include an increased signal inside the tendon in a linear or circular shape, a synovial sheath with excessive fluid, bone edema in the lateral wall of the calcaneal, or hypertrophy of the peroneal trochlea [72, 73]. Additionally, loss of homogeneity can be seen on MRI, with discontinuity of the tendon or with fracture and/or an increase of intensity of the signal in the os peroneum [60].

Treatment

Conservative Treatment

Despite the fact that conservative treatment in patients with chronic peroneal tendon injuries has shown a failure rate of up to 50%, particularly in peroneal tendon instability [16, 74].

Several conditions should be taken into consideration: chronicity of the injury, the moment of the injury, associated clinical findings, level of activity, and patients' expectations [75]. Conservative treatment includes nonsteroidal anti-inflammatory drugs (NSAIDs), ice, compression, physiotherapy with stretching, strengthening and proprioception exercises, modification of the activity, and variable methods of immobilization. In refractory cases, rigid ankle braces and/or orthotics with ankle mobility restriction (CAM-boot) can be used.

Injections with NSAIDs or corticosteroids inside the synovial sheath of the tendon can be diagnostic and therapeutic. However, infiltration with corticosteroids should be limited to avoid iatrogenic tears of the peroneal tendons [37, 41].

Surgical Treatment

Pain persisting after a prolonged conservative treatment after a minimum of 3 months and imaging study evidence of tendinopathy of the peroneal tendons are indications of surgical management [21, 38, 41].

Tendinopathy

Surgical treatment implies debridement of the affected tendon, and tenosynovectomy can be performed with open or endoscopic procedures. For the open procedure, a lateral incision is made, starting 1 cm back from the tip of the fibula and extends to distal following the course of the peroneal tendons until 1 cm proximal to the base of the fifth metatarsal. During this approach, special care should be taken not to damage the sural nerve, of which is located in the retromalleolar zone between the lateral malleolus and the Achilles tendon. The synovial sheath of the peroneal tendons is opened longitudinally, and each tendon is inspected if there is evidence of erythema, attenuation, synovitis, and/or granulatory tissue that must be debrided. The peroneus longus tendon should be explored distally up to the cuboid groove. If it is evident, a peroneal quartus tendon or a peroneal brevis of low insertion must be resected (Fig. 6.4).

Associated split tears must be repaired firstly with the tubularization technique; however, it is reported that tears of 30% or less of the thickness of the tendon are resected since they correspond to areas of tendinosis [76]. The authors prefer to resect the affected segment and not to tubularize the remaining to maintain an adequate excursion of the tendon. The postoperative management includes a period of brief initial immobilization with the foot in plantar flexion and eversion, which will allow for the correct healing of the peroneal tendons.

Indication for tendoscopy in the peroneal tendons is pain caused by an inflammatory process related with the peroneal and their synovial sheath [4, 5]. The tenosynovitis of the peroneal tendons is often associated with recurring sprains of the ankle or chronic lateral instability of the ankle [60]. As the peroneal muscles act as lateral stabilizers of the ankle as greater stress falls on them in cases of recurring sprains, microinstability or greater chronic instability resulting in tenosynovitis (Fig. 6.5).

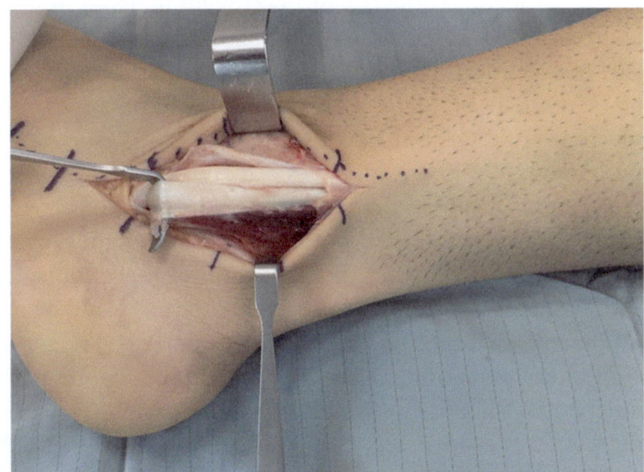

Fig. 6.4 Lateral approach for accessing the peroneal tendons. Identifies a muscle belly of low insertion in the peroneus brevis tendon, which should be resected

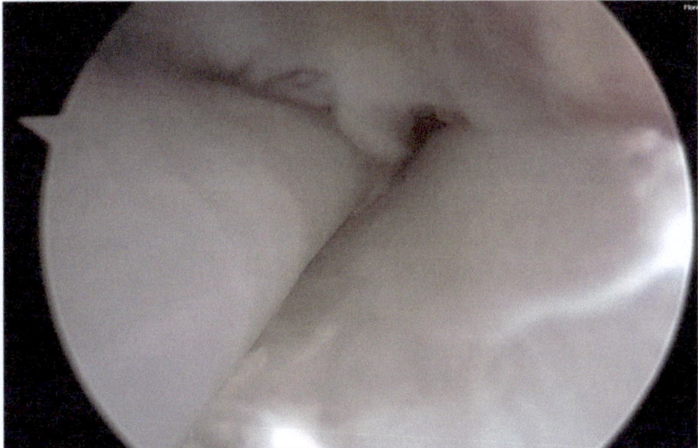

Fig. 6.5 Tendoscopy of the peroneal tendons. A tenosynovitis of both tendons can be observed, without evidence of tears. The mechanical debridement of the synovitis is performed through the middle portal

Instability

Incompetent Superior Peroneal Retinaculum

In these patients, incompetence of the superior peroneal retinaculum determines that the peroneal tendons are dislocated outside of the retromalleolar groove. Surgical treatment is usually indicated in young patients and athletes that have presented acute episodes or recurrences of subluxation [77]. Many surgical procedures have been described, including (1) anatomical reconstruction of the retinaculum, (2) bone-block technique, (3) reinforcement of the superior peroneal retinaculum with transference of adjacent soft tissue, and (4) deepening of the retromalleolar groove [58]. Independently from the selected procedure, all associated pathologic findings with debridement of the low muscle belly of the peroneal brevis or the presence of a peroneus quartus should be addressed. The anatomical reinsertion of the superior peroneal retinaculum is the procedure of choice in acute injuries, since it allows to primarily return the containment of the peroneal tendons [58].

The procedure consists of making an incision in line with the peroneal tendons approximately at 6 cm proximal and 2 cm distal to the tip of the fibula. The superior peroneal retinaculum is elevated from the posterolateral aspect of the fibula, and a rongeur is utilized to expose cancellous bone for healing. Three drill holes in the posterolateral border of the fibula are performed to reinsert the retinaculum with transosseous suture. Alternatively, suture anchors can used into the posterolateral border of the fibula to reinsert the retinaculum. Non-reabsorbable, high-resistance sutures are used to approximate the superior peroneal retinaculum to the bone [78, 79]. Adachi et al. [79] did not report episodes of subluxation with this technique after a follow-up period of 3 years, and Maffuli et al. [78] reported that all patients returned to their previous activity levels. In general, the authors concomitantly perform a groove deepening procedure as described by Anderson [80], independently of the peroneal groove morphology. Recently most authors are moving out from groove deepening procedures into retinaculum tightening with similar good results and apparently less pain and recovery time. This approach is based in studies showing that there is no relation between groove shape and peroneal tendon dislocation [81]. Kelly et al. [82] originally described the bone-block technique that consists of a sagittal osteotomy of the distal fibula, followed by a posterior displacement of this lateral fragment that serves as a mechanical block to the subluxation of the peroneal tendons. Nonunion, tendon irritation, and adherence to the subjacent bony fragment are reasons not to consider this modality the treatment of choice.

Patients that present with recurrent subluxation of the peroneal tendons frequently are associated to insufficiency or attenuation of the superior peroneal retinaculum. Many types of tissue transfer have been described, including the plantaris tendon and the peroneus brevis tendon to reinforce the superior peroneal retinaculum [60, 79].

Deepening of the retromalleolar groove is another procedure used for the treatment of the recurrent dislocation of the peroneal tendons. Open techniques can be done by impaction of the posterior fibular after elevating the peroneal tendons, and an osteotomy of the posterior fibular wall is performed maintaining a hinge on medial side. Cancellous bone is removed until a 5 mm deepening is reached, and the osseous flap is reduced and impacted. The peroneal tendons are reduced, and the superior peroneal retinaculum is repaired [60, 78].

The endoscopic deepening of the peroneal groove is a noninvasive procedure to address chronic subluxation of the peroneal tendons [5, 83]. Under endoscopic control, the groove is easily deepened with the use of a burr [83]. In those cases in which there exists a concave surface of the peroneal groove, the endoscopic reparation of the superior peroneal retinaculum will be indicated, as described by Lui et al. [84].

Competent Superior Peroneal Retinaculum: Intrasheath Dislocation

In this subgroup an injury of the superior peroneal retinaculum is not observed, and the patients describe pain in the retromalleolar zone without clinically dislocation. This clinical entity includes a flat or convex peroneal groove and/or the added presence of an anatomical structure occupying the space that includes a low muscle belly of the peroneus brevis or a peroneus quartus [78, 85, 86]. The surgical treatment through endoscopic or open approach includes the resection of the occupying added structures of evident space, and in those patients without structure occupying space, deepening of the peroneal groove can solve the subluxations [5, 86].

Tears

Sobet et al. [6] classified tears of the peroneus brevis tendon by severity: (I) widening of the tendon, (II) tears of partial thickness < 1 cm of diameter, (III) complete tear of thickness of 1–2 cm of diameter, and (IV) complete tear of thickness > 2 cm of diameter. Then Krause and Brodsky [47] designed an alternative classification to guide surgical management according to the area of cross section of the viable tendon: (I) compromise of the tendon <50% and (II) compromise of the tendon >50%. Likewise, tears compromising <50% of the cross section area should be treated with excision of the affected area and tubularization of the remaining tendon. If the normal anatomical shape of the peroneus brevis tendon is flat, tubularization should not be indicated. Those tears that compromise >50% should be treated with tenodesis to the peroneus longus tendon.

Despite a low incidence of tears of the peroneal tendons, repairing and debridement and tubularization of the tendon have been proposed as the best option for treatment [44, 45, 73]. However, although the evidence available comprises of a series of cases [35, 49, 70, 87], expert opinions [14, 88], or case reports [89], it has not been demonstrated that the normal biomechanics of the ankle and foot are restored with these surgeries. The problem that arises with these pioneer studies is that there were no established guidelines of what can be considered a remnant of adequate and viable, susceptible to repair. Tenodesis of a severely damaged peroneal tendon to the adjacent tendon or even transfer to the cuboid or calcaneus has been reported as a salvage option for the tears of the peroneus longus tendon [90] and for the tears of the peroneus brevis tendon [35].

Although tenodesis is a relatively simple surgical procedure and less demanding from technical point of view, there are still questions about its functional results. It is estimated that at least 50% of the patients who submitted to this surgical technique were not able to resume their previous levels of activity, while approximately two-thirds reported pain related with the activity [47].

To preserve the continuity of the muscle-tendon unit, Mook et al. [88] described bridging the defect with an intercalary segment of allograft tendon. In each case, the allograft was integrated into the distal end of the native tendon with a Pulvertaft type suture, or in case of distal end inadequately fusing, it is sutured with anchors of 3.5 mm at the base of the fifth metatarsal. After appropriately adjusting the tension of the muscle-tendon unit, another Pulvertaft suture is used to integrate the proximal segment of the allograft in the healthy remnant of the native tendon.

Tears of both peroneal tendons have been rarely documented, and the great majority of studies correspond to case studies [24, 49] or small retrospective series [34, 87, 91, 92]. And the presence of irreparable tears of both tendons is even rarer; consequently, its treatment is controversial.

Another valid alternative for reconstructing irreparable tears of both peroneal tendons is tendon transfer. Borton et al. [55] initially described the transference of the flexor digitorum longus tendon (FDL) as a method of reconstruction for concomitant irreparable tears of the peroneal tendons. Redfern and Myerson [34] subsequently reported the use of FDL transference in four patients with type IIIa concomitant tears. In a series of seven patients with chronic tears and both irreparable tendons, Wapner et al. [91] reported good results with the use of a Hunter Bar and then a transference of the flexor hallucis longus (FHL), as a procedure of salvage in two stages.

Tendoscopy treatment of peroneal tendon tears is possible for the majority of patients when tendon tear is localized in the retromalleolar zone. On the other hand, when the diagnosis for peroneal tendon tears is not possible through means of image, tendoscopy of the peroneal is indicated as diagnosis [2–5].

The endoscopic debridement in partial tendon tears is possible in all zones. The possibility of endoscopic resection of the smallest tendinous lip must be considered in those split-type complete longitudinal tears [11]. However, the reparation and endoscopic suture in total or partial longitudinal tears is a technically possible procedure in the retromalleolar zone, but not in other zones where an open or mini-open procedure is suggested [5].

In some cases of peroneal tendon tears, some additional tendoscopic techniques such as the deepening of the peroneal groove or the resection of a low muscle belly of a peroneus quartus can be carried out.

Literature Review

Mercer et al. performed a systematic review conducted according to PRISMA (Preferred Reporting Items for Systematic Reviews and Meta-Analyses) guidelines on MEDLINE, EMBASE, and The Cochrane Library databases in August 2020 with combination of search terms of peroneal tendon *or* peroneal tear *or* peroneal tendon tear [93]. As a result of the search findings, nine articles evaluating a total of 336 patients were included in this systematic review with six articles being retrospective studies and three being case series. The systematic review demonstrated improvement in functional outcomes (AOFAS, FAAM, VAS, SF, LEFS, and SMFA scores) after surgical treatment intervention for peroneal tendon tears, which showed significant improvement from baseline for each surgical intervention consisting of primary repair with and without tenodesis, FDL/FHL tendon transfer, and allograft reconstruction, and no statistical significance was identified between each surgical treatment modality [93]. The systematic review found that overall the most common concomitant pathologies found during arthroscopic evaluation were peroneal synovitis and lateral ankle instability, and the complication rate for patients who underwent primary repair without tenodesis was associated with a higher rate of complications [93].

Conclusion

Disorders of the peroneal tendons are infrequent but at the same time underdiagnosed as pain and lateral dysfunction of the ankle. For the correct diagnosis, a detailed clinical history should be performed as a complete physical exam, as well as understanding the mechanisms of injury and the anatomical variants that can predispose to said injury. MRI is the gold standard for the evaluation of the pathology of the peroneal tendons. Dynamic MRI is a new available and useful option. Although there exists diverse alternative of surgical treatment, there does not exist sufficient evidence to recommend one treatment over the other in irreparable tears of the peroneal tendons. The tenodesis is an easy and reproducible procedure that should be reserved for patients with less functional demand. The reconstruction with allograft should be reserved for those patients with higher demand that preserves muscular excursion and maintains the functional muscle-tendon unit. In the presence of irreparable tears of both peroneal tendons without muscular excursion, a tendon transfer should be considered as a salvage procedure (Fig. 6.6).

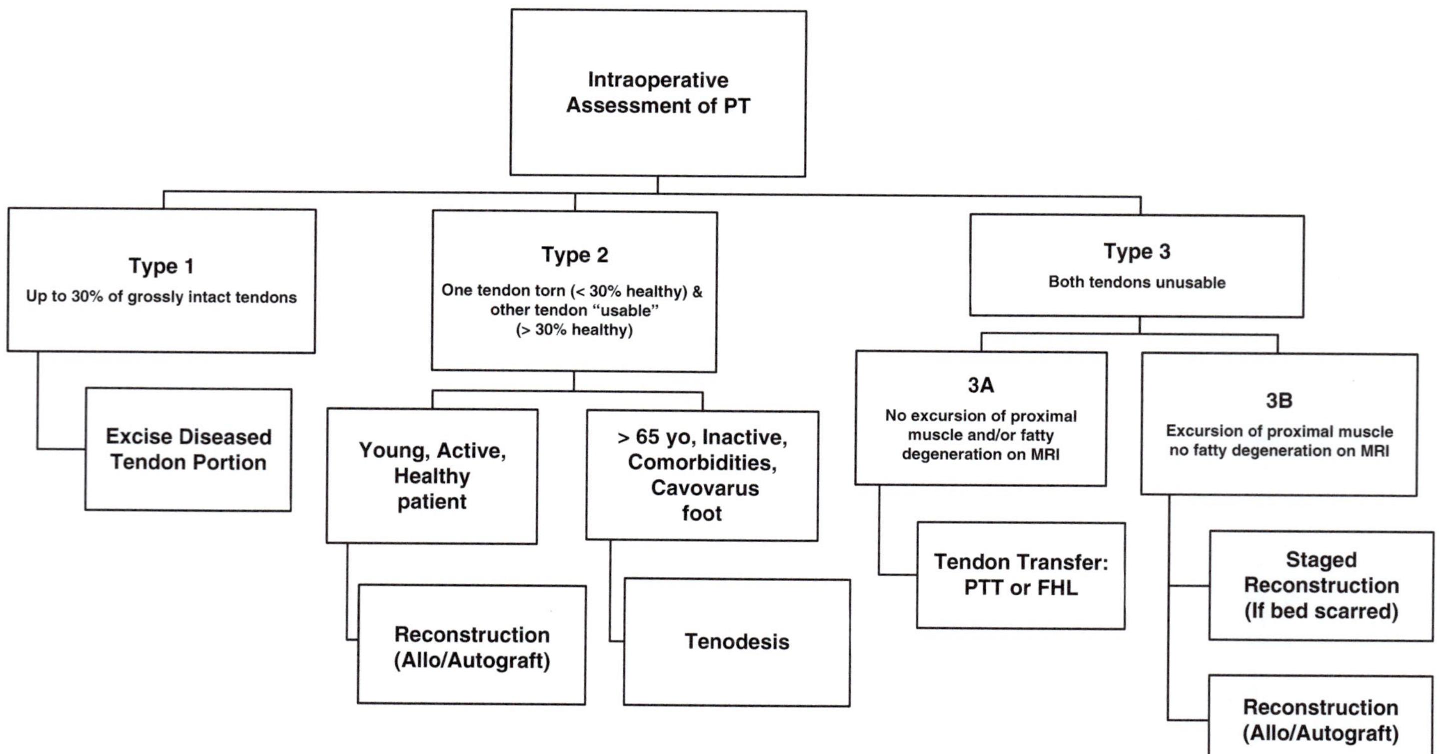

Fig. 6.6 Treatment algorithm recommended by the authors for peroneal tendon disorders

References

1. Demetracopoulos CA, Vineyard JC, Kiesau CD, Nunley JA. Long-term results of debridement and primary repair of peroneal tendon tears. Foot Ankle Int. 2014;35(3):252–7.
2. van Dijk CN, Kort N. Tendoscopy of the peroneal tendons. Arthroscopy. 1998;14:471–8.
3. Lui TH. Arthroscopy and endoscopy of the foot and ankle: indications for new techniques. Arthroscopy. 2007;23:889–902.
4. Panchbhavi VK, Trevino SG. The technique of peroneal tendoscopy and its role in management of peroneal tendón anomalies. Tech Foot Ankle Surg. 2003;2:192–8.
5. Vega J, Golanó P, Batista JP, Malagelada F, Pellegrino A. Tendoscopic procedure associated with peroneal tendons. Tech Foot Ankle. 2013;12:39–48.
6. Freccero DM, Berkowitz MJ. The relationship between tears of the peroneus brevis tendon and the distal extent of its muscle belly: an MRI study. Foot Ankle Int. 2006;27:236–9.
7. Lamm BM, Myers DT, Dombek M, Mendicino RW, Catanzariti AR, Saltrick K. Magnetic resonance imaging and surgical correlation of peroneus brevis tears. J Foot Ankle Surg. 2004;43:30–6.
8. Cheung YY, Rosenberg ZS, Ramsinghani R, Beltran J, Jahss MH. Peroneus quartus muscle: MR imaging features. Radiology. 1997;202:745–50.
9. Sobel M, Levy ME, Bohne WH. Congenital variations of the peroneus quartus muscle: an anatomic study. Foot Ankle. 1990;11:81–9. Erratum in: Foot Ankle. 1991;11:342.
10. Zammit J, Singh D. The peroneus quartus muscle. Anatomy and clinical relevance. J Bone Joint Surg Br. 2003;85:1134–7.
11. Molloy R, Tisdel C. Failed treatment of peroneal tendon injuries. Foot Ankle Clin. 2003;8:115–29. ix
12. Brage ME, Hansen ST Jr. Traumatic subluxation/dislocation of the peroneal tendons. Foot Ankle. 1992;13:423–31.
13. Roster B, Michelier P, Giza E. Peroneal tendon disorders. Clin Sports Med. 2015;34(4):625–41.
14. Edwards ME. The relations of the peroneal tendons to the fibula, calcaneus, and cuboideum. Am J Anat. 1928;42:213–53.
15. Kumai T, Benjamin M. The histological structure of the malleolar groove of the fibula in man: its direct bearing on the displacement of peroneal tendons and their surgical repair. J Anat. 2003;203:257–62.
16. Eckert WR, Davis EA Jr. Acute rupture of the peroneal retinaculum. J Bone Joint Surg Am. 1976;58:670–2.
17. Sobel M, Geppert MJ, Olson EJ, Bohne WH, Arnoczky SP. The dynamics of peroneus brevis tendon splits: a proposed mechanism, technique of diagnosis, and classification of injury. Foot Ankle. 1992;13(7):413–22.
18. Adachi N, Fukuhara K, Kobayashi T, et al. Morphologic variations of the fibular malleolar groove with recurrent dislocation of the peroneal tendons. Foot Ankle Int. 2009;30(6):540–4.
19. Davis WH, Sobel M, Deland J, Bohne WH, Patel MB. The superior peroneal retinaculum: an anatomic study. Foot Ankle Int. 1994;15:271–5.
20. Anatomical Society. Collective investigations, sesamoids in the gastrocnemius and peroneus longus. J Anat Physiol. 1897;32:182–6.
21. Sobel M, Pavlov H, Geppert MJ, Thompson FM, DiCarlo EF, Davis WH. Painful os peroneum syndrome: a spectrum of conditions responsible for plantar lateral foot pain. Foot Ankle Int. 1994;15:112–24.
22. Burman M. Stenosing tendovaginitis of the foot and ankle. Arch Surg. 1953;67:686–98.
23. Sobel M, Geppert MJ, Warren RF. Chronic ankle instability as a cause of peroneal tendon injury. Clin Orthop Relat Res. 1993;296:187–91.
24. Wind WM, Rohrbacher BJ. Peroneus longus and brevis rupture in a collegiate athlete. Foot Ankle Int. 2001;22:140–3.
25. Petersen W, Bobka T, Stein V, Tillmann B. Blood supply of the peroneal tendons: injection and immunohistochemical studies of cadaver tendons. Acta Orthop Scand. 2000;71:168–74.

26. Sobel M, Geppert MJ, Hannafin JA, Bohne WH, Arnoczky SP. Microvascular anatomy of the peroneal tendons. Foot Ankle. 1992;13:469–72.
27. van Dijk PA, Madirolas FX, Carrera A, Kerkhoffs GM, Reina F. Peroneal tendons well vascularized: results from a cadaveric study. Knee Surg Sports Traumatol Arthrosc. 2016;24(4):1140–7.
28. Maffulli N, Longo U, Loppini M, Spiezia F, Denaro V. New options in the management of tendinophaty. Open Access J Sports Med. 2010;1:29–37.
29. Abraham E, Stirnaman JE. Neglected rupture of the peroneal tendons causing recurrent sprains of the ankle. Case report. J Bone Joint Surg Am. 1979;61:1247–8.
30. Bonnin M, Tavernier T, Bouysset M. Split lesions of the peroneus brevis tendon in chronic ankle laxity. Am J Sports Med. 1997;25:699–703.
31. Karlsson J, Brandsson S, Kalebo P, Eriksson BI. Surgical treatment of concomitant chronic ankle instability and longitudinal rupture of the peroneus brevis tendon. Scand J Med Sci Sports. 1998;8:42–9.
32. Rosenberg ZS, Feldman F, Singson RD. Peroneal tendon injuries: CT analysis. Radiology. 1986;161:743–8.
33. Gray JM, Alpar EK. Peroneal tenosynovitis following ankle sprains. Injury. 2001;32:487–9.
34. Redfern D, Myerson M. The management of concomitant tears of the peroneus longus and brevis tendons. Foot Ankle Int. 2004;25:695–707.
35. Dombek MF, Lamm BM, Saltrick K, Mendicino RW, Catanzariti AR. Peroneal tendon tears: a retrospective review. J Foot Ankle Surg. 2003;42:250–8.
36. Alanen J, Orava S, Heinonen OJ, Ikonen J, Kvist M. Peroneal tendon injuries. Report of thirty-eight operated cases. Ann Chir Gynaecol. 2001;90(1):43–6.
37. Philbin T, Landis G, Smith B. Peroneal tendon injuries. J Am Acad Orthop Surg. 2009;17:306–17.
38. Bruce WD, Christofersen MR, Phillips DL. Stenosing tenosynovitis and impingement of the peroneal tendons associated with hypertrophy of the peroneal tubercle. Foot Ankle Int. 1999;20:464–7.
39. Boles MA, Lomasney LM, Demos TC, Sage RA. Enlarged peroneal process with peroneus longus tendon entrapment. Skelet Radiol. 1997;26:313–5.
40. Pierson JL, Inglis AE. Stenosing tenosynovitis of the peroneus longus tendon associated with hypertrophy of the peroneal tubercle and an os peroneum. A case report. J Bone Joint Surg Am. 1992;74:440–2.
41. Taki K, Yamazaki S, Majima T, Ohura H, Minami A. Bilateral stenosing tenosynovitis of the peroneus longus tendon associated with hypertrophied peroneal tubercle in a junior soccer player: a case report. Foot Ankle Int. 2007;28:129–32.
42. Brandes CB, Smith RW. Characterization of patients with primary peroneus longus tendinopathy: a review of twenty-two cases. Foot Ankle Int. 2000;21:462–8.
43. DiGiovanni BF, Fraga CJ, Cohen BE, et al. Associated injuries found in chronic lateral ankle instability. Foot Ankle Int. 2000;21(10):809–15.
44. Bassett FH 3rd, Speer KP. Longitudinal rupture of the peroneal tendons. Am J Sports Med. 1993;21:354–7.
45. Munk RL, Davis PH. Longitudinal rupture of the peroneus brevis tendon. J Trauma. 1976;16:803–6.
46. Cerrato RA, Myerson MS. Peroneal tendon tears, surgical management and its complications. Foot Ankle Clin. 2009;14(2):299–312.
47. Krause JO, Brodsky JW. Peroneus brevis tendon tears: pathophysiology, surgical reconstruction, and clinical results. Foot Ankle Int. 1998;19(5):271–9.
48. Sammarco GJ. Peroneal tendon injuries. Orthop Clin North Am. 1994;25:135–45.
49. Pelet S, Saglini M, Garofalo R, Wettstein M, Mouhsine E. Traumatic rupture of both peroneal longus and brevis tendons. Foot Ankle Int. 2003;24:721–3.
50. Hyer CF, Dawson JM, Philbin TM, Berlet GC, Lee TH. The peroneal tubercle: description, classification, and relevance to peroneus longus tendon pathology. Foot Ankle Int. 2005;26:947–50.

51. Grant TH, Kelikian AS, Jereb SE, McCarthy RJ. Ultrasound diagnosis of peroneal tendon tears. A surgical correlation. J Bone Joint Surg Am. 2005;87:1788–94.
52. Tehranzadeh J, Stoll DA, Gabriele OM. Case report 271. Posterior migration of the os peroneum of the left foot, indicating a tear of the peroneal tendon. Skelet Radiol. 1984;12:44–7.
53. Peacock KC, Resnick EJ, Thoder JJ. Fracture of the os peroneum with rupture of the peroneus longus tendon. A case report and review of the literature. Clin Orthop Relat Res. 1986;202:223–6.
54. Bianchi S, Abdelwahab IF, Tegaldo G. Fracture and posterior dislocation of the os peroneum associated with rupture of the peroneus longus tendon. Can Assoc Radiol J. 1991;42:340–4.
55. Borton DC, Lucas P, Jomha NM, et al. Operative reconstruction after transverse rupture of the tendons of both peroneus longus and brevis. Surgical reconstruction by transfer of the flexor digitorum longus tendon. J Bone Joint Surg Br. 1998;80(5):781–4.
56. Safran MR, O'Malley D Jr, Fu FH. Peroneal tendon subluxation in athletes: new exam technique, case reports, and review. Med Sci Sports Exerc. 1999;31(7 Suppl):S487–92.
57. Zoellner G, Clancy W Jr. Recurrent dislocation of the peroneal tendon. J Bone Joint Surg Am. 1979;61:292–4.
58. Maffulli N, Ferran NA, Oliva F, Testa V. Recurrent subluxation of the peroneal tendons. Am J Sports Med. 2006;34:986–92.
59. Geppert MJ, Sobel M, Bohne WH. Lateral ankle instability as a cause of superior peroneal retinacular laxity: an anatomic and biomechanical study of cadaveric feet. Foot Ankle. 1993;14:330–4.
60. Selmani E, Gjata V, Gjika E. Current concepts review: peroneal tendon disorders. Foot Ankle Int. 2006;27:221–8.
61. Purnell ML, Drummond DS, Engber WD, Breed AL. Congenital dislocation of the peroneal tendons in the calcaneovalgus foot. J Bone Joint Surg Br. 1983;65:316–9.
62. Altchek DW, DiGiovanni CW, Dines JS, et al. Foot and ankle sports medicine. Philadelphia: LippinCott Williams & Wilkins; 2013.
63. Rosenberg ZS, Feldman F, Singson RD, Price GJ. Peroneal tendon injury associated with calcaneal fractures: CT findings. AJR Am J Roentgenol. 1987;149:125–9.
64. Truong DT, Dussault RG, Kaplan PA. Fracture of the os peroneum and rupture of the peroneus longus tendon as a complication of diabetic neuropathy. Skelet Radiol. 1995;24:626–8.
65. Sharma P, Maffulli N. Tendon injury and tendinopathy: healing and repair. J Bone Joint Surg Am. 2005;87:187–202.
66. Church CC. Radiographic diagnosis of acute peroneal tendon dislocation. AJR Am J Roentgenol. 1977;129:1065–8.
67. Mitchell M, Sartoris DJ. Magnetic resonance imaging of the foot and ankle: an updated pictorial review. J Foot Ankle Surg. 1993;32:311–42.
68. Major NM, Helms CA, Fritz RC, Speer KP. The MR imaging appearance of longitudinal split tears of the peroneus brevis tendon. Foot Ankle Int. 2000;21:514–9.
69. Wang XT, Rosenberg ZS, Mechlin MB, Schweitzer ME. Normal variants and diseases of the peroneal tendons and superior peroneal retinaculum: MR imaging features. Radiographics. 2005;25:587–602. Erratum in: Radiographics. 2005;25:1436. Radiographics. 2006;26:640
70. Squires N, Myerson MS, Gamba C. Surgical treatment of peroneal tendon tears. Foot Ankle Clin. 2007;12(4):675–95. vii
71. Lee SJ, Jacobson JA, Kim SM, et al. Ultrasound and MRI of the peroneal tendons and associated pathology. Skelet Radiol. 2013;42(9):1191–200.
72. Rademaker J, Rosenberg ZS, Delfaut EM, Cheung YY, Schweitzer ME. Tear of the peroneus longus tendon: MR imaging features in nine patients. Radiology. 2000;214:700–4.
73. Khoury NJ, el-Khoury GY, Saltzman CL, Kathol MH. Peroneus longus and brevis tendon tears: MR imaging evaluation. Radiology. 1996;200:833–41.
74. Stover CN, Bryan DR. Traumatic dislocation of the peroneal tendons. Am J Surg. 1962;103:180–6.

75. Chiodo CP. Acute and chronic tendon injury. In: Richardson EG, editor. Orthopaedic knowledge update: foot and ankle 3. Rosemont, IL: American Academy of Orthopaedic Surgeons; 2003. p. 81–9.

76. Roser B, Michelier P, Giza E. Peroneal tendon disorders. Clin Sports Med. 2015;34(4):625–41.

77. Porter D, McCarroll J, Knapp E, Torma J. Peroneal tendon subluxation in athletes: fibular groove deepening and retinacular reconstruction. Foot Ankle Int. 2005;26:436–41.

78. Raikin SM, Elias I, Nazarian LN. Intrasheath subluxation of the peroneal tendons. J Bone Joint Surg Am. 2008;90:992–9.

79. Adachi N, Fukuhara K, Tanaka H, Nakasa T, Ochi M. Superior retinaculoplasty for recurrent dislocation of peroneal tendons. Foot Ankle Int. 2006;27:1074–8.

80. Anderson R, Shawen S. Indirect groove deepening in the management of chronic peroneal tendon dislocation. Tech Foot Ankle Surg. 2004;3(2):118–25.

81. Title CI, Jung HG, Parks BG, Schon LC. The peroneal groove deepening procedure: a biomechanical study of pressure reduction. Foot Ankle Int. 2005;26:442–8.

82. Kelly RE. An operation for the chronic dislocation of the peroneal tendons. Br J Surg. 1920;7:502–4.

83. Vega J, Batista JP, Golanó P, Dalmau A, Viladot R. Tendoscopic groove deepening for chronic subluxation of the peroneal tendons. Foot Ankle Int. 2013;34:832–40.

84. Lui TH. Endoscopic peroneal retinaculum reconstruction. Knee Surg Sports Traumatol Arthrosc. 2006;14:478–81.

85. Thomas JL, Lopez-Ben R, Maddox J. A preliminary report on intrasheath peroneal tendón subluxation: a prospective review of 7 patients with ultrasound verification. J Foot Ankle Surg. 2009;48:323–9.

86. Vega J, Golanó P, Dalmau A, Viladot R. Tendoscopic treatment of intrasheath subluxation of the peroneal tendons. Foot Ankle Int. 2011;32:1147–51.

87. Kollias SL, Ferkel RD. Fibular grooving for recurrent peroneal tendon subluxation. Am J Sports Med. 1997;25:329–35.

88. Mook WR, Parekh SG, Nunley JA. Allograft reconstruction of peroneal tendons: operative technique and clinical outcomes. Foot Ankle Int. 2013;34(9):1212–20.

89. Cooper ME, Selesnick FH, Murphy BJ. Partial peroneus longus rupture in professional basketball players: a report of 2 cases. Am J Orthop. 2002;31(12):691–4.

90. Sammarco GJ. Peroneus longus tendon tears: acute and chronic. Foot Ankle Int. 1995;16:245–53.

91. Wapner KL, Taras JS, Lin SS, et al. Staged reconstruction for chronic rupture of both peroneal tendons using hunter rod and flexor hallucis longus tendon transfer: a long-term followup study. Foot Ankle Int. 2006;27(8):591–7.

92. Saxena A, Cassidy A. Peroneal tendon injuries: an evaluation of 49 tears in 41 patients. J Foot Ankle Surg. 2003;42(4):215–20.

93. Mercer NP, Gianakos AL, Mercurio AM, Kennedy JG. Clinical outcomes of Peroneal tendon tears: a systematic review. J Foot Ankle Surg. 2021;60(5):1008–13. https://doi.org/10.1053/j.jfas.2021.03.003.

Posterior Tibial Tendon Injuries

7

Michael F. Levidy, Lea Bach, Nicholas Genovese, Adam Weiner, and Sheldon S. Lin

Anatomy/Biomechanics

The posterior tibial tendon (PTT) is continuous with the posterior tibial muscle. The muscle originates from the proximal third of the tibia and interosseous membrane in the deep compartment of the calf (see Fig. 7.1). The PTT lies posterior to the medial malleolus, coursing posterior to the axis of the ankle and medial to the axis of the subtalar joint. The tendon then continues distally toward the medial side of the navicular and splits to form attachments to the navicular tuberosity and the plantar aspects of the medial cuneiform and second–fourth metatarsals.

The anatomy of the PTT demonstrates its function: elevation and maintenance of the medial longitudinal arch of the foot. Loss of this function helps explain a common presentation of posterior tibial tendon dysfunction – a flattened arch with stretching and weakening of associated soft tissue structures. PTTD is also commonly associated with inability to perform a single-leg heel rise. This results from loss of a different function of the PTT, namely, inversion of the subtalar joint and the resultant "locking" of the transverse tarsal. Without this locking action, the foot lacks the rigidity required for the push of phase of gait, as well as the mechanical advantage required by the gastrocnemius-soleus complex to perform the heel rise test. The PTT is also indirectly involved in supporting the calcaneus.

Etiology/Risk Factors

PTTD has multiple direct etiologies. Typically, PTTD begins as an inflammatory synovitis related to overuse. Two areas of the tendon are particularly at risk. Proximally, this involves the first area of tendon about 1 cm distal to the medial

M. F. Levidy · L. Bach · N. Genovese · A. Weiner · S. S. Lin (✉)
Department of Orthopaedics, Rutgers New Jersey Medical School, Newark, NJ, USA
e-mail: mfl55@njms.rutgers.edu; ng503@njms.rutgers.edu; atw39@njms.rutgers.edu

© Springer Nature Switzerland AG 2022
J. D. Cain, M. V. Hogan (eds.), *Tendon and Ligament Injuries of the Foot and Ankle*,
https://doi.org/10.1007/978-3-031-10490-9_7

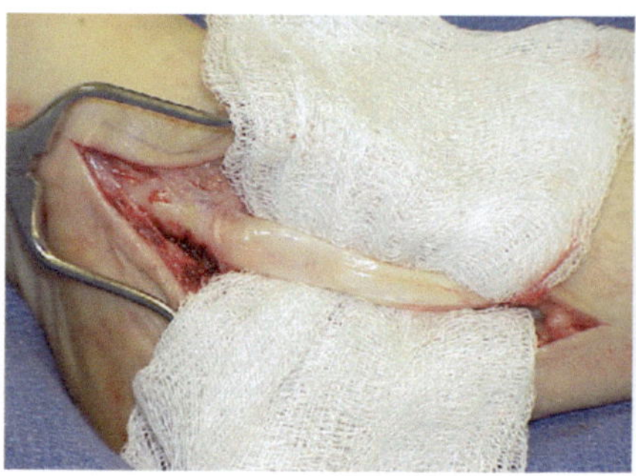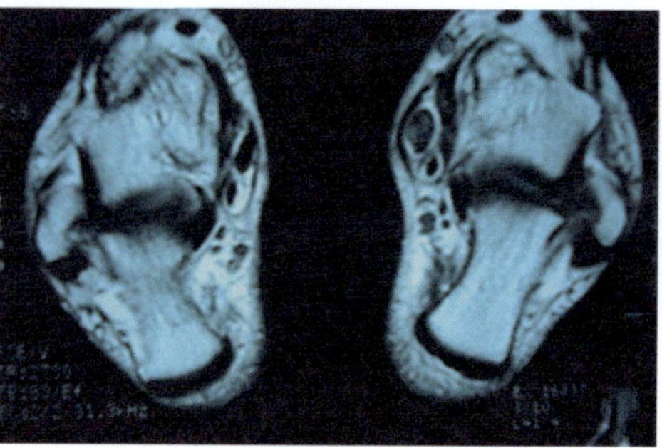

Fig. 7.1 Left: Intraoperative view of PTT showing pathology. Right: T2 weight axial section MRI showing healthy and torn PTT. Photo courtesy of Dr. Terry Philbin of the Orthopedic Foot and Ankle Center

malleolus. This phenomenon was best explained by Frey and Sherrif, who demonstrated a zone of hypovascularity 1.5 cm distal to the medial malleolus. Distal synovitis can also occur at the PTT insertion points, although it is less common. Slip 1 issues typically involve the tuberosity of the navicular, the inferior aspect of the naviculocuneiform capsule, or the medial cuneiform, while slip 2 issues involve the plantar surface of the cuneiform, cuboid, or base of the metatarsals. PTTD can rarely occur from acute trauma. Trauma cases may involve dislocation of the ankle with incarceration, untreated Lisfranc fracture-dislocations, or Charcot arthropathy. Steroids have been implicated in PTTD, too, with higher dosages being correlated with more PTTD. Structures interrupting the passage of the PTT, such as an accessory navicular or exostosis, can also play a role in PTTD by irritating the tendon itself. Very rarely, a neoplastic cause is the root of the problem, as in PVNS.

Risk factors for PTTD are numerous, but key pathognomonic among them are the "four Fs" – fat, female, over forty, and fertile. Additional factors include hypertension, obesity, diabetes, prior surgery or trauma in the area, steroids, and seronegative inflammatory disorders like ankylosing spondylitis, Reiter syndrome, and psoriasis. History takers must keep these in mind when working up a suspected PTTD case so as not to miss an underlying cause.

Diagnosis/Clinical Evaluation

History – While PTTD symptoms vary with severity of disease, patients will typically complain of medial ankle pain, fatigue, or swelling along the course of the tendon, with more diffuse pain occurring as the disease progresses. Onset is usually gradual, so patients may not be able to recall an inciting event. Symptoms are often experienced during normal daily activities like walking on uneven ground or hurrying to catch a bus. At later stages, pain may be reported on the lateral side of the ankle, too, as the calcaneus begins to impinge on the fibula. Secondary dysfunctions may also accompany later stages of disease, including equinus deformity, horizontal orientation of the subtalar joint, valgus orientation of the heel, calcaneus impingement on fibula, hallux elevatus, and Achilles contracture.

Visual – As PTTD progresses, visual signs become easier to notice. Chief among them is the progressive collapse of the medial longitudinal arch as a result of a diminished arch maintenance force from the PTTD. Loss of dynamic forces from PTT leads to stretching of the static ligaments of the medial foot. Simultaneously, subtalar eversion takes place, resulting in a loss of secondary soft tissue support from the deltoid ligament, talonavicular capsule, and spring ligament. The heel then assumes valgus positioning, and the foot abducts at the talonavicular joint, resulting in the "too-many-toes" sign. Visual examination of more severe cases may also reveal forefoot abduction from the neutral positioning observed in less severe cases, as well as fixed supination deformity. During surgery, hypertrophy of the PTT may also be noted.

Physical – Physical examination of PTTD includes the single-leg heel rise test. Patients lose the ability to perform this test as the disease progresses; thus the results are helpful in staging. Additionally, physical examination should involve testing of the various muscle groups of the lower leg, notably including the posterior tibial muscle, by asking the patient to plantarflex and invert against resistance. It is also crucial to evaluate the subtalar, ankle, and transverse tarsal joints for range of motion. As disease progresses, mobility of the subtalar joint is reduced, and again, this finding is particularly useful in staging. Finally, the Achilles should be assessed for presence of a contracture, as it is a common concomitant finding in patients with PTTD.

Radiographic – Radiographic studies typically include ankle and foot series. It is important to emphasize that radiographic studies be performed in a weight-bearing position to ensure proper alignment and joint spacing. The AP view of the foot in AAFD will show abduction of the forefoot via the transverse tarsal joint, as well as uncovering of navicular or talonavicular joint. The lateral view will show a decrease in the talometatarsal angle, which may range +10 to −10 in normal patients, but negative in PTTD patients. Lateral views may also reveal a decreased distance from the medial cuneiform floor. Typically, this distance is from 15 to 25 mm. Finally, the lateral view may also show a break in Meary's line, the lateral line from the talo-first metatarsal. MRI is not typically required to make a diagnosis and is not helpful in the planning of treatment.

Histology – Although a biopsy is not recommended, it should be noted that histology of PTTD shows degenerative changes in the tendon.

Staging

Staging of PTTD is important, as it informs treatment. The predominant classification system was that of Johnson and Strom, which only includes three stages, which has since been modified by Myerson to include a fourth stage. Still others suggest that the second stage is too generalized and would benefit from subdivision into classes IIA, IIB, and IIC. See chart below for detailed descriptions of each stage (Table 7.1).

Table 7.1 PTTD staging [1]

Stage	Tendon	Deformity	Pain	Single-heel rise test	Too-many-toes sign	Valgus/arthritis of the ankle
Stage I	Tenosynovitis, degeneration	Absent	Medial	Mild weakness, normal hindfoot inversion	No	No
Stage II	Elongation, degeneration	Flexible, reducible	Medial and/or lateral	Marked weakness or no hindfoot inversion	Yes	No
Stage III	Elongation, degeneration	Fixed, irreducible	Medial and/or lateral	Unable	Yes	No
Stage IV	Elongation, degeneration	Fixed, irreducible	Medial and/or lateral	Unable	Yes	Yes

Nonoperative Treatments by Stage

Nonsurgical interventions may be an option for patients with PTTD stage I or II while the deformity is still flexible, with its purpose being symptomatic relief through eliminating pronation and restoring the medial arch. Before initial treatments for PTTD are started, decreasing posteromedial hindfoot forces through weight loss and improvement of footwear as well as lifestyle and activity modifications are attempted. NSAIDs can be used simultaneously for pain. When lifestyle modifications do not work, patients can be fitted for a CAM walker boot or short leg cast. If symptoms are relieved, an orthotic device should be the mainstay of treatment. If symptoms worsen or persist, surgical management should be considered. There are many reasons a doctor or a patient would want to avoid surgery, particularly when there are factors such as underlying health risk or advanced age that raise the risk level. Nonoperative treatments consist of shoe inserts with medial heel and sole shoe wedge, UCBL orthotics, ankle orthoses devices, and physical therapy.

Medial Heel and Sole Shoe Wedge Insert – These shoe inserts are used to support the medial part of the foot in order to stabilize the whole foot and attempt to maintain the most optimum position possible for normal functioning. With a neutral position of the foot, symptoms of PTTD are lessened or nonexistent, making it possible to return to active hobbies.

UCBL [2] – UCBL orthotic is a rigid custom-made insert that fully encompasses the heel. It is used for controlling postural flexible deformities by maintaining a neutral position in the hindfoot by locking the tarsal joints and keeping the calcaneus in a neutral position, thus limiting forefoot abduction and pronation. The use of UCBL orthosis has been shown to be 77% successful for the conservative management of stage II PTTD based on several criteria [3]. UCBL use criteria consisted of flexible deformity, less than a 10-degree forefoot varus, and not being clinically obese.

Arizona Brace – Ankle-foot orthoses (AFO) are another type of orthotic intervention that can be used. Unlike foot orthoses which span the intrinsic joints of the foot, AFOs extend above the ankle. One such device is the Arizona AFO (see Fig. 7.2), a brace that starts proximally at the mid-shaft of the tibia and extends distally to the metatarsal heads. It is designed to minimize hindfoot valgus alignment, lateral calcaneal displacement, and ankle collapse by way of a three-point fixation. Augustin describes the boot being fitted with the calcaneus reduced to its "proper anatomic alignment underneath the tibia and talus" [4]. Augustin and colleagues found that patients that used the Arizona AFO had a 90% improvement in their symptoms based on questionnaires and physician evaluation.

Orthotic + Exercise – Physical therapy is seen to be a successful form of non-operative treatment of PTTD stages I and II. Alvarez et al. utilized a combination of orthotic and specific strengthening exercises for the peroneal, posterior and anterior tibial, and triceps surae muscles [2]. Exercises consisted of isokinetic exercises, exercise band, double- and single-support heel rises (DSHR, SSHR), and toe walking. Pain was monitored with a visual analogue scale (VAS), and functionality and strength were assessed throughout the rehabilitation process. Participants were given one of two types or orthotic devices: a short articulated ankle-foot orthosis

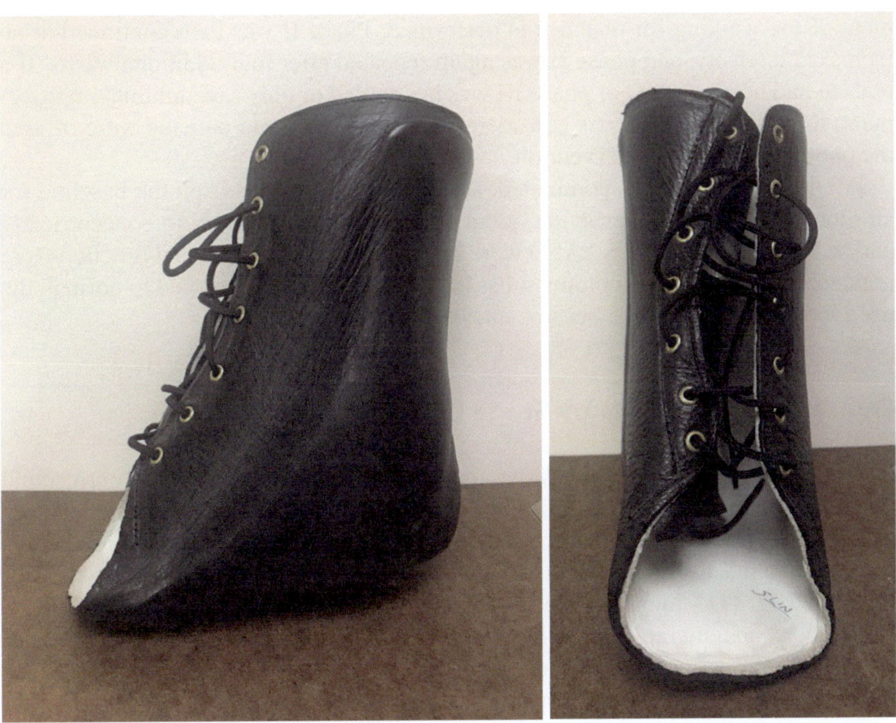

Fig. 7.2 The Arizona ankle-foot orthosis

(SAAFO) is used if there was posterior tibial tendon pain for more than 3 months or the patient could not perform a single-support heel rise or walk more than one block, and a foot orthosis (FO) was given if a patient had posterior tibial tendon pain for less than 3 months, could perform at least one SSHR, and could walk more than one block. A strength discrepancy of more than 10% between a patient's feet is considered clinically significant.

The physical rehabilitation treatment consists of a pretreatment phase followed by three treatment phases of increasing difficulty and strength. The pretreatment phase consists of seated sole-to-sole exercises, which continue until the patient can successfully do 300 with ease. Phase 1 consists of an office evaluation and institution of another home exercise program consisting of 200 repetitions of dorsiflexion, inversion, and eversion with a red exercise band, and a controlled eccentric phase without any leg rotation was required. Phase II consists of the addition of isokinetic workout. Inversion and eversion exercises of 6 degrees with gradual addition of resistance, starting at 2 pounds, were started, and it was seen how many repetitions could be done in a 20–25-min time frame and increased as tolerated. For the home exercise program, exercise band resistance was increased. Weight-bearing SSHR, working toward 50 repetitions, as well as toe walking working toward 100 yards, and Biomechanical Ankle Platform System (BAPS) (Jelaga, Inc., Jasper, MI) were started. Phase III consists of another evaluation of isokinetic strength and assessment of toe walking for distance is performed. Phase II was then continued at an increased intensity, and phase II was again repeated after four additional visits. If a plateau had been reached or phase III was not passed or only saw minimal improvement, then the treatment was considered to have failed, and patients were offered the option of operative intervention.

After the program was completed, strength was improved from the baseline for all directions (inversion, eversion, plantarflexion, dorsiflexion) both concentrically and eccentrically. FO and SAAFO were important while strength and function were regained. However, as symptoms subsided and functionality returned to normal, the need for an orthotic device became unessential.

Operative Treatments by Stage (See Table 7.2)

Operative treatment of PTTD varies, but treatment options generally correspond well to disease stage. In this section we will bring clarity to which treatment is best in each case. It is important to note that cases should be individualized, and there is no "one size fits all" approach to PTTD.

Stage I PTTD – Stage I can be treated conservatively. NSAIDs, immobilization, ice, and physical therapy are sufficient to stop progression and even reverse symptoms. For this reason, surgical procedures at this stage may be considered only after failure of nonoperative management.

Stage II PTTD – Stage II can be broken out into three substages: IIA, IIB, and IIC. Many variations of treatment options exist for this stage than in others. In stage IIA, MDCO with concurrent FDL transfer is recommended. These procedures form

Table 7.2 PTTD treatments by stage

Stage	Surgical techniques
I	N/A
IIA	Tenosynovectomy, MDCO, and FDL transfer
IIB	MDCO, FDL transfer, spring ligament repair, LCL, and/or Achilles lengthening
IIC	Similar to stages IIA and IIB with a medial column procedure such as a cotton osteotomy, Lapidus, or naviculocuneiform arthrodesis to correct forefoot supination varus
Stage III	Triple arthrodesis
Stage IV	Triple arthrodesis and/or total ankle reconstruction or TTC

the basis of all stage II surgical treatments. In stage IIB, MDCO and FDL transfer are still recommended, but so too are additional procedures that bolster overall stability and biomechanics. These include a spring ligament repair, lateral column lengthening procedure, and Achilles lengthening. Stage IIC addresses relatively dorsiflexed medial column and loss of tripod by yet another procedure to IIB, just as IIB added to IIA. In stage IIC, a medial column procedure, like Cotton osteotomy, Lapidus procedure, and/or naviculocuneiform arthrodesis, is recommended in addition to those recommended for stage IIB.

Stage III PTTD – For a rigid pes planovalgus deformity of the type seen in stage III PTTD, the subtalar and transverse tarsal joints are often arthritic and require realignment fusion-type procedure. Surgical treatment for stage III PTTD is generally confined to triple arthrodesis. Unfortunately, this surgery results in a severe limitation to ankle mobility.

Stage IV PTTD – Stage IV PTTD involves instability spreading to the ankle. It mirrors stage III surgical treatment in the use of a triple arthrodesis, but adds additional ankle reconstructions to address the ankle instability, which may include deltoid ligament reconstruction. Because of valgus ankle arthrosis, a total ankle replacement may also be indicated. Traditional concepts utilizes pantalar fusion.

Details of Major Surgical Interventions

Surgical intervention for PTTD was first described in 1893 by Gleich, who outlined a medial/plantar wedge to address medial arch flattening. Since then, a number of surgical interventions have proven themselves useful in the treatment of PTTD. In this section, we will describe those procedures and provide detail on indications, contraindications, and complications. We begin with discussion of the most common surgeries and later discuss the secondary procedures that often accompany PTT surgical treatment.

Tenosynovectomy of PTT – *After standard prepping and draping in supine position, prominences of the navicular tuberosity are identified. Skin incision is made from the navicular tuberosity proximal to the medial malleolus. Care is taken to longitudinally open the PTT sheath with inspection for any tears* *(especially at the level of medial malleolus), with possible repair and/or debridement of PTT if needed. One should also inspect the spring ligament as well as FDL tendon which is plantar to the PTT. This initial step forms the basis for other surgical procedures.*

The purpose of the tenosynovectomy is to dispose of any inflammatory tissue that may contribute to further degeneration of the PTT at a later date.

Indications/Contraindications for Tenosynovectomy – Tenosynovectomy is somewhat unique in that it forms the basis of most surgical PTTD interventions. As such, it is almost always indicated in cases where surgery is indicated. Specifically, this includes stages II and up, whenever conservative treatment attempts during that stage have failed.

Complications of tenosynovectomy can include infection and structural compromise of the tendon itself. Notably, tenosynovectomy is not always sufficient to prevent progression of disease, with many patients suffering continuing or worsening symptoms afterward. It is due to this shortcoming that the first stage of PTTD is treated conservatively instead of operatively.

FDL Transfer – FDL transfer involves attaching the flexor digitorum longus to the navicular, thus adding support to the existing PTT *(see* Fig. 7.3). *Care is taken to follow the FDA distally and harvest the FDL tendon beyond the navicular tuberosity, followed by running suture tuberlization. I used the guidewire from either 6.5 or 7.3 mm cannulated screw system from dorsal to plantar in the medial third of the navicular, followed by drill bit to create the osseous tunnel. Care must be taken not to be so medial to break the bone as a bridge. Initially, a curette is used to remove any loose bone debris. This step facilitates passage of the free harvested FDL to be transferred going from plantar to dorsal in the navicular osseous tunnel. One may secure FDL by either sewing back to itself or using a biotenodesis screw.*

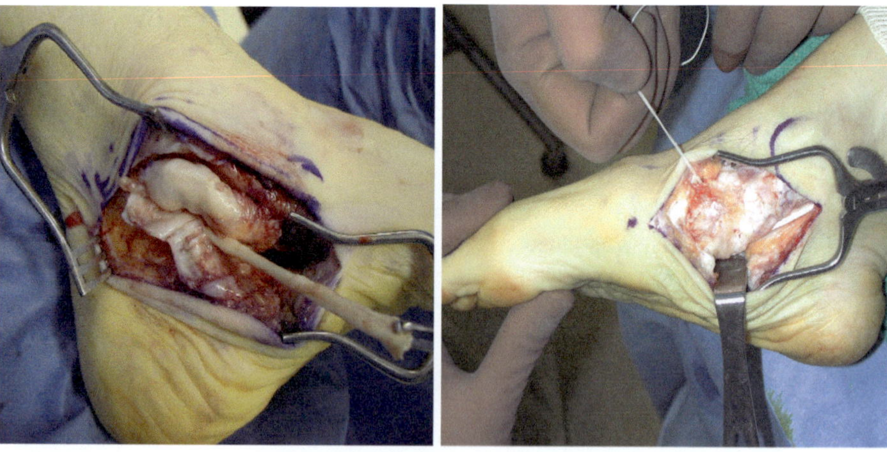

Fig. 7.3 Left: Medial view showing inflamed PTT and harvested FDL. Right: FDL transferred to the dorsum via navicular. Photo courtesy of Dr. Terry Philbin of the Orthopedic Foot and Ankle Center

Complications – FDL transfer can lead to weakness in plantarflexion of the toes, owing to the loss of FDL tension. Failure at the site of insertion is also possible, particularly when other procedures that reduce load are not also performed.

Medial Displacement Calcaneal Osteotomy – *Care is taken to use a metal wire to localize the skin incision on the lateral calcaneus. I aim to be between the posterior aspect of subtalar joint and superior tuberosity of the calcaneus. An incision is made with care to avoid the sural nerve. We placed human retractors at the dorsal and plantar aspect of calcaneus along the planned osteotomy. A small micro-sagittal saw is used to perform the calcaneal osteotomy with care to avoid plunging. I often gently place the micro-sagittal to the far cortex and finish the osteotomy of the far cortex with dull osteotome. I will place a laminar spreader and stretch the soft tissue 1 cm. Next, holding the foot, I perform a medial translation of distal calcaneus 6–10 mm relative to size of the patient. Using my thumb to maintain the medial translation on lateral distal calcaneal fragment, I will place a guidewire for either a 4.5, 6.5, or 7.3 cannulated screw to a point just plantar to subtalar joint beyond the angle of Gissane, followed by checking placement of wire using lateral and axial Harris view. We then used countersink followed by screw placement (see* Fig. 7.4*).*

Medial displacement calcaneal osteotomy (MDCO), also known as "calcaneal slide," is a technique first described by Koutsogiannis in 1971. The technique serves to shift the biomechanical axis laterally, realigning it to reduce valgus and improve

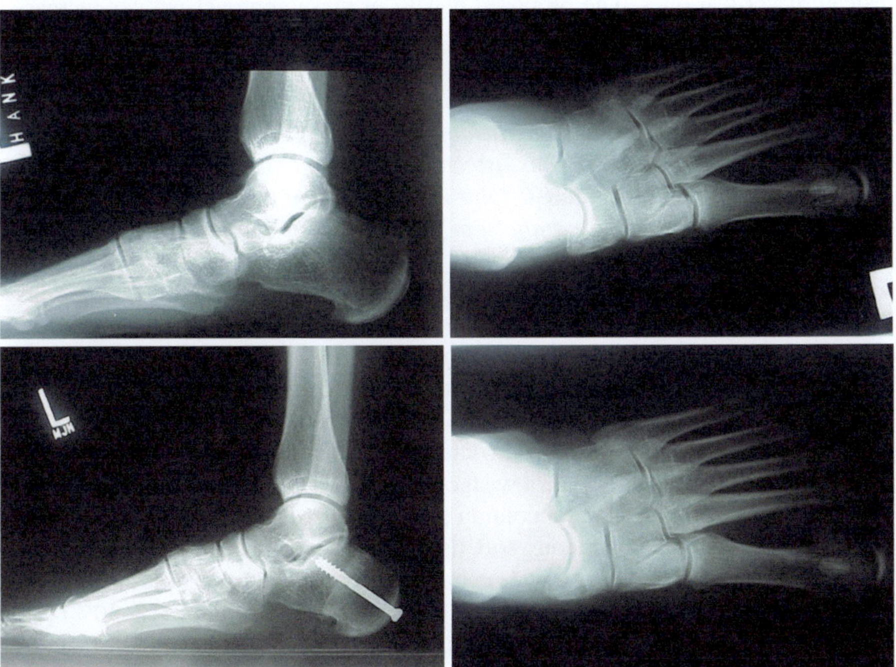

Fig. 7.4 Top row: Pre-op MDCO. Bottom row: Post-Op MDCO. Photo courtesy of Dr. Terry Philbin of the Orthopedic Foot and Ankle Center

medial arch. The MDCO also produces benefits by repositioning the Achilles tendon relative to the rest of the foot, rendering it a stronger invertor and decreasing stresses on other structures. Post-MDCO, improvement should be apparent on radiograph with an improved T-N coverage ratio. Major benefits to the MDCO approach include retention of flexibility in the foot and protection of the FDL transfer site, which permits another common surgical intervention for PTTD (the FDL transfer).

Indications/contraindications for MDCO include the following: MDCO is used when a patient has stage II PTTD and conservative approaches have failed. Its usage is more highly indicated with increased pain, hindfoot valgus, and obesity. MDCO is contraindicated in cases of fixed deformity, especially subtalar, which often precludes its use in later stages of disease. It is also not advisable in cases of severe forefoot abduction and degenerative joint disease of the subtalar joint.

Complications of MDCO include medial plantar nerve paresthesia, sural nerve neuritis, and disease progression. Overcorrection is possible, but more frequently, an issue exists with undercorrection, taking the form of persistent forefoot abduction. Postsurgical calf atrophy has been reported, but is not a common complication. Notably, nonunion of the displaced segments of the calcaneus is not a major concern (see Table 7.3).

Variants on the traditional MDCO do exist, although they are relatively recent developments, involving creating stepped, Z-shaped, or *scarf* cuts in the calcaneus instead of vertical ones. The proposed benefit of these approaches cites increased stability due to the geometry of the cut as well as increased surface area of healing of the osteotomy.

Lateral Column Lengthening – *If significant forefoot abduction still exists, options include lateral column lengthening by either an Evans calcaneal osteotomy or calcaneal cuboid fusion. Evans osteotomy is a joint sparing procedure, with a bone cut 1 cm proximal to the CC joint with placement of either tri-cortical iliac autograft, allograft wedge, or trabecular metal. I like to pin the calcaneal cuboid joint prior to placement of the distracting wedge to avoid loss of alignment of distal fragment of the calcaneus. The calcaneal cuboid fusion is a joint-sacrificing procedure performed with placement of either tri-cortical iliac autograft, allograft wedge, or trabecular metal, with either screw or plate fixation.*

Another common group of surgical interventions for PTTD is the lateral column lengthening procedures. This includes the Evans procedure, also known as an extra-articular lateral column procedure or lateral wedge procedure. As the name suggests, it involves the insertion of a wedge along the lateral longitudinal arch of the foot. The wedge provides lateral column support, corrects the talonavicular uncoverage, and prevents simultaneous soft tissue reconstructions from stretching. As with the MDCO, T-N coverage and arch both improve. These procedures are particularly attractive, thanks to the minimal loss of subtalar motion (18–30%) [10]. Another option to perform lateral column lengthening is through fusion of the calcaneocuboid joint.

Indications/Contraindications for LCL – Lateral column procedures are indicated in stage II disease, particularly in cases where correction of talonavicular

Table 7.3 Collected surgical outcomes for MDCO with FDL transfer – note the absence of nonunions

Name	Follow-up	Avg age (years)	# feet	Post-op AOFAS	Complication rate	Complications/ follow-ups required	Patient satisfaction
Wacker 2002 [5]	51 months	–	44	88.5	4.5%	4.5% CC fusion	97% good to excellent for pain and function
Fayazi 2002 [6]	35 months	56	23	89	4.3%	4.3% DVT	96% "better" or "much better" 4% "same"
Myerson 2004 [7]	62.4 months	55	129	79	9.3%	0.8% severe valgus deformity	92% entirely satisfied
						1.6% heel varus	97% had relief of pain
						2.3% sural neuritis	87% improvement of function
						0.8% calf muscle atrophy	
						3.9% median plantar nerve distribution numbness	
Schuh 2013 [8]	48 months	59.9	73	91	4.1%	1.4% hindfoot varus	N/A
						2.7% sural nerve injury	
Chadwick 2015 [9]	15.2 years	54.3	31	90.3	12.9%	6.45% CC fusion	87.1% totally satisfied
						3.2% talonavicular fusion	9.6% satisfied with reservation
						3.2% triple fusion	3.2% unsatisfied

uncoverage is desired. Evans osteotomy is contraindicated in cases with minimal forefoot hindfoot alignment, fixed pes planovalgus deformity or hypermobility, DJD or severe subtalar arthritis, and neuromuscular diseases and in the relatively obese and elderly.

Complications of Lateral Column Lengthening – Pain is often reported where the bone graft is sourced from the hip, although this is not a concern in cases where an allograft is used. The osteotomy may violate anterior and/or middle calcaneal facets, leading to arthritis and pain, and both of which are relatively common complications of the surgery. It has been postulated that the arthritis complication is the result of increased C-C joint pressure. Conflicting studies by Cooper, Momberger, and Xia show increased pressure, decreased pressure, and a decrease followed by an increase for the C-C joint, respectively [11–13]. In cases where calcaneocuboid fusion is chosen as the LCL procedure, there is a high risk of nonunion, overload, and pain, along with a slight loss of motion. Lastly, pain due to hardware is a common complication, and hardware removal surgery is often required after an Evans osteotomy (see Fig. 7.5) (see Table 7.4).

Medial Column Procedures – *Cotton procedure: A dorsal incision is made proximal at the level of the medial cuneiform or over medial column of the first tarsometatarsal joint depending upon the planned procedure. For the joint-sparing procedure, an opening wedge osteotomy of 6–10 mm is made at middle of the medial cuneiform with placement of dorsal wedge of bone with care to align the forefoot cascade and plantarflex the medial column. This is followed by fixation of the bone wedge with either screw or plate.*

Just as the lateral column can be targeted in the surgical treatment of PTTD, so too can the medial column, although it is a less common and usually reserved for more advanced forefoot supination with varus alignment to recreate the "tripod." Medial column procedures include the Lapidus procedure, naviculocuneiform arthrodesis, or a plantarflexion cuneiform osteotomy (also known as a Cotton osteotomy after the doctor who first described it in 1936) (see Fig. 7.6). In either case, the goal is to address the loss of tripod by increasing support along the medial arch of the foot. The Cotton osteotomy is particularly useful in correcting forefoot supination, while Lapidus is best suited for cases where hallux elevatus has become apparent. Lapidus procedure involves plantarflexion fusion of the proximal aspect of the first metatarsal to the medial cuneiform.

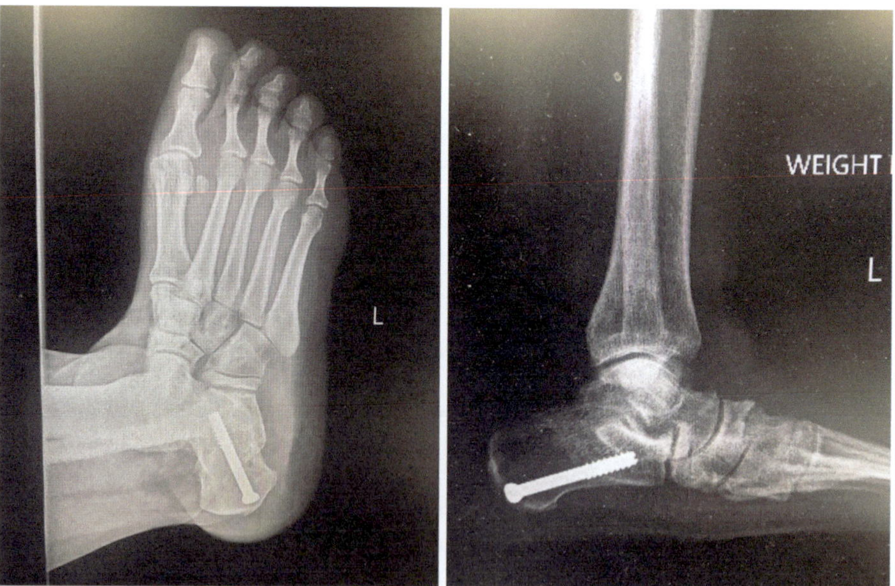

Fig. 7.5 Lateral column collapse due to allograft collapse (also with MDCO). Photo courtesy of Dr. Terry Philbin of the Orthopedic Foot and Ankle Center

Table 7.4 Collected surgical outcomes of LCL procedures

Author	Procedure	Follow-up (months)	Avg age	# feet	AOFAS	Complication rate	Complications/ follow-ups	Nonunion risk?	Patient satisfaction
Dolan 2007 [14]	LCL	3	57	33	N/A	6%	6% autograft hip donor site pain	No	N/A
Saunders 2018 [15]	Evans	24	58	65	72.88* FAOS	66%	8% nonunion 58% hardware pain leading to removal	Yes	N/A
	Stepcut lengthening calcaneal osteotomy		54	78	74.2* FAOS	42%	1% nonunion 41% hardware pain leading to removal		
Beat 1999 [16]	LCL	23.4	53	19	91.1	21%	5.3% nonunion 5.3% wound dehiscence leading to posterior CO 5.3% CC arthritis 5.3% graft dislocation	Yes	79% complete relief of pain 16% minor pain 5% moderate pain
Haeseker 2010 [17]	LCL by CC distraction arthrodesis	42.4	–	16	72	12.5%	6.25% nonunion 6.25% wound complication	Yes	100% satisfaction
	LCL by calcaneal osteotomy	15.8	–	19	85		68.4% mild calcaneocuboid subluxation 5.2% nonunion 5.2% wound complication	Yes	89.5% satisfaction
Kobayas 2017 [18]	CC distraction arthrodesis	32.76	65	13	85.46	15.40%	7.7% nonunion 7.7% hardware pain with subsequent removal	Yes	92.3% relief of pain and improvement in walking ability

(continued)

Table 7.4 (continued)

Author	Procedure	Follow-up (months)	Avg age	# feet	AOFAS	Complication rate	Complications/ follow-ups	Nonunion risk?	Patient satisfaction
R L Thomas 2001 [19]	Evans	52	45	10	87.9		17.6% failures 11.8% dorsal displacement 5.9% Achilles contracture 5.9% iliac seroma 5.9% tender iliac scar	No	88.9% very satisfied 11.1% satisfied with reservations 88.9% would have surgery again
	CC distraction arthrodesis	24.7		17	80.9		11.8% nonunion 17.6% delayed unions 17.6% graft stress fractures 5.9% fifth MT stress fracture 17.6% residual supination 17.6% three screw fractures	Yes	80% very satisfied 20% satisfied with reservations 100% would have surgery again
Grier 2010 [20]	Evans CC distraction arthrodesis	20	57	18 33	N/A	47%	5.9% rural neuritis 25.4% hardware issues 7.8% harvest site issues 11.7% superficial wound infection	Yes 5.6% Yes 21.2%	N/A

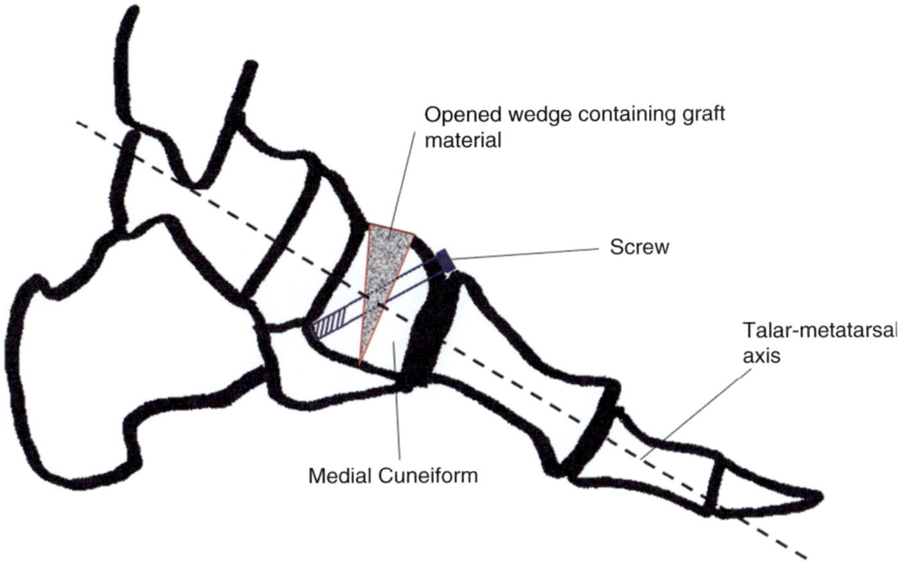

Fig. 7.6 Medial cuneiform or "Cotton" osteotomy

Indications/contraindications for a medial column procedure include advanced stage II PTTD, usually with first TMT hypermobility, instability, or arthritis. It is important to note that while disease is advanced, it is still stage II, and as such the forefoot is not yet in a fixed deformity. Fixed forefoot supination and varus are in fact contraindications to the surgery, as they may lead to an overload of the lateral border of the foot.

Complications – Undercorrection and delayed union are possible with a Cotton osteotomy, as is displacement of the graft. Hardware-induced pain is also a possible complication.

The "All American" or "Around the World" or "Double Osteotomy"

The "All American" or "Around the World" or "double osteotomy" combines the previously described MDCO with a lateral column lengthening procedure. The surgery captures benefits from each, with strong results.

Indications/Contraindications – This procedure is indicated when there is a severe loss of height due to severe pes planus and forefoot abduction.

Complications – The major complication associated with this surgery is pain at the site of hardware. Moseir-LaClair et al. found that 35% of patients experience a sufficiently high level of pain to necessitate hardware removal. A separate study by Boffeli et al. found that sural neuritis is a possible complication, likely associated with the incision it requires; although this complication isn't unique to the All American, it is worth noting. Calcaneocuboid arthritis has also been noted, as has talonavicular joint degeneration (see Table 7.5).

Table 7.5 Collected surgical outcomes of the "All American"

Name	Follow-up (months)	Avg age	# feet	AOFAS (SF-36)	Complication rate	Complication	Patient satisfaction
S Moseir-LaClair 2001 [21]	60	49	28	90	14%	CC arthritis	81% near to complete resolution of symptoms
Boffeli 2015 [22]	11.4	38	11	N/A	9%	Sural neuritis	N/A
Pomeroy 1997 [23]	17.5	43	20	82.8 (ankle-hindfoot)	5% asymptomatic recurrence 5% talonavicular joint degeneration 5% broken screw 10% sural nerve distribution numbness 20% hardware pain resulting in removal		90% AOFAS score improvement
Oh I 2011 [24]	62.4	16	16	93.4 (55.1 physical)	6.25%	6.25% adhesions around PTT and FDL	93.75% excellent 6.25% good
Silva 2014 [25]	24	46	43	85.6 (midfoot). 83.3 (hindfoot) (73)	5%	2.3% sural nerve entrapment 2.3% implant removal following infection	N/A

Triple Arthrodesis – *The order of joint to be fused in triple arthrodesis consists of subtalar joint followed by calcaneal cuboid and then talonavicular joint. First, a modified Ollie skin incision is made from the tip of fibula to the base of fourth-fifth metatarsal base. The EDB is elevated to expose the CC joint as well as subtalar joint. Care is taken to make dorsal incision from medial aspect of EHL over the talonavicular joint. Care is taken to prepare the three joints to achieve raw bleeding bone bed, with care to look for severe preexisting pes planovalgus deformity. One may have add accommodative large medially based wedge allograft to restore hindfoot alignment to achieve 5 degree hindfoot valgus. The corrected hindfoot alignment is fixated by placement of one/two subtalar screws, followed by lateral column lengthening by autograft/allograft/trabecular wedge for the calcaneal cuboid joint (with either screw or plate fixation). This is followed by talonavicular fixation (see* Fig. 7.7*).*

Indications/Contraindications – Triple arthrodesis is generally reserved for more severe cases of PTTD, especially those that involve a rigid flatfoot deformity. The surgery involves fixation of the talonavicular, subtalar, and calcaneocuboid joints. Not surprisingly, ankle mobility is severely restricted by this surgery. Triple arthrodesis is generally only indicated in stages III and IV of PTTD, as it imposes serious restrictions on movement and lifestyle. Specifically, triple arthrodesis is indicated in cases of stage IV PTTD with passively correctable ankle valgus.

Complications of triple arthrodesis may occur due to the malrotation or malunion of the proposed procedure, owing largely to the fact that the surgery is only pursued in more advanced cases of PTTD. Nonunion is a relatively common complication, specifically of the talonavicular joint, and likely contributes to another common complication: progression of deformity. Post-op collapse has also been reported in some cases (see Table 7.6).

Total Ankle Arthroplasty – In a total ankle arthroplasty, the entire joint between the talus and the tibia/fibula is replaced. The opposing surfaces of each of these bones are cut, and a manufactured insert is inserted. The new insert provides stability to PTTD sufferers.

Indications/Contraindications – Total ankle arthroplasty is only reserved for the most severe cases of PTTD.

Complications – The most common complications of this surgery are a progression of the deformity due to valgus tilt in the ankle joint, collapse of the medial arch, and nonunion. Avascular necrosis of the talus is a rare but serious complication of this technique and may present alongside damage to the deltoid ligament [27].

Variants – Numerous systems exist for the total ankle arthroplasty, although most follow a similar procedure.

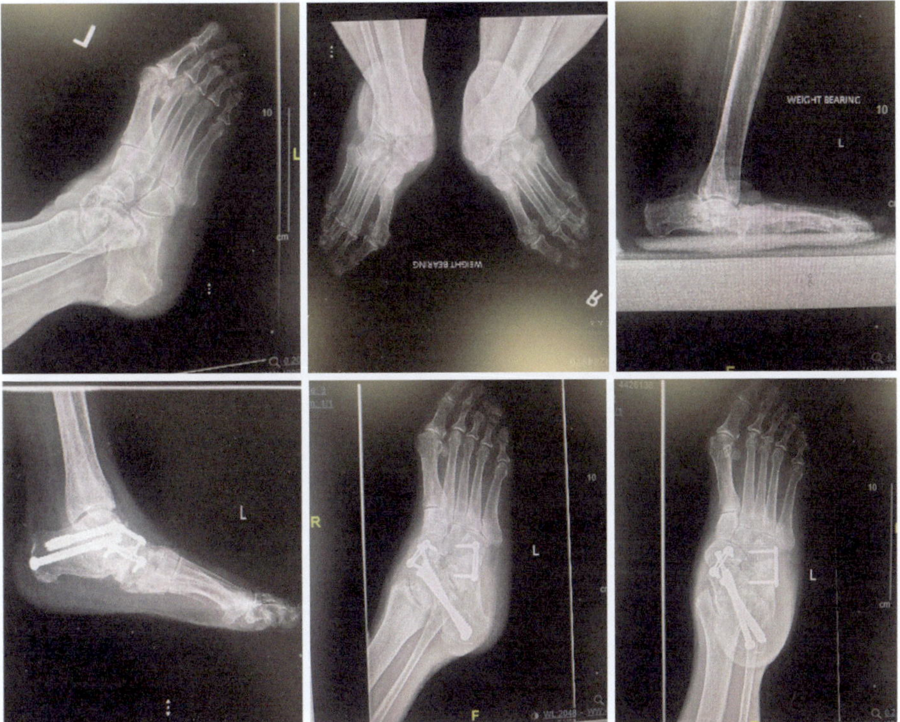

Fig. 7.7 Top row: imaging pre-triple arthrodesis. Bottom row: post-triple arthrodesis. Photo courtesy of Dr. Terry Philbin of the Orthopedic Foot and Ankle Center

Table 7.6 Selected surgical outcomes of triple arthrodesis

Name	Follow-up	Avg age	# feet	AOFAS	Complication rate	Complication	Nonunion?	Patient satisfaction
Chou 2007 [26]	12 weeks	55	13	87 (ankle-hindfoot) and 85 (mid-foot)	7.70%	Nonunion	Yes	100.00%
Röhm 2015 [27]	56 months	66	96	67 (hindfoot)	14.70%	6.25% nonunion 2% avascular necrosis 5.2% progression of deformity and arthritis 1% symptomatic overcorrection	Yes	"Very good" in 31% "good" in 35% "moderate" in 18% "bad" in 16% of cases
Graves 1993 [28]	42 months	66	18	—		16.7% nonunion 38.9% progressive degeneration involving the ankle 38.9% progressive degeneration of mobile joints in the foot 5.56% post-op collapse 5.56% removal of hardware due to pain	Yes	77.78% satisfied

Details of Standard Concurrent Procedures

As previously mentioned, PTTD is often accompanied by damage to soft tissues. For that reason, surgical interventions often include repair of these damaged structures alongside one of the "major" procedures described in the preceding section. Below are some of the soft tissue repairs commonly undertaken during surgery for PTTD. The choice of which of the following procedures should be done is generally done on a patient-by-patient basis, although certain combinations are common, such as MDCO with FDL transfer.

Cobb Procedure – Also known as an anterior tibial tendon transfer, this procedure is when the medial half of the anterior tibial tendon is attached to the medial cuneiform or navicular. This is almost always done alongside an osseous procedure such as an Evans osteotomy. It can also be done alongside an FDL transfer.

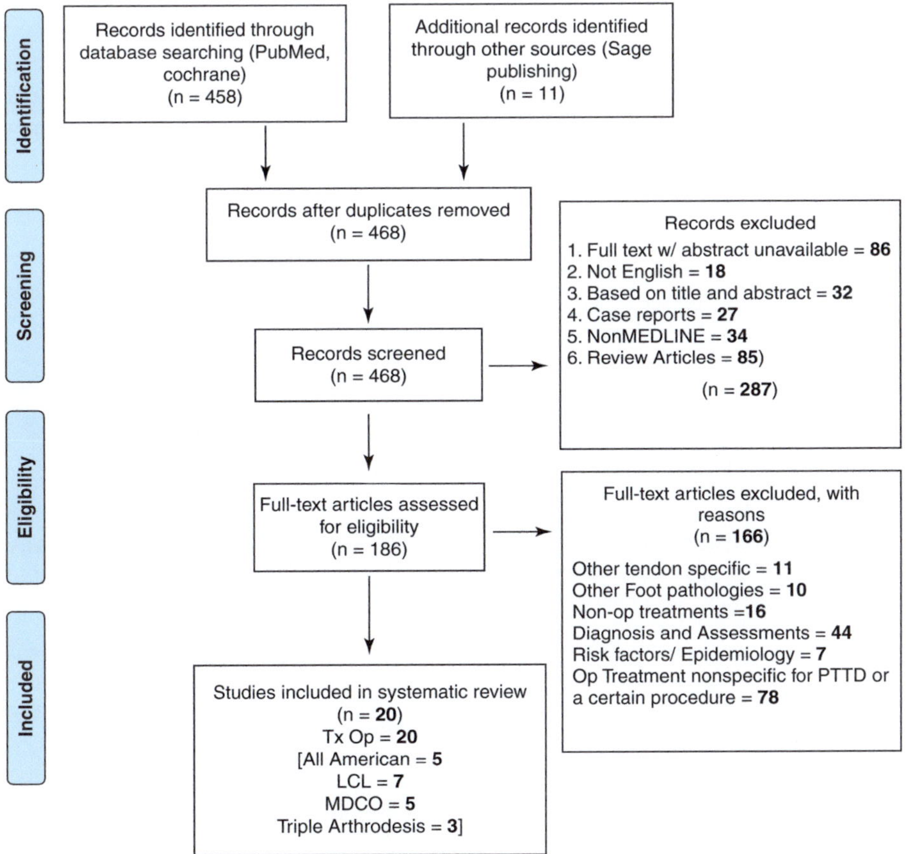

Fig. 7.8 PRISMA flow for literature review

Spring Ligament Repair – *A medial incision is made from the tip of the medial malleolus to 2 cm distal to the navicular to inspect the posterior tibial tendon and expose the spring ligament complex by retracting the tendon. Often the tear is obviously seen or soft tissue attenuation commonly is present. Nondegradable suture is used to sew this soft tissue defect and reconstruct the spring ligament.*

Tendo-Achilles Lengthening – *Tendo-Achilles lengthening is performed by either triple hemisection method of Hoke or more proximal gastrocnemius slide depending upon the Silfverskiold test.*

Evidence-Based/Critical Appraisal of the Literature

A comprehensive literature search conforming to PRISMA statement was performed. See Fig. 7.8 for details (Fig. 7.8).

Final Treatment Algorithm

Using the information discussed in this chapter, an overall treatment algorithm can be generated (Table 7.7). It is important to note that every patient is different, and these serve broadly as guidelines. Treatment should always be tailored to the specific needs of the patient.

Table 7.7 Final treatment algorithm

Stage	Nonsurgical	Surgical
Tenosynovitis	NSAID for 6–8 Weeks, CAM boot	N/A
	If symptoms improve, ankle stirrup brace	
	If symptoms do not improve, UCBL/Arizona	
	If still no improvement, proceed to surgical treatment	
Stage I	Medial heel and sole shoe wedge, hinged ankle-foot orthosis, orthotic arch supports as stated above	N/A
Stage II	Medial heel and sole shoe wedge, stuff orthotic support, hinged ankle-foot orthosis as stated above	Stage IIA: MDCO and FDL transfer
		Stage IIB: MDCO, FDL transfer ± spring ligament repair, LCL, and Achilles lengthening
		Stage IIC: Similar as stages IIA and IIB with a medial column procedure to correct supinated forefoot varus (cotton, Lapidus, or naviculocuneiform arthrodesis)
Stage III	Rigid ankle-foot orthosis	Triple arthrodesis
Stage IV	Rigid ankle-foot orthosis	Triple arthrodesis + total ankle reconstruction OR TTC fusion

References

1. Johnson K, Strom D. Tibialis posterior tendon dysfunction. Clin Orthop Relat Res. 1989;239:196–206.
2. Alvarez R, Marini A, Schmitt C, Saltzman C. Stage I and II posterior tibial tendon dysfunction treated by a structured nonoperative management protocol: an orthosis and exercise program. Foot Ankle Int. 2006;27(1):2–8.
3. Chao W, Wapner K, Lee T, Adams J, Hecht P. Nonoperative management of posterior tibial tendon dysfunction. Foot Ankle Int. 1996;17(12):736–41.
4. Augustin J, Lin S, Berberian W, Johnson J. Nonoperative treatment of adult acquired flat foot with the Arizona brace. Foot Ankle Clin. 2003;8(3):491–502.
5. Wacker J, Hennessy M, Saxby T. Calcaneal osteotomy and transfer of the tendon of flexor digitorum longus for stage-II dysfunction of tibialis posterior. J Bone Joint Surg Br. 2002;84-B(1):54–8.
6. Fayazi A, Nguyen H, Juliano P. Intermediate term follow-up of calcaneal osteotomy and flexor digitorum longus transfer for treatment of posterior tibial tendon dysfunction. Foot Ankle Int. 2002;23(12):1107–11.
7. Myerson M, Badekas A, Schon L. Treatment of stage II posterior tibial tendon deficiency with flexor digitorum longus tendon transfer and calcaneal osteotomy. Foot Ankle Int. 2004;25(7):445–50.
8. Schuh R, Gruber F, Wanivenhaus A, Hartig N, Windhager R, Trnka H. Flexor digitorum longus transfer and medial displacement calcaneal osteotomy for the treatment of stage II posterior tibial tendon dysfunction: kinematic and functional results of fifty one feet. Int Orthop. 2013;37(9):1815–20.
9. Chadwick C, Whitehouse S, Saxby T. Long-term follow-up of flexor digitorum longus transfer and calcaneal osteotomy for stage II posterior tibial tendon dysfunction. Bone Joint J. 2015;97-B(3):346–52.
10. Deland J, Otis J, Lee K, Kenneally S. Lateral column lengthening with calcaneocuboid fusion: range of motion in the triple joint complex. Foot Ankle Int. 1995;16(11):729–33.
11. Cooper P, Nowak M, Shaer J. Calcaneocuboid joint pressures with lateral column lengthening (Evans) procedure. Foot Ankle Int. 1997;18(4):199–205.
12. Momberger N, Morgan J, Bachus K, West J. Calcaneocuboid joint pressure after lateral column lengthening in a cadaveric planovalgus deformity model. Foot Ankle Int. 2000;21(9):730–5.
13. Xia J, Zhang P, Yang Y, Zhou J, Li Q, Yu G. Biomechanical analysis of the calcaneocuboid joint pressure after sequential lengthening of the lateral column. Foot Ankle Int. 2013;34(2):261–6.
14. Dolan C, Henning J, Anderson J, Bohay D, Kornmesser M, Endres T. Randomized prospective study comparing tri-cortical iliac crest autograft to allograft in the lateral column lengthening component for operative correction of adult acquired flatfoot deformity. Foot Ankle Int. 2007;28(1):8–12.
15. Saunders S, Ellis S, Demetracopoulos C, Marinescu A, Burkett J, Deland J. Comparative outcomes between step-cut lengthening calcaneal osteotomy vs traditional Evans osteotomy for stage IIB adult-acquired flatfoot deformity. Foot Ankle Int. 2017;39(1):18–27.
16. Hintermann B, Valderrabano V, Kundert H. Lengthening of the lateral column and reconstruction of the medial soft tissue for treatment of acquired flatfoot deformity associated with insufficiency of the posterior tibial tendon. Foot Ankle Int. 1999;20(10):622–9.
17. Haeseker G, Mureau M, Faber F. Lateral column lengthening for acquired adult flatfoot deformity caused by posterior tibial tendon dysfunction stage II: a retrospective comparison of calcaneus osteotomy with calcaneocuboid distraction arthrodesis. J Foot Ankle Surg. 2010;49(4):380–4.
18. Kobayashi H, Kageyama Y, Shido Y. Calcaneocuboid distraction arthrodesis with synthetic bone grafts: preliminary results of an innovative bone grafting procedure in 13 patients. J Foot Ankle Surg. 2017;56(6):1223–31.
19. Thomas R, Wells B, Garrison R, Prada S. Preliminary results comparing two methods of lateral column lengthening. Foot Ankle Int. 2001;22(2):107–19.

20. Grier K, Walling A. The use of Tricortical autograft versus allograft in lateral column lengthening for adult acquired flatfoot deformity: an analysis of union rates and complications. Foot Ankle Int. 2010;31(9):760–9.
21. Moseir-LaClair S, Pomeroy G, Manoli A. Intermediate follow-up on the double osteotomy and tendon transfer procedure for stage II posterior tibial tendon insufficiency. Foot Ankle Int. 2001;22(4):283–91.
22. Boffeli T, Abben K. Double calcaneal osteotomy with percutaneous Steinmann pin fixation as part of treatment for flexible flatfoot deformity: a review of consecutive cases highlighting our experience with pin fixation. J Foot Ankle Surg. 2015;54(3):478–82.
23. Pomeroy G, Manoli A. A new operative approach for flatfoot secondary to posterior tibial tendon insufficiency: a preliminary report. Foot Ankle Int. 1997;18(4):206–12.
24. Oh I, Williams B, Ellis S, Kwon D, Deland J. Reconstruction of the symptomatic idiopathic flatfoot in adolescents and young adults. Foot Ankle Int. 2011;32(3):225–32.
25. Silva M, Tan S, Chong H, Su H, Singh I. Results of operative correction of grade IIB tibialis posterior tendon dysfunction. Foot Ankle Int. 2014;36(2):165–71.
26. Chou L, Halligan B. Treatment of severe, painful pes planovalgus deformity with hindfoot arthrodesis and wedge-shaped tricortical allograft. Foot Ankle Int. 2007;28(5):569–74.
27. Röhm J, Zwicky L, Horn Lang T, Salentiny Y, Hintermann B, Knupp M. Mid- to long-term outcome of 96 corrective hindfoot fusions in 84 patients with rigid flatfoot deformity. Bone Joint J. 2015;97-B(5):668–74.
28. Graves S, Mann R, Graves K. Triple arthrodesis in older adults. Results after long-term follow-up. J Bone Joint Surg Am. 1993;75(3):355–62.

Plantar Fascia Injuries

8

Korey DuBois and Jacob Wynes

Introduction

The plantar fascia is a soft tissue structure on the plantar aspect of the foot that is critically relevant to foot function and pathophysiology. It originates from the plantar-medial tubercle of the calcaneus, spanning the plantar foot to insert on the metatarsophalangeal joints and their associated toes. Injuries to the plantar fascia result in over 1 million medical encounters in the United States each year, with many patients requiring more than one visit [1, 2]. The natural history of plantar fascia injuries encompasses a wide spectrum, from mild and self-limiting to severe and debilitating. Risk factors for plantar fasciitis include high body mass index, occupational risks such as prolonged standing, overtraining, physical inactivity, foot structure (such as pes valgus or pes cavus), and biomechanical or gait abnormalities [3, 4]. Although uncommon, rupture of the plantar fascia can occur and requires accurate diagnosis by the treating clinician to achieve successful treatment [5]. Treatment of plantar fasciitis is usually amenable to conservative methods, but due to the prevalence of these injuries, clinicians will encounter patients recalcitrant to such noninvasive methods.

K. DuBois
Limb Preservation and Deformity Correction Fellowship, University of Maryland School of Medicine, Baltimore, MD, USA

J. Wynes (✉)
Department of Orthopaedics, University of Maryland School of Medicine, Baltimore, MD, USA

© Springer Nature Switzerland AG 2022
J. D. Cain, M. V. Hogan (eds.), *Tendon and Ligament Injuries of the Foot and Ankle*,
https://doi.org/10.1007/978-3-031-10490-9_8

Anatomy

The plantar fascia is an organization of connective tissue that originates from a fibrocartilaginous attachment at the plantar-medial tuberosity of the calcaneus and extends across the sole of the foot to the toes. Grossly, it is described as having a medial, central, and lateral band with the central aponeurosis being the most robust [6]. The medial band is thin and courses superficial to the fascia of the abductor hallucis muscle. The lateral band extends from the calcaneal tuberosity to the abductor digiti minimi fascia and the fifth metatarsal base. The central band is much more distinct, it courses distally, and at the metatarsal level, it divides into five separate components that ultimately find various insertions on each respective plantar plate and associated phalanx. The plantar fascia is composed primarily of type I collagen, but a small amount of type III and type IV collagen has been identified. Collagen fibers are generally oriented in a longitudinal proximal to distal direction. Histologically, the plantar fascia appears to be made up of a central "core" tissue with dense, primarily type I collagen bundles, and a "sheath" tissue consisting primarily of loose type IV collagen [7].

During gait, extension of the metatarsophalangeal joints causes tension of the plantar fascia, which results in elevation of the medial longitudinal arch of the foot and inverts the hindfoot. This is known as the windlass mechanism and was originally described by Hicks [8]. Following heel strike, tension on the plantar fascia gradually increases, peaking at approximately 80% of midstance [9]. The plantar fascia is capable of withstanding very high tensile loads, with reported failure loads averaging 1189 N [10].

The inception of plantar fasciitis is believed to be repetitive microtrauma resulting in collagen injury. If the causative etiology is not managed, continued stress may inhibit healing and lead to the chronic form of the disease, which is more appropriately characterized as a degenerative process [11, 12]. Zhang et al. [7] found increased inflammatory modulators and induction of aberrant stem cell differentiation in the setting of simulated in vivo mechanical overload [7].

Recently, it has been shown that physiological mechanical loading of the plantar fascia increases differentiation of stem cells into fibroblasts, which helps in maintaining plantar fascia structure. However elevated nonphysiologic loading resulted in gene expression for adipogenesis, osteogenesis, and chondrogenesis, which may explain evidence for degenerative changes identified in surgical pathology [7, 12].

Approximately 15% of people exhibit a plantar calcaneal spur. The anatomy, histology, and etiology were closely studied by Kirkpatrick et al. [13], and they report spurring is more prevalent in patients with plantar fasciitis/heel pain, patients with elevated BMI, patients with arthritides, the elderly, and patients with abnormal foot biomechanics [13]. Kumai et al. [14] found that the spur could not be a traction spur, as they generally form deep to the plantar fascia and the trabecular pattern is consistent with a vertically oriented force, rather than a horizontal traction force [14].

Diagnosis/Clinical Evaluation

Plantar Fasciitis

In plantar fasciitis, the classic presentation is a patient reporting a sharp pain with the first steps of a day. This pain usually evolves to become less severe with low-impact activity, but with prolonged activity or high-impact exercise, the symptoms may become exacerbated and more severe. Differential diagnoses include metabolic causes such as gout, neurogenic causes such as lumbar radiculopathy or entrapment of the first branch of the lateral plantar nerve, traumatic causes such as calcaneal fracture or contusion, and rheumatic causes such as seronegative spondyloarthropathy, rheumatoid arthritis, or reactive arthritis [15].

The patient will often present with limping and/or guarding of the affected extremity. Evaluating the patient in stance is useful in identifying structural foot deformity such as pes plano valgus or pes cavus. Palpation of the plantar calcaneal tubercle will reproduce symptoms of plantar fasciitis. A calcaneal squeeze test is useful in ruling out calcaneal stress fracture. Palpation of the course of the plantar fascia should be performed to assess for plantar fascia rupture or pain associated with plantar fibroma formation. A Silfverskiold test should be performed to assess calf muscle-tendon tightness. Percussion of the tarsal tunnel should be performed, and if it reproduces symptoms, a neurogenic component such as tarsal tunnel syndrome should be considered. Weakness or atrophy of the abductor digiti minimi should be accessed, as entrapment of the first branch of the lateral plantar nerve is known to cause heel pain as well as weakness to this muscle, which it innervates.

In patients with atraumatic heel pain, plain film radiographs are rarely indicated on the initial visit [16]. It is important to consider atypical causes of heel pain that may indicate early imaging. Examples include pain with calcaneal squeeze examination, which may represent a calcaneal stress fracture, or nocturnal pain, which may represent neoplasm. Multiple studies have found ultrasonography to be clinically useful in the diagnosis of plantar fasciitis [17–23]. Patients with symptomatic plantar fasciitis generally exhibit thickening on ultrasound in comparison to asymptomatic patients [19]. It is commonly accepted that plantar fascia thickness greater than 4.0 mm is considered pathologic [17, 19]. MRI is a valuable resource for the diagnosis of plantar fasciitis. MRI of symptomatic patients commonly exhibit perifascial edema, which is characterized as a poorly differentiated area of increased STIR signal intensity within the tissue superficial and deep to the plantar fascia (Fig. 8.1). Increased STIR signal intensity within the fascia may represent partial fascial tearing. Fascia thickening greater than 5.0 mm is common in symptomatic patients.

Acute Plantar Fascia Rupture

Patients presenting with an acute plantar fascia rupture exhibit similar histories and physical symptoms to patients with plantar fasciitis, but key differences will allow

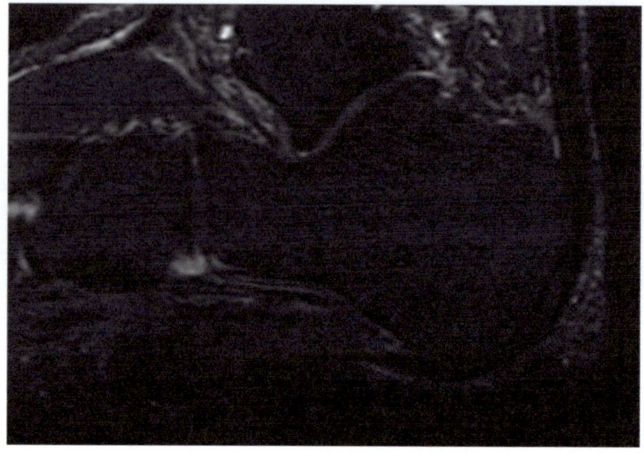

Fig. 8.1 MRI T2-weighted image demonstrating perifascial edema and plantar fascia thickening in a 52-year-old male patient

for accurate diagnosis and appropriate treatment. Most plantar fascia ruptures occur in the setting of chronic degenerative plantar fasciitis, and a history of corticosteroid injection for the treatment of plantar fasciitis is associated with most plantar fascia tears [24–28]. Examination often shows acute plantar heel pain and ecchymosis. It is important to engage the windlass mechanism and compare plantar fascia tension to the contralateral foot, as decreased plantar fascia tension is diagnostic [28]. MRI or ultrasound may be utilized for accurate diagnosis of partial or complete plantar fascia tears [29].

Treatment

Plantar Fasciitis

A comprehensive literature search was performed, with no time limit to maximize the pool of work available, conforming to the PRISMA statement. The databases used were PubMed, CINAHL, and EMBASE. The search found a literature review of plantar fascia injuries, which provided further articles that were included for evaluation of nonoperative and operative treatments.

Nonoperative Management

The treatment plan should be tailored to each patient's etiology, activity level, and disease course. The American College of Foot and Ankle Surgeons [30] has classified plantar fasciitis into three stages. Acute plantar fasciitis refers to the initial 4 to 6 weeks after the onset of an inflammatory event due to mechanical overload. Subacute plantar fasciitis is present when symptoms have persisted for approximately 6 to 12 weeks. Chronic plantar fasciitis occurs when the symptoms have been present for greater than 3 months [30]. At this stage, degenerative changes may be present within the plantar fascia, and treatment is much more difficult.

Stretching Exercises and Physical Therapy

Multiple studies have shown that a tight calf muscle/tendon group resulting in limited ankle dorsiflexion is a common pathologic force in the development of plantar fasciitis [11, 31–37]. Lack of anatomic ankle dorsiflexion results in increased pronatory moments at the subtalar joint and midtarsal joints, which is believed to increase strain on the medial longitudinal arch and plantar fascia [11]. Stretching exercises are a critical element of most initial treatment protocols and have been shown to be an effective modality in both acute and chronic plantar fasciitis [31–37]. The goal of stretching exercises is to increase ankle dorsiflexion, thereby reducing abnormal hindfoot motion and the resulting plantar fascia stress. Digiovanni et al. [36] compared the outcomes of a plantar fascia-specific stretching protocol to outcomes of an Achilles tendon stretching protocol. They concluded that a fascia-specific stretching regiment was critical in treating chronic plantar fasciitis [36]. Engkananuwat et al. [32] prospectively evaluated outcomes between an Achilles tendon-only stretching protocol and a simultaneous Achilles tendon and plantar fascia stretching protocol. They found the simultaneous Achilles tendon and plantar fascia stretching protocol to be significantly more effective than Achilles-only stretching following a 4-week treatment period [32].

Night Splints

Night splints are most commonly prescribed as an adjunctive treatment for acute or chronic plantar fasciitis. Probe et al. [38] evaluated 116 patients randomized to two groups. Group one was treated with 1 month of oral anti-inflammatory medication, Achilles tendon stretching exercises, and shoe recommendations. Group two received the same treatment with the addition of a night splint. At 12 weeks there was no difference in improvement between the two groups [38]. Powell et al. [39] performed a crossover study of 37 patients with chronic plantar fasciitis. The first group utilized a night splint in month one of the study, and the second group in month two. Both groups discontinued use of the night splint over the next 4 months. No other treatment modality was utilized. Both groups showed significant improvement after 1 month of splinting [39].

Taping and Strapping

Taping can offer short-term symptomatic relief in patients with plantar fasciitis [40–43]. Taping is effective in reducing mechanical strain on the plantar fascia, thereby reducing symptoms. Landorf et al. [42] compared 65 patients with plantar fasciitis who underwent a stretching routine and low-dye taping for 3 to 5 days to a group of 40 patients who underwent only stretching. The group undergoing taping showed a significant improvement in pain as compared to the control group [42]. Radford et al. [43] performed a randomized trial comparing low-dye taping with sham ultrasound to outcomes in patients undergoing sham ultrasound alone. They found taping provided a small improvement in "first-step" pain compared to the sham intervention [43].

Foot Orthoses

Both custom and prefabricated foot orthoses are prescribed for treatment of plantar fasciitis. The goal of orthoses in this setting is to stabilize the foot and reduce tissue stress secondary to biomechanical abnormalities. Kogler et al. [44] showed that some foot orthoses could reduce plantar fascia strain in a "static stance" cadaver model [44]. Whitaker et al. [45] performed a systematic review and meta-analysis of studies accessing foot orthoses for plantar heel pain. They found moderate evidence that foot orthoses were more effective than sham orthoses in reducing pain in the medium term, which they defined as 7 to 12 weeks [45]. Gross et al. [46] assessed the ability of plantar fasciitis patients to walk 100 meters with and without custom semirigid orthotics. They found a reduction in pain during walking when the patients utilized orthoses [46]. Redmond et al. [47] found there was no significant difference in plantar pressures when comparing patients with flatfoot utilizing custom orthoses to patients with flatfoot utilizing prefabricated orthoses [47]. Landorf et al. [48] found that custom and prefabricated orthoses provided mild short-term improvement in pain and function, but did not produce long-term significant differences in comparison to sham orthotics [48].

Anti-inflammatories

Anti-inflammatory medications are utilized in most treatment plans for plantar fasciitis. Options include oral nonsteroidal anti-inflammatories (NSAIDs), topical NSAIDs, oral steroid anti-inflammatories, and corticosteroid injections. Donley et al. [49] performed a randomized, prospective, placebo-controlled trial to access the efficacy of oral NSAIDs in treatment of plantar fasciitis. They evaluated 29 patients with plantar fasciitis who received a conservative treatment plan that included heel cups, heel-cord stretching, and night splinting. Half of the patients also received an NSAID regimen (celecoxib 200 mg once a day for 30 days), and half received a placebo. They concluded that the addition of an NSAID to conservative treatment protocols may increase pain relief and decrease disability [49].

The use of oral corticosteroids is common in the treatment of plantar fasciitis. However, there are no studies evaluating the efficacy of oral corticosteroids in the treatment of plantar fasciitis. They are most commonly prescribed as a methylprednisolone dose pack or a prednisone taper. Long-term use of oral corticosteroids have well-known adverse effects, most notably adrenal suppression [50]. Short-term oral corticosteroids are commonly prescribed for a number of inflammatory conditions. However, recent evidence shows that even short-term oral corticosteroids lead to an increased risk of serious adverse events, such as infection, venous thromboembolism, and fracture [51].

Corticosteroids are anti-inflammatory and can provide significant symptomatic relief. Multiple studies have shown that corticosteroid injections can greatly reduce pain, especially in the short term [52–54]. Unfortunately, there are a number of adverse effects associated with corticosteroid injections; therefore their use is controversial [55, 56]. Corticosteroids have been shown to cause connective soft tissue breakdown secondary to collagen degeneration [57, 58]. Lee et al. [5] reported that among 35 patients with plantar fascia rupture, 33 had received steroid injections, and steroid injection was the only variable associated with plantar fascia rupture in their study [5]. Sellman [26] reported on a series of 37 patients who suffered plantar fascia rupture following corticosteroid injection for plantar fasciitis. He noted some patients developed long-term sequelae, including lateral column pain, metatarsal stress fractures, and arch pain [26]. Acevedo et al. [25] reported a series of 765 patients with plantar fasciitis. Fifty-two patients were diagnosed with plantar fascia rupture, and of those, 44 patients had previously undergone at least one corticosteroid plantar fascia injection. These patients also exhibited longer-term symptoms including midfoot pain, lateral column pain, hammertoe development, and neurologic symptoms localized to the lateral plantar nerve [25]. Despite these serious adverse effects, corticosteroids are still utilized as a central component of many treatment programs. Johannsen et al. [59] evaluated the effect of corticosteroid injections combined with a strength training and stretching program. They found that the addition of corticosteroid injections had superior short- and long-term outcomes in the treatment of plantar fasciitis [59].

Utilization of ultrasound for guidance during corticosteroid injection has gained popularity. Tsai et al. [60] compared a group of patients undergoing ultrasound-guided injection to a group undergoing palpation-guided injection. They found use of the ultrasound was associated with a lower recurrence of heel pain. Both groups exhibited significant pain improvement and decreased plantar fascia thickness [60].

Pro-inflammatory Modalities

Extracorporeal shockwave therapy is used to cause extracellular responses that lead to an inflammatory response, resulting in neovascularization and tissue regeneration [61]. Multiple studies have shown that shockwave therapy is a safe therapy that can be effective in treating plantar fasciitis [62–64]. Gollwitzer et al. [63] performed a prospective, multicenter, double-blind, randomized, placebo-controlled trial to assess effectiveness of shockwave therapy in relieving chronic heel pain secondary to plantar fasciitis. The treatment arm received focused extracorporeal shockwave therapy (0.25 mJ/mm^2) with 3 treatments of 2000 impulses in weekly intervals. They found shockwave therapy to be superior to the placebo with treatment success rates between 50% and 65% [63].

Platelet-Rich Plasma

Platelet-rich plasma is an autologous concentration of platelets suspended within autologous plasma [65, 66]. Platelets release growth factors and cytokines responsible for angiogenesis, collagen production, and fibroblast upregulation. PRP allows for the delivery of large amounts of platelets and associated growth factors/cytokines to the site of injury with the goal of inducing tissue repair. Multiple studies have suggested that PRP is safe and can be effective in reducing pain and symptoms of plantar fasciitis [67–71]. Monto [67] performed a level I prospective and randomized study comparing a single ultrasound-guided PRP injection to a 40 mg Depo-Medrol corticosteroid injection. At 3 months, the corticosteroid group showed improvement in AOFAS scores, but AOFAS scores declined from that point until the final 24-month follow-up. He concluded that PRP was more effective than corticosteroid treatment in treatment of chronic plantar fasciitis [67]. Jain et al. [70] performed a similar level II, prospective, randomized comparative study between one group receiving a corticosteroid injection and a second group receiving PRP. Both groups showed improvement, but at 6 months there was no significant difference between the two groups [70].

Amniotic/Chorionic/Placental Membrane Injection

Micronized dehydrated human amniotic/chorionic membrane (mDHACM) is hypothesized to deliver growth factors to facilitate regeneration of degenerative tissue [72]. Zelen et al. [72] performed a level I, prospective, randomized study with 45 patients. Each arm received an injection of 2 cc 0.5% Marcaine plain. The control arm received a 1.25 cc saline injection, and the two treatment arms received 0.5 cc mDHACM or 1.25 cc mDHACM. They noted significant reduction in AOFAS hindfoot scores at 1 week and 8 weeks in comparison to the control arm. There were no significant outcome differences between the groups receiving 0.5 cc mDHACM and 1.25 cc mDHACM [72]. Cazzell et al. [73] performed a multicenter, prospective, single-blinded, randomized control trial of mDHACM in comparison to a saline placebo in patients with plantar fasciitis. At 3 months postinjection, data showed statistically significant reduction in pain and improvement in function for the mDHACM treatment arm [73]. Hanselmann et al. [74] performed a randomized, controlled, double-blinded trial comparing cryopreserved human amniotic membrane (c-hAM) injection to corticosteroid injection for treatment of plantar fasciitis. Fourteen patients received a corticosteroid injection and nine received c-hAM injection. In their study, c-HAM was found to be "safe and comparable" to corticosteroid injection. These studies present preliminary data, with the longest duration of follow-up being 3 months. Their results are therefore speculative, and further studies are needed to access for long-term efficacy and safety [74].

Operative Management

Operative treatment is reserved for recalcitrant plantar fasciitis that fails to respond to conservative treatment for at least 6 to 12 months. Successful outcomes of various surgical treatments for plantar fasciitis range from 40th percentile to the 90th percentile [75–82]. Due to the unpredictable nature of surgical treatment, nonoperative treatment is favored. Even so, due to the high prevalence of plantar fasciitis, most surgeons who treat plantar fasciitis will encounter patients who ultimately require surgical management.

Open Plantar Fasciotomy

Open plantar fasciotomy is a commonly performed procedure for treatment of recalcitrant plantar fasciitis. This procedure is often combined with heel spur resection, gastrocnemius recession, tarsal tunnel release, or external neurolysis of the first branch of the lateral plantar nerve. Multiple studies have evaluated the biomechanical consequences of performing a plantar fasciotomy [83–88]. Associated complications of plantar fasciotomy include lateral column overload, medial arch fatigue, midfoot pain, and forefoot overload. The risks of these complications are

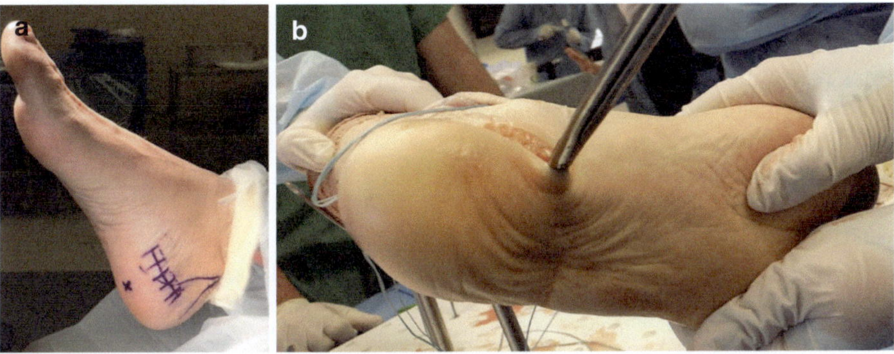

Fig. 8.2 (**a**) Incisional approach for partial open plantar fasciotomy along the medial glabrous skin junction with appropriate preoperative marking of the patient's point of maximal tenderness and distribution of the tibial nerve. (**b**) Cadaveric representation of dissection through the interval of the abductor hallucis fascia and plantar fascia with insertion of a curved mayo scissor to demonstrate a "pucker" correlating with the interval just below the plantar fascia in preparation for partial open fasciotomy

greater if more than 50% of the fascia is released; therefore some authors recommend release of no more than 1/3 of the fascia [83–89]. A significant weakness of performing an isolated plantar fascia release is failure to address the biomechanical etiology of the symptoms (Fig. 8.2).

Endoscopic Plantar Fasciotomy (EPF)

Endoscopic plantar fasciotomy gained popularity with the use of smaller incisions that will result in a more rapid recovery with less morbidity [80, 90]. In a cadaveric study of 13 feet, Hofmeister et al. [91] found that the average amount of plantar fascia released was 81% and the flexor digitorum brevis muscle was injured in 6 of the 13 feet. In their study they reported the approach does not risk damage to underlying neurovascular structures [91]. Hawkins et al. [92] performed a cadaveric study of 18 cadaver specimens. They attempted a 75% fascial release and found the average release was 82% of the width of the plantar fascia. Again they noted no injury to the first branch of the lateral plantar nerve [77, 92]. Morton et al. [93] reported a series of 105 patients undergoing an EPF utilizing a medial uniportal approach. They reported complete pain relief in 80.9% of their patients and no significant complications [93]. Chou et al. [94] compared a series of 28 open plantar fasciotomies to 14 endoscopic plantar fasciotomies. They found superior short-term outcomes for the EPF group, reporting significantly greater AOFAS scores, SF-36 scores, and lower pain scores at 3 months [94]. Malahias et al. [95] performed a systematic review of endoscopic plantar fasciotomy clinical outcomes. Fifteen studies met their criteria with a total of 576 feet in 535 patients. Their review showed improvement in clinical and subjective outcomes with a postoperative complication rate of 11%. They noted the overall quality of studies was low and concluded there is weak evidence to support EPF as a safe and effective treatment for plantar fasciitis [95]. In a multi-center prospective study of 25 providers who had successfully completed a cadaveric training and certification, 652 cases were performed with 599 successful interventions without complication. The most common complications were reported in 25 cases as lateral column destabilization resulting in calcaneal cuboid and midtarsal joint pain. Medical destabilization was found to result in central arch pain and intrinsic myositis in 3 and 4 patients, respectively. With respect to general outcomes 19 of 652 patients still had persistent heel pain [96].

Gastrocnemius Recession

Calf tightness is a common biomechanical etiology of plantar fasciitis [4, 11, 31–39, 97–100]. Calf tightness results in altered foot mechanics, leading to increased strain on the plantar fascia [11]. Calf muscle-tendon lengthening can be approached at different levels (zones) of the triceps surae with different effects (Fig. 8.3) [99]. Zone 1 is from the femoral origin of the gastrocnemius muscle and extends to the conclusion of medial gastrocnemius muscle belly. The Baumann and Strayer procedures are performed within this zone, and they are considered to be the most mechanically stable lengthening procedures. Zone 2 courses from the distal aspect of the medial gastrocnemius muscle belly to the conclusion of the soleus muscle belly. The Baker and Vulpius procedures are performed at this level. Zone 3 extends from the conclusion of the soleus muscle to the insertion of the Achilles tendon on the calcaneus. Appropriately performed lengthenings in zone 1 or 2 can allow for protected weightbearing [99]. In patients with a positive Silfverskiold in the setting of plantar fasciitis, posterior muscle group lengthening has been proposed as a treatment option in patients recalcitrant to conservative management [31, 97–101]. Monteagudo et al. [101] compared gastrocnemius recession to plantar fascia release in patients with chronic plantar fasciitis. Patients undergoing gastrocnemius release showed 95% postoperative satisfaction in comparison to 60% satisfaction among patients undergoing plantar fascia release. They concluded gastrocnemius recession produced better results with less morbidity in comparison to open plantar fasciotomy [101]. Abbassian et al. [97] performed a proximal medial gastrocnemius recession on 21 feet of 17 patients. They reported complete pain relief in 17 of 21 (81%)

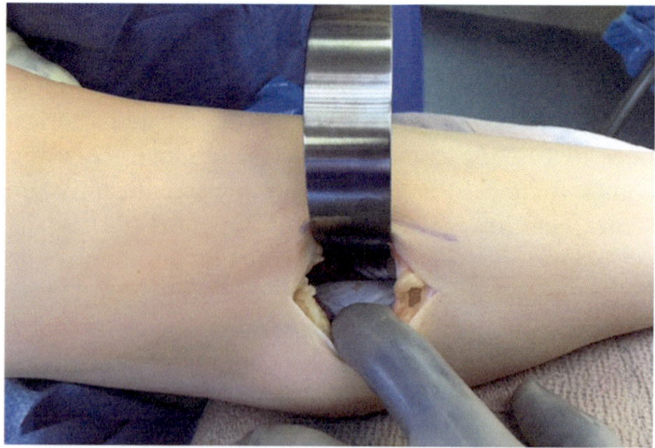

Fig. 8.3 Incisional approach for Baumann gastrocnemius recession where this provides visibility of both the gastrocnemius fascia and soleus fascia along the medial mid-calf region

of the procedures and reported no major complications. Mulhern et al. performed a combination of an open gastrocnemius recession and endoscopic plantar fasciotomy for 25 consecutive patients who met their inclusion criteria. They reported significant improvements in pain and ankle range of motion at 3.7-month follow-up [97]. Molund et al. [98] evaluated postoperative outcomes of gastrocnemius recession in 73 patients with various lower extremity ailments, including plantar fasciitis. They reported good or excellent results in 14 of 18 patients who underwent gastrocnemius recession for management of plantar fasciitis [98].

Bipolar Radiofrequency Microdebridement

Bipolar radiofrequency coblation microdebridement is affecting induction of angiogenesis to the degenerative plantar fascia in the treatment of chronic plantar fasciitis [101–108]. The proposed physiologic mechanism for this procedure has been elucidated in several investigations. In a rabbit model, the technique has been shown to increase angiogenesis, but showed no significant difference in healing of degenerative Achilles tendon in comparison to a control group [105]. Weil et al. [102] first published the use of the technique for management of plantar fasciosis. They prospectively reviewed ten patients who underwent percutaneous microtenotomy and found improved AOFAS scores, VAS scores, and patient satisfaction scores at 6 months and 1 year. Sorensen et al. performed a similar case series of 21 patients, with 18 patients (86%) subjectively rating their outcome as excellent or good [102]. Tay et al. [103] reported a prospective, nonrandomized trial comparing open plantar fasciotomy to radiofrequency coblation. In their study of 48 patients and 59 feet, they found improvement in both arms of their study, but more significant improvement in patients undergoing the open procedure [103].

Botulinum Injection

Botulinum toxin A blocks the release of acetylcholine at the neuromuscular junction, resulting in skeletal muscle paralysis. It also may reduce inflammatory and pain mediators and has been utilized successfully in the treatment of myofascial pain [109–111]. Babcock et al. [109] performed a prospective, randomized, controlled, double-blinded study accessing the use of botulinum toxin A in the treatment of chronic plantar fasciitis. In their study both the most tender site of the medial heel and the most tender site of the arch were injected. They reported statistically significant improvement for the treatment group in pain and foot function at 3 and 8 weeks [109]. A similar trial with 50 patients was performed by Ahmad [110]. They again showed significantly better improvement for the treatment group [110]. Abbassian et al. [112] performed a level I, prospective, randomized control trial accessing the outcomes of ultrasound-guided medial gastrocnemius head injection with botulinum toxin for treatment of chronic plantar fasciitis. They reported statistically significant improvements in pain and foot function for the treatment group at 1 year [112]. Elizondo-Rodriguez et al. [111] performed a level I study comparing gastrocnemius botulinum A injection to plantar heel corticosteroid injection in treatment of plantar fasciitis. In their study, the botulinum A injection group showed faster and longer-lasting results in comparison to the corticosteroid injection group [111].

Plantar Fascia Rupture

The vast majority of plantar fascia ruptures respond to conservative management. Most studies recommend immobilization via a rigid-soled device, such as a CAM walker. Length of immobilization varies, but is generally between 2 and 4 weeks. Immobilization is usually discontinued once the patient is able to ambulate without pain in normal shoes. Debus et al. [24] performed a systematic review of the standard of care for rupture of the plantar fascia. They reported poor quality of available data [24]. To our knowledge there is only one reported case series of surgical repair of acute plantar fascia rupture. Schaarup et al. [113] reported a case series of five complete plantar fascia ruptures in athletes participating in high-demand, explosive sports. Two athletes were treated surgically and three were treated nonoperatively. They noted morphological differences between the operative and nonoperative groups, assessed on ultrasound, the foot posture index, and measurement of foot length. They also reported the operative group had no complaints according to the Foot Function Index, whereas the nonoperative group had impairments in activities of daily living. They concluded surgical repair of acute plantar fascia ruptures is feasible in high-impact athletes [113].

Conclusion

The plantar fascia is a band of connective tissue that spans the plantar foot. The central band is the most robust and is believed to be the most functionally and clinically relevant portion. The plantar fascia functions to stabilize the medial longitudinal arch and undergoes tensile stress during the stance phase of gait. Plantar fascia injuries are common in many populations, but are especially prevalent in highly active individuals and high BMI individuals. Chronic plantar fasciitis is much more common than acute plantar fascia rupture and occurs secondary to overuse and mechanical overload, resulting in partial tearing at the origin of the plantar fascia. The inflammatory phase of plantar fasciitis represents the most critical window of treatment, as successful treatment is much more difficult if the disease progresses to the chronic stage. The chronic stage appears to represent cycles of acute inflammation inciting progressive degeneration of the plantar fascia. Despite the complexity of the disease process, for many the natural history is self-limiting. Treatment for symptomatic patients should be tailored to match the etiology, which is often multifactorial. Due to the difficulty in treating patients

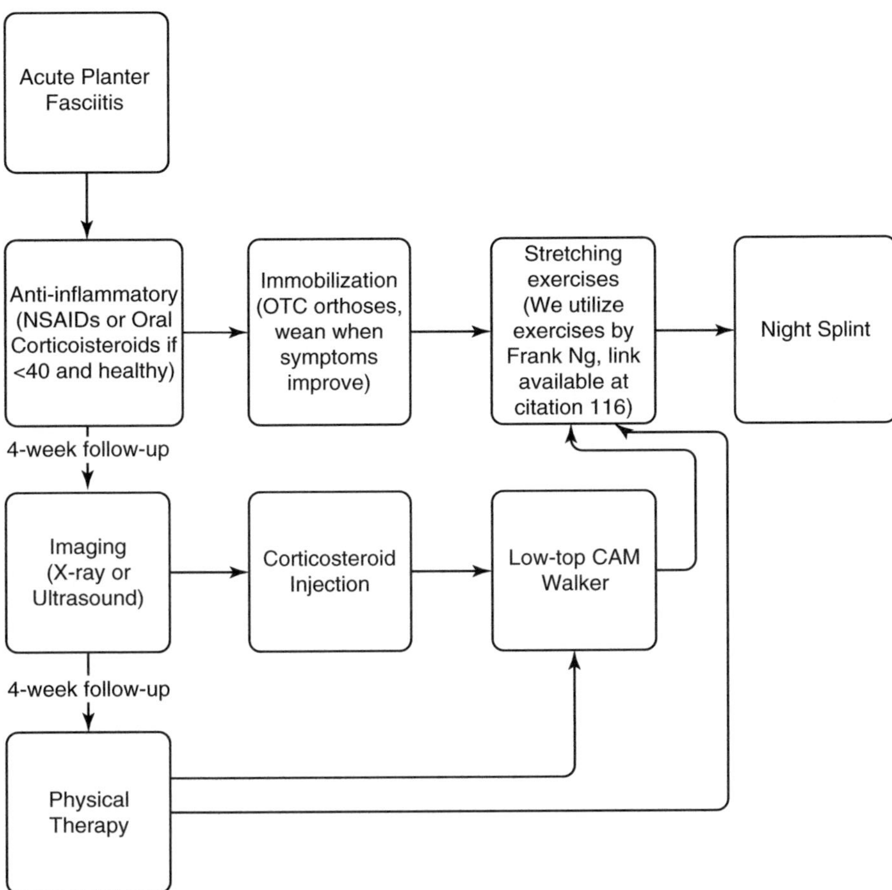

Fig. 8.4 Conservative treatment options for *acute* plantar fascia pain presented as an algorithmic approach

who progress to chronic plantar fasciitis, there are many treatment modalities. Unfortunately the evidence for most treatments is relatively poor. There are very few level I studies with large patient populations. Even treatments that have been shown to be successful, such as stretching exercises, are debated in terms of techniques and practices. Surgical management is reserved for those who experience symptoms recalcitrant to conservative methods. A treatment algorithm for acute and chronic plantar fascia injury is represented below in keeping with the authors' experience and is based on available evidence noted in the studies reported in this chapter (Figs. 8.4 and 8.5).

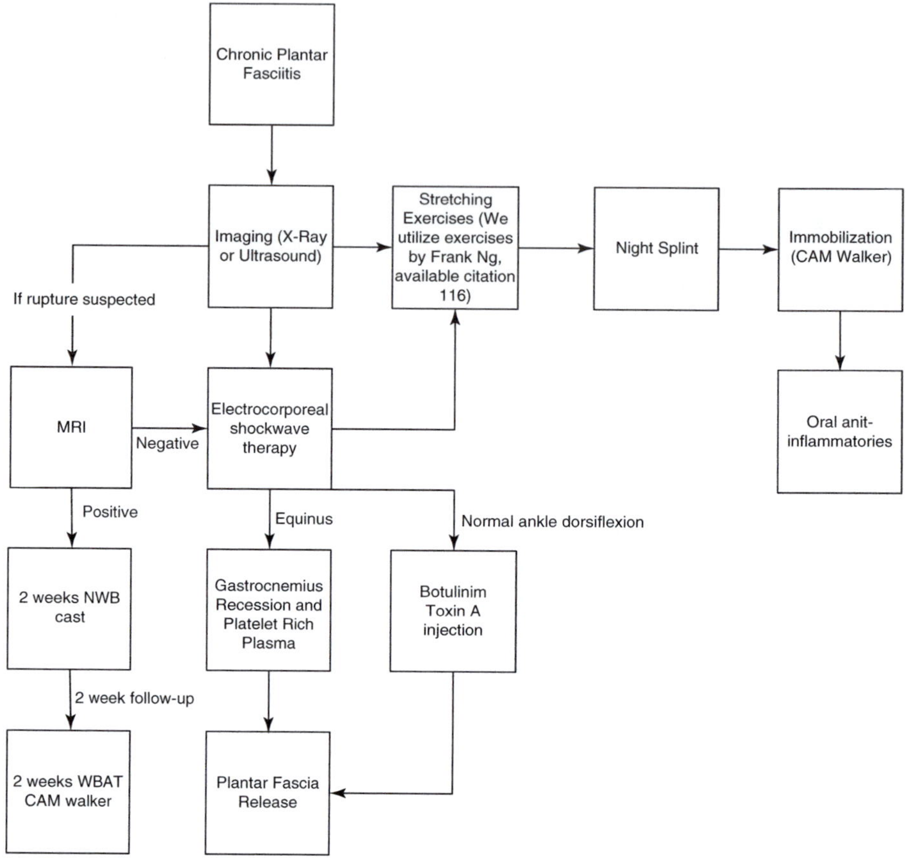

Fig. 8.5 Treatment algorithm is presented for the conservative and surgical management of *chronic* plantar fascia injury

Final Treatment Algorithm

References

1. Riddle DL, Schappert SM. Volume of ambulatory care visits and patterns of Care for Patients Diagnosed with plantar fasciitis: a National Study of medical doctors. Foot Ankle Int. 2004;25(5):303–10. https://doi.org/10.1177/107110070402500505.
2. Nahin RL. Prevalence and pharmaceutical treatment of plantar fasciitis in United States adults. J Pain. 2018;19(8):885–96. https://doi.org/10.1016/j.jpain.2018.03.003.
3. van Leeuwen KDB, Rogers J, Winzenberg T, et al. Higher body mass index is associated with plantar fasciopathy/'plantar fasciitis': systematic review and meta-analysis of various clinical and imaging risk factors. Br J Sports Med. 2016;50:972–81.
4. Riddle DL, Pulisic M, Pidcoe P, Johnson RE. Risk factors for plantar fasciitis: a matched case-control study. J Bone Joint Surg Am. 2003;85(5):872–7. https://doi.org/10.2106/00004623-200305000-00015.

5. Lee HS, Choi YR, Kim SW, Lee JY, Seo JH, Jeong JJ. Risk factors affecting chronic rupture of the plantar fascia. Foot Ankle Int. 2014;35(3):258–63. https://doi.org/10.1177/1071100713514564.
6. Sarrafian SK. Anatomy of the foot and ankle. Descriptive, topographic, functional. Philadelphia: J.B. Lippincott; 2011.
7. Zhang J, Nie D, Rocha JL, Hogan MV, Wang JH. Characterization of the structure, cells, and cellular mechanobiological response of human plantar fascia. J Tissue Eng. 2018;9:2041731418801103. https://doi.org/10.1177/2041731418801103.
8. Hicks JH. The mechanics of the foot, II: the plantar aponeurosis and the arch. J Anat. 1954;88:25–30.
9. Erdemir A, Hamel AJ, Fauth AR, Piazza SJ, Sharkey NA. Dynamic loading of the plantar aponeurosis in walking. J Bone Joint Surg Am. 2004;86(3):546–52. https://doi.org/10.2106/00004623-200403000-00013.
10. Kitaoka HB, Luo ZP, Growney ES, Berglund LJ, An KN. Material properties of the plantar aponeurosis. Foot Ankle Int. 1994;15(10):557–60. https://doi.org/10.1177/107110079401501007.
11. Wearing SC, Smeathers JE, Urry SR, Hennig EM, Hills AP. The pathomechanics of plantar fasciitis. Sports Med. 2006;36(7):585–611. https://doi.org/10.2165/00007256-200636070-00004.
12. Lemont H, Ammirati KM, Usen N. Plantar fasciitis: a degenerative process (fasciosis) without inflammation. J Am Podiatr Med Assoc. 2003;93(3):234–7. https://doi.org/10.7547/87507315-93-3-234.
13. Kirkpatrick J, Yassaie O, Mirjalili SA. The plantar calcaneal spur: a review of anatomy, histology, etiology and key associations. J Anat. 2017;230(6):743–51. https://doi.org/10.1111/joa.12607.
14. Kumai T, Benjamin M. Heel spur formation and the subcalcaneal enthesis of the plantar fascia. J Rheumatol. 2002;29(9):1957–64.
15. Lareau CR, Sawyer GA, Wang JH, DiGiovanni CW. Plantar and medial heel pain: diagnosis and management. J Am Acad Orthop Surg. 2014;22(6):372–80. https://doi.org/10.5435/JAAOS-22-06-372.
16. Levy JC, Mizel MS, Clifford PD, Temple HT. Value of radiographs in the initial evaluation of nontraumatic adult heel pain. Foot Ankle Int. 2006;27(6):427–30. https://doi.org/10.1177/107110070602700607.
17. McMillan AM, Landorf KB, Barrett JT, Menz HB, Bird AR. Diagnostic imaging for chronic plantar heel pain: a systematic review and meta-analysis. J Foot Ankle Res. 2009;2:32. https://doi.org/10.1186/1757-1146-2-32.
18. Karabay N, Toros T, Hurel C. Ultrasonographic evaluation in plantar fasciitis. J Foot Ankle Surg. 2007;46(6):442–6. https://doi.org/10.1053/j.jfas.2007.08.006.
19. Mahowald S, Legge BS, Grady JF. The correlation between plantar fascia thickness and symptoms of plantar fasciitis. J Am Podiatr Med Assoc. 2011;101(5):385–9. https://doi.org/10.7547/1010385.
20. Hall MM, Finnoff JT, Sayeed YA, Smith J. Sonographic evaluation of the plantar heel in asymptomatic endurance runners. J Ultrasound Med. 2015;34(10):1861–71. https://doi.org/10.7863/ultra.14.12073.
21. Sabir N, Demirlenk S, Yagci B, Karabulut N, Cubukcu S. Clinical utility of sonography in diagnosing plantar fasciitis. J Ultrasound Med. 2005;24(8):1041–8. https://doi.org/10.7863/jum.2005.24.8.1041.
22. Wall JR, Harkness MA, Crawford A. Ultrasound diagnosis of plantar fasciitis. Foot Ankle. 1993;14(8):465–70. https://doi.org/10.1177/107110079301400807.
23. Akfirat M, Sen C, Günes T. Ultrasonographic appearance of the plantar fasciitis. Clin Imaging. 2003;27(5):353–7. https://doi.org/10.1016/s0899-7071(02)00591-0.
24. Debus F, Eschbach D, Ruchholtz S, Peterlein CD. Rupture of plantar fascia: current standard of therapy: a systematic literature review. Foot Ankle Surg. 2020;26(4):358–62. https://doi.org/10.1016/j.fas.2019.05.006.

25. Acevedo J, Beskin J. Complications of plantar fascia rupture associated with corticosteroid injection. Foot Ankle Int. 1998;19:91–7.
26. Sellman JR. Plantar fascia rupture associated with corticosteroid injection. Foot Ankle Int. 1994;15:376–81.
27. Saxena A, Fullem B. Plantar fascia ruptures in athletes. Am J Sports Med. 2004;32(3):662–5. https://doi.org/10.1177/0363546503261727.
28. Ahstrom JP Jr. Spontaneous rupture of the plantar fascia. Am J Sports Med. 1988;16(3):306–7. https://doi.org/10.1177/036354658801600319.
29. Sichting F, Holowka NB, Ebrecht F, Lieberman DE. Evolutionary anatomy of the plantar aponeurosis in primates, including humans. J Anat. 2020;237:85–104. https://doi.org/10.1111/joa.13173.
30. Schneider HP, Baca JM, Carpenter BB, Dayton PD, Fleischer AE, Sachs BD. American College of Foot and Ankle Surgeons Clinical Consensus Statement: diagnosis and treatment of adult acquired infracalcaneal heel pain. J Foot Ankle Surg. 2018;57(2):370–81. https://doi.org/10.1053/j.jfas.2017.10.018.
31. Molund M, Husebye EE, Hellesnes J, Nilsen F, Hvaal K. Proximal medial gastrocnemius recession and stretching versus stretching as treatment of chronic plantar heel pain. Foot Ankle Int. 2018;39(12):1423–31. https://doi.org/10.1177/1071100718794659.
32. DiGiovanni CW, Kuo R, Tejwani N, et al. Isolated gastrocnemius tightness. J Bone Joint Surg Am. 2002;84(6):962–70. https://doi.org/10.2106/00004623-200206000-00010.
33. Engkananuwat P, Kanlayanaphotporn R, Purepong N. Effectiveness of the simultaneous stretching of the Achilles tendon and plantar fascia in individuals with plantar fasciitis. Foot Ankle Int. 2018;39(1):75–82. https://doi.org/10.1177/1071100717732762.
34. Bolívar YA, Munuera PV, Padillo JP. Relationship between tightness of the posterior muscles of the lower limb and plantar fasciitis. Foot Ankle Int. 2013;34(1):42–8. https://doi.org/10.1177/1071100712459173.
35. DiGiovanni BF, Nawoczenski DA, Lintal ME, et al. Tissue-specific plantar fascia-stretching exercise enhances outcomes in patients with chronic heel pain. A prospective, randomized study. J Bone Joint Surg Am. 2003;85(7):1270–7. https://doi.org/10.2106/00004623-200307000-00013.
36. Digiovanni BF, Nawoczenski DA, Malay DP, et al. Plantar fascia-specific stretching exercise improves outcomes in patients with chronic plantar fasciitis. A prospective clinical trial with two-year follow-up. J Bone Joint Surg Am. 2006;88(8):1775–81. https://doi.org/10.2106/JBJS.E.01281.
37. Porter D, Barrill E, Oneacre K, May BD. The effects of duration and frequency of Achilles tendon stretching on dorsiflexion and outcome in painful heel syndrome: a randomized, blinded, control study. Foot Ankle Int. 2002;23(7):619–24. https://doi.org/10.1177/107110070202300706.
38. Probe RA, Baca M, Adams R, Preece C. Night splint treatment for plantar fasciitis. A prospective randomized study. Clin Orthop Relat Res. 1999;368:190–5.
39. Powell M, Post WR, Keener J, Wearden S. Effective treatment of chronic plantar fasciitis with dorsiflexion night splints: a crossover prospective randomized outcome study. Foot Ankle Int. 1998;19(1):10–8. https://doi.org/10.1177/107110079801900103.
40. Dye RW. A strapping. 1939. J Am Podiatr Med Assoc. 2007;97(4):282–4. https://doi.org/10.7547/0970282.
41. Verbruggen LA, Thompson MM, Durall CJ. The effectiveness of low-dye taping in reducing pain associated with plantar fasciitis. J Sport Rehabil. 2018;27(1):94–8. https://doi.org/10.1123/jsr.2016-0030.
42. Landorf KB, Radford JA, Keenan AM, Redmond AC. Effectiveness of low-dye taping for the short-term management of plantar fasciitis. J Am Podiatr Med Assoc. 2005;95(6):525–30. https://doi.org/10.7547/0950525.
43. Radford JA, Landorf KB, Buchbinder R, Cook C. Effectiveness of low-dye taping for the short-term treatment of plantar heel pain: a randomised trial. BMC Musculoskelet Disord. 2006;7:64. https://doi.org/10.1186/1471-2474-7-64.

44. Kogler GF, Solomonidis SE, Paul JP. Biomechanics of longitudinal arch support mechanisms in foot orthoses and their effect on plantar aponeurosis strain. Clin Biomech (Bristol, Avon). 1996;11(5):243–52. https://doi.org/10.1016/0268-0033(96)00019-8.

45. Whittaker GA, Munteanu SE, Menz HB, Tan JM, Rabusin CL, Landorf KB. Foot orthoses for plantar heel pain: a systematic review and meta-analysis. Br J Sports Med. 2018;52(5):322–8. https://doi.org/10.1136/bjsports-2016-097355.

46. Gross MT, Byers JM, Krafft JL, Lackey EJ, Melton KM. The impact of custom semirigid foot orthotics on pain and disability for individuals with plantar fasciitis. J Orthop Sports Phys Ther. 2002;32(4):149–57. https://doi.org/10.2519/jospt.2002.32.4.149.

47. Redmond AC, Landorf KB, Keenan AM. Contoured, prefabricated foot orthoses demonstrate comparable mechanical properties to contoured, customised foot orthoses: a plantar pressure study. J Foot Ankle Res. 2009;2:20. https://doi.org/10.1186/1757-1146-2-20.

48. Landorf KB, Keenan AM, Herbert RD. Effectiveness of foot orthoses to treat plantar fasciitis: a randomized trial. Arch Intern Med. 2006;166(12):1305–10. https://doi.org/10.1001/archinte.166.12.1305.

49. Donley BG, Moore T, Sferra J, Gozdanovic J, Smith R. The efficacy of oral nonsteroidal anti-inflammatory medication (NSAID) in the treatment of plantar fasciitis: a randomized, prospective, placebo-controlled study. Foot Ankle Int. 2007;28(1):20–3. https://doi.org/10.3113/FAI.2007.0004.

50. Price DB, Trudo F, Voorham J, et al. Adverse outcomes from initiation of systemic corticosteroids for asthma: long-term observational study. J Asthma Allergy. 2018;11:193–204. https://doi.org/10.2147/JAA.S176026.

51. Waljee AK, Rogers MA, Lin P, et al. Short term use of oral corticosteroids and related harms among adults in the United States: population based cohort study. BMJ. 2017;357:j1415. https://doi.org/10.1136/bmj.j1415.

52. Ball EM, McKeeman HM, Patterson C, et al. Steroid injection for inferior heel pain: a randomised controlled trial. Ann Rheum Dis. 2013;72(6):996–1002. https://doi.org/10.1136/annrheumdis-2012-201508.

53. McMillan Andrew M, Landorf Karl B, Gilheany Mark F, Bird Adam R, Morrow Adam D, Menz Hylton B, et al. Ultrasound guided corticosteroid injection for plantar fasciitis: randomised controlled trial. BMJ. 2012;344:e3260.

54. Crawford F, Atkins D, Young P, Edwards J. Steroid injection for heel pain: evidence of short-term effectiveness. A randomized controlled trial. Rheumatology (Oxford). 1999;38(10):974–7. https://doi.org/10.1093/rheumatology/38.10.974.

55. Brinks A, Koes BW, Volkers AC, Verhaar JA, Bierma-Zeinstra SM. Adverse effects of extra-articular corticosteroid injections: a systematic review. BMC Musculoskelet Disord. 2010;11:206. https://doi.org/10.1186/1471-2474-11-206.

56. Anderson SE, Lubberts B, Strong AD, Guss D, Johnson AH, DiGiovanni CW. Adverse events and their risk factors following intra-articular corticosteroid injections of the ankle or subtalar joint. Foot Ankle Int. 2019;40(6):622–8. https://doi.org/10.1177/1071100719835759.

57. Wei AS, Callaci JJ, Juknelis D, et al. The effect of corticosteroid on collagen expression in injured rotator cuff tendon. J Bone Joint Surg Am. 2006;88(6):1331–8. https://doi.org/10.2106/JBJS.E.00806.

58. Haraldsson BT, Langberg H, Aagaard P, et al. Corticosteroids reduce the tensile strength of isolated collagen fascicles. Am J Sports Med. 2006;34(12):1992–7. https://doi.org/10.1177/0363546506290402.

59. Johannsen FE, Herzog RB, Malmgaard-Clausen NM, Hoegberget-Kalisz M, Magnusson SP, Kjaer M. Corticosteroid injection is the best treatment in plantar fasciitis if combined with controlled training. Knee Surg Sports Traumatol Arthrosc. 2019;27(1):5–12. https://doi.org/10.1007/s00167-018-5234-6.

60. Tsai WC, Hsu CC, Chen CP, Chen MJ, Yu TY, Chen YJ. Plantar fasciitis treated with local steroid injection: comparison between sonographic and palpation guidance. J Clin Ultrasound. 2006;34(1):12–6. https://doi.org/10.1002/jcu.20177.

61. Wang CJ. Extracorporeal shockwave therapy in musculoskeletal disorders. J Orthop Surg Res. 2012;7:11. https://doi.org/10.1186/1749-799X-7-11.

62. Malay DS, Pressman MM, Assili A, et al. Extracorporeal shockwave therapy versus placebo for the treatment of chronic proximal plantar fasciitis: results of a randomized, placebo-controlled, double-blinded, multicenter intervention trial. J Foot Ankle Surg. 2006;45(4):196–210. https://doi.org/10.1053/j.jfas.2006.04.007.

63. Gollwitzer H, Saxena A, DiDomenico LA, et al. Clinically relevant effectiveness of focused extracorporeal shock wave therapy in the treatment of chronic plantar fasciitis: a randomized, controlled multicenter study. J Bone Joint Surg Am. 2015;97(9):701–8. https://doi.org/10.2106/JBJS.M.01331.

64. Gerdesmeyer L. Extracorporeal shock wave therapy for chronic painful heel syndrome: a prospective, double blind, randomized trial assessing the efficacy of a new electromagnetic shock wave device. J Foot Ankle Surg. 2007;46(5):348–57. https://doi.org/10.1053/j.jfas.2007.05.011.

65. Marx RE. Platelet-rich plasma: evidence to support its use. J Oral Maxillofac Surg. 2004;62(4):489–96. https://doi.org/10.1016/j.joms.2003.12.003.

66. Wasterlain AS, Braun HJ, Harris AH, Kim HJ, Dragoo JL. The systemic effects of platelet-rich plasma injection. Am J Sports Med. 2013;41(1):186–93. https://doi.org/10.1177/0363546512466383.

67. Monto RR. Platelet-rich plasma efficacy versus corticosteroid injection treatment for chronic severe plantar fasciitis. Foot Ankle Int. 2014;35(4):313–8. https://doi.org/10.1177/1071100713519778.

68. Martinelli N, Marinozzi A, Carnì S, Trovato U, Bianchi A, Denaro V. Platelet-rich plasma injections for chronic plantar fasciitis. Int Orthop. 2013;37(5):839–42. https://doi.org/10.1007/s00264-012-1741-0.

69. Akşahin E, Doğruyol D, Yüksel HY, et al. The comparison of the effect of corticosteroids and platelet-rich plasma (PRP) for the treatment of plantar fasciitis. Arch Orthop Trauma Surg. 2012;132(6):781–5. https://doi.org/10.1007/s00402-012-1488-5.

70. Jain SK, Suprashant K, Kumar S, Yadav A, Kearns SR. Comparison of plantar fasciitis injected with platelet-rich plasma vs corticosteroids. Foot Ankle Int. 2018;39(7):780–6. https://doi.org/10.1177/1071100718762406.

71. Acosta-Olivo C, Elizondo-Rodriguez J, Lopez-Cavazos R, Vilchez-Cavazos F, Simental-Mendia M, Mendoza-Lemus O. Plantar fasciitis-a comparison of treatment with intralesional steroids versus platelet-rich plasma a randomized, blinded study. J Am Podiatr Med Assoc. 2017;107(6):490–6. https://doi.org/10.7547/15-125.

72. Zelen CM, Poka A, Andrews J. Prospective, randomized, blinded, comparative study of injectable micronized dehydrated amniotic/chorionic membrane allograft for plantar fasciitis—a feasibility study. Foot Ankle Int. 2013;34(10):1332–9.

73. Cazzell S, Stewart J, Agnew PS, et al. Randomized controlled trial of micronized dehydrated human amnion/chorion membrane (dHACM) injection compared to placebo for the treatment of plantar fasciitis. Foot Ankle Int. 2018;39(10):1151–61. https://doi.org/10.1177/1071100718788549.

74. Hanselman AE, Tidwell JE, Santrock RD. Cryopreserved human amniotic membrane injection for plantar fasciitis: a randomized, controlled, double-blind pilot study. Foot Ankle Int. 2015;36(2):151–8. https://doi.org/10.1177/1071100714552824.

75. Davies MS, Weiss GA, Saxby TS. Plantar fasciitis: how successful is surgical intervention? Foot Ankle Int. 1999;20(12):803–7. https://doi.org/10.1177/107110079902001209.

76. Brown JN, Roberts S, Taylor M, Paterson RS. Plantar fascia release through a transverse plantar incision. Foot Ankle Int. 1999;20(6):364–7. https://doi.org/10.1177/107110079902000604.

77. O'Malley MJ, Page A, Cook R. Endoscopic plantar fasciotomy for chronic heel pain. Foot Ankle Int. 2000;21(6):505–10. https://doi.org/10.1177/107110070002100610.

78. Fishco WD, Goecker RM, Schwartz RI. The instep plantar fasciotomy for chronic plantar fasciitis. A retrospective review. J Am Podiatr Med Assoc. 2000;90(2):66–9. https://doi.org/10.7547/87507315-90-2-66.

79. Woelffer KE, Figura MA, Sandberg NS, Snyder NS. Five-year follow-up results of instep plantar fasciotomy for chronic heel pain. J Foot Ankle Surg. 2000;39(4):218–23. https://doi.org/10.1016/s1067-2516(00)80003-4.

80. Boyle RA, Slater GL. Endoscopic plantar fascia release: a case series. Foot Ankle Int. 2003;24(2):176–9. https://doi.org/10.1177/107110070302400213.

81. Gibbons R, Mackie KE, Beveridge T, Hince D, Ammon P. Evaluation of long-term outcomes following plantar fasciotomy. Foot Ankle Int. 2018;39(11):1312–9. https://doi.org/10.1177/1071100718788546.

82. Wheeler P, Boyd K, Shipton M. Surgery for patients with recalcitrant plantar fasciitis: good results at short-, medium- and long-term follow-up. Orthop J Sports Med. 2014;2(3):1–6.

83. Sharkey NA, Ferris L, Donahue SW. Biomechanical consequences of plantar fascial release or rupture during gait: part I—disruptions in longitudinal arch conformation. Foot Ankle Int. 1998;19(12):812–20. https://doi.org/10.1177/107110079801901204.

84. Sharkey NA, Donahue SW, Ferris L. Biomechanical consequences of plantar fascial release or rupture during gait. Part II: alterations in forefoot loading. Foot Ankle Int. 1999;20(2):86–96. https://doi.org/10.1177/107110079902000204.

85. Thordarson DB, Kumar PJ, Hedman TP, Ebramzadeh E. Effect of partial versus complete plantar fasciotomy on the windlass mechanism. Foot Ankle Int. 1997;18(1):16–20. https://doi.org/10.1177/107110079701800104.

86. Murphy GA, Pneumaticos SG, Kamaric E, Noble PC, Trevino SG, Baxter DE. Biomechanical consequences of sequential plantar fascia release. Foot Ankle Int. 1998;19(3):149–52. https://doi.org/10.1177/107110079801900306.

87. Cheung JT, An KN, Zhang M. Consequences of partial and total plantar fascia release: a finite element study. Foot Ankle Int. 2006;27(2):125–32. https://doi.org/10.1177/107110070602700210.

88. Anderson DJ, Fallat LM, Savoy-Moore T. Computer-assisted assessment of lateral column movement following plantar fascial release: a cadaveric study. J Foot Ankle Surg. 2001;40(2):62–70. https://doi.org/10.1016/s1067-2516(01)80047-8.

89. Brugh AM, Fallat LM, Savoy-Moore RT. Lateral column symptomatology following plantar fascial release: a prospective study. J Foot Ankle Surg. 2002;41(6):365–71. https://doi.org/10.1016/s1067-2516(02)80082-5.

90. Bader L, Park K, Gu Y, O'Malley MJ. Functional outcome of endoscopic plantar fasciotomy. Foot Ankle Int. 2012;33(1):37–43. https://doi.org/10.3113/FAI.2012.0037.

91. Hofmeister EP, Elliott MJ, Juliano PJ. Endoscopic plantar fascia release: an anatomical study. Foot Ankle Int. 1995;16(11):719–23. https://doi.org/10.1177/107110079501601109.

92. Hawkins BJ, Langermen RJ Jr, Gibbons T, Calhoun JH. An anatomic analysis of endoscopic plantar fascia release. Foot Ankle Int. 1995;16(9):552–8. https://doi.org/10.1177/107110079501600907.

93. Morton TN, Zimmerman JP, Lee M, Schaber JD. A review of 105 consecutive uniport endoscopic plantar fascial release procedures for the treatment of chronic plantar fasciitis. J Foot Ankle Surg. 2013;52(1):48–52. https://doi.org/10.1053/j.jfas.2012.10.011.

94. Chou AC, Ng SY, Koo KO. Endoscopic plantar fasciotomy improves early postoperative results: a retrospective comparison of outcomes after endoscopic versus open plantar fasciotomy. J Foot Ankle Surg. 2016;55(1):9–15. https://doi.org/10.1053/j.jfas.2015.02.005.

95. Malahias MA, Cantiller EB, Kadu VV, Müller S. The clinical outcome of endoscopic plantar fascia release: a current concept review. Foot Ankle Surg. 2020;26(1):19–24. https://doi.org/10.1016/j.fas.2018.12.006.

96. Barrett SL, Day SV, Pignetti TT, Robinson LB. Endoscopic plantar fasciotomy: a multi-surgeon prospective analysis of 652 cases. J Foot Ankle Surg. 1995;34(4):400–6. https://doi.org/10.1016/S1067-2516(09)80011-2.

97. Abbassian A, Kohls-Gatzoulis J, Solan MC. Proximal medial gastrocnemius release in the treatment of recalcitrant plantar fasciitis. Foot Ankle Int. 2012;33(1):14–9. https://doi.org/10.3113/FAI.2012.0014.

98. Molund M, Paulsrud Ø, Ellingsen Husebye E, Nilsen F, Hvaal K. Results after gastrocnemius recession in 73 patients. Foot Ankle Surg. 2014;20(4):272–5. https://doi.org/10.1016/j.fas.2014.07.004.

99. Firth GB, McMullan M, Chin T, et al. Lengthening of the gastrocnemius-soleus complex: an anatomical and biomechanical study in human cadavers. J Bone Joint Surg Am. 2013;95(16):1489–96. https://doi.org/10.2106/JBJS.K.01638.

100. Mulhern JL, Protzman NM, Summers NJ, Brigido SA. Clinical outcomes following an open gastrocnemius recession combined with an endoscopic plantar fasciotomy. Foot Ankle Spec. 2018;11(4):330–4. https://doi.org/10.1177/1938640017733097.

101. Monteagudo M, Maceira E, Garcia-Virto V, Canosa R. Chronic plantar fasciitis: plantar fasciotomy versus gastrocnemius recession. Int Orthop. 2013;37(9):1845–50. https://doi.org/10.1007/s00264-013-2022-2.

102. Weil L Jr, Glover JP, Weil LS Sr. A new minimally invasive technique for treating plantar fasciosis using bipolar radiofrequency: a prospective analysis. Foot Ankle Spec. 2008;1(1):13–8. https://doi.org/10.1177/1938640007312318.

103. Tay KS, Ng YC, Singh IR, Chong KW. Open technique is more effective than percutaneous technique for TOPAZ radiofrequency coblation for plantar fasciitis. Foot Ankle Surg. 2012;18(4):287–92. https://doi.org/10.1016/j.fas.2012.05.001.

104. Sorensen MD, Hyer CF, Philbin TM. Percutaneous bipolar radiofrequency microdebridement for recalcitrant proximal plantar fasciosis. J Foot Ankle Surg. 2011;50(2):165–70. https://doi.org/10.1053/j.jfas.2010.11.002.

105. Gunes T, Bilgic E, Erdem M, et al. Effect of radiofrequency microtenotomy on degeneration of tendons: an experimental study on rabbits. Foot Ankle Surg. 2014;20(1):61–6. https://doi.org/10.1016/j.fas.2013.11.003.

106. Tasto JP, Cummings J, Medlock V, Hardesty R, Amiel D. Microtenotomy using a radiofrequency probe to treat lateral epicondylitis. Arthroscopy. 2005;21(7):851–60. https://doi.org/10.1016/j.arthro.2005.03.019.

107. Morrison RJM, Brock TM, Reed MR, Muller SD. Radiofrequency microdebridement versus surgical decompression for Achilles tendinosis: a randomized controlled trial. J Foot Ankle Surg. 2017;56(4):708–12. https://doi.org/10.1053/j.jfas.2017.01.049.

108. Blakey CM, O'Donnell J, Klaber I, et al. Radiofrequency microdebridement as an adjunct to arthroscopic surgical treatment for recalcitrant gluteal tendinopathy: a double-blind, randomized controlled trial. Orthop J Sports Med. 2020;8(1):2325967119895602. https://doi.org/10.1177/2325967119895602.

109. Babcock MS, Foster L, Pasquina P, Jabbari B. Treatment of pain attributed to plantar fasciitis with botulinum toxin a: a short-term, randomized, placebo-controlled, double-blind study. Am J Phys Med Rehabil. 2005;84(9):649–54. https://doi.org/10.1097/01.phm.0000176339.73591.d7.

110. Ahmad J, Ahmad SH, Jones K. Treatment of plantar fasciitis with botulinum toxin. Foot Ankle Int. 2017;38(1):1–7. https://doi.org/10.1177/1071100716666364.

111. Elizondo-Rodriguez J, Araujo-Lopez Y, Moreno-Gonzalez JA, Cardenas-Estrada E, Mendoza-Lemus O, Acosta-Olivo C. A comparison of botulinum toxin a and intralesional steroids for the treatment of plantar fasciitis: a randomized, double-blinded study. Foot Ankle Int. 2013;34(1):8–14. https://doi.org/10.1177/1071100712460215.

112. Abbasian M, Baghbani S, Barangi S, et al. Outcomes of ultrasound-guided gastrocnemius injection with botulinum toxin for chronic plantar fasciitis. Foot Ankle Int. 2020;41(1):63–8. https://doi.org/10.1177/1071100719875220.

113. Schaarup SO, Burgaard P, Johannsen FE. Surgical repair of complete plantar fascia ruptures in high-demand power athletes: an alternative treatment option. J Foot Ankle Surg. 2020;59(1):195–200. https://doi.org/10.1053/j.jfas.2019.07.018.

Medial Deltoid Ligament Injuries

Nacime Salomão Barbachan Mansur, Elijah Auch,
Eli Lerner Schmidt, and Cesar de Cesar Netto

Introduction

Deltoid ligament repairs are usually performed for acute lesions of this complex, whether there are additional lesions or not. Despite the lack of quality data in the literature to support this approach, its indication is advocated in order to prevent unfortunate outcomes such as ankle arthritis, medial ankle instability, and collapsing foot deformity [1–3].

Ankle fractures are the most common scenario resulting in acute deltoid ruptures; however, they may also occur with syndesmosis injuries, with lateral ligament lesions, or in isolation [4, 5]. Partial ruptures with no signs of instability or combined conditions may first undergo nonsurgical treatment with an immobilization and non-weight-bearing regimen [6]. Complete and conjoined ruptures can be repaired by arthroscopic or open techniques [7, 8].

Two indications for deltoid reconstruction include failure in deltoid ligament healing after ankle trauma leading to medial instability or deltoid ligament degeneration secondary to progressive collapsing foot deformity (PCFD) [1, 9]. These conditions are usually demanding for the patient, causing gradual ankle incapacity

N. S. B. Mansur (✉)
Department of Orthopaedic and Rehabilitation, Carver College of Medicine, University of Iowa, Iowa City, IA, USA

Departamento de Ortopedia e Traumatologia, Escola Paulista de Medicina, Universidade Federal de São Paulo, São Paulo, Brazil
e-mail: nacime@nacime.com.br

E. Auch · E. L. Schmidt · C. de Cesar Netto
Department of Orthopaedic and Rehabilitation, Carver College of Medicine, University of Iowa, Iowa City, IA, USA
e-mail: elijah-auch@uiowa.edu; eli-schmidt@uiowa.edu; cesar-netto@uiowa.edu

© Springer Nature Switzerland AG 2022
J. D. Cain, M. V. Hogan (eds.), *Tendon and Ligament Injuries of the Foot and Ankle*,
https://doi.org/10.1007/978-3-031-10490-9_9

and articular destruction [10]. Many techniques have been described for chronic deltoid ruptures, but none of them have established a standard of care [11]. Reconstruction and/or reinforcement are the current first choices for this condition, as repair alone has been shown to be associated with recurrence due the ligament quality [12].

Anatomy

Recent studies picture the deltoid complex in two main portions: the superficial layer and the deep layer. Four ligaments are described superficially: tibionavicular, tibiospring, tibiocalcaneal, and tibiotalar. The strongest of the four is the tibionavicular portion which is also the most important stabilizer with the ankle in external rotation. The tibiocalcaneal ligament is responsible for abduction, and the tibiospring ligament reaches the plantar calcaneonavicular ligament, adding strength to the medial arch (Fig. 9.1). All these structures emerge from the anterior colliculus [13–16].

The deep deltoid layer has two distinct portions: anterior and posterior. Anterior deep deltoid is the main medial talar restraint which prevents translation. The posterior portion, even though smaller, was found to be more prevalent in the general population according to recent publications. Proximal attachments of this layer are located in the intercollicular groove (Fig. 9.2).

A literature review by Yammine et al. in 2017 explored the incidence and characteristics of each deltoid portion, concluding that the deep posterior (100%), tibiospring (94%), tibionavicular (90%), tibiocalcaneal (85%), tibiotalar (80%), and deep anterior (63%) had an overall high prevalence in the population as demonstrated by the percentages for each. The tibionavicular ligament was found to be the longest and thinnest component of the entire medial deltoid complex [17].

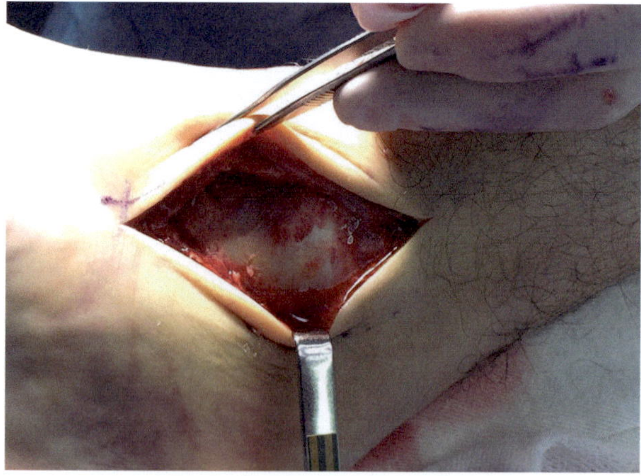

Fig. 9.1 Deltoid superficial layer

Fig. 9.2 Deltoid deep layer, visible after posterior tibial tendon retraction

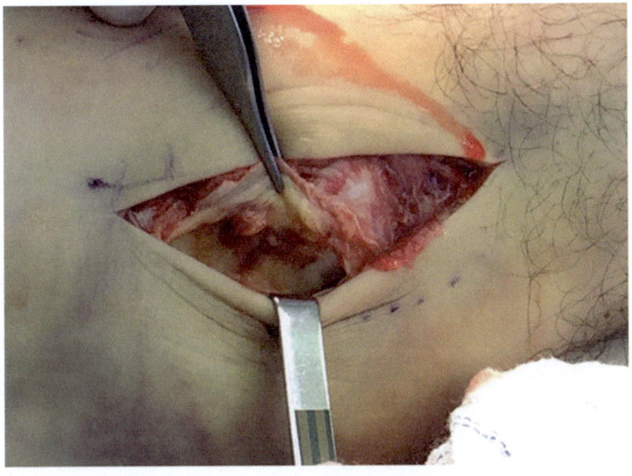

Clinical Evaluation

Acute

The majority of acute deltoid injuries occur in the ankle fracture scenario, usually in conjunction with malleolar fractures and/or syndesmosis lesions [18, 19]. Rotational traumas, combined with some degree of axial forces, cause an external spin and eversion movement to the talus [20, 21]. Inversion forces have the potential to cause a rupture to the deltoid as well. Ankle sprains, most often with eversion, may injure the deltoid, but lateral sprains can as well, adding more structures that may be combined to this particular situation [1, 22].

Clinical suspicion for deltoid injury increases when medial edema and ecchymosis are present, though these signs have a low positive predictive value for this injury [23]. Tenderness over the medial gutter and at the inframalleolar area are moderate indicators of deltoid injury [24]. Three classical maneuvers are described for deltoid ruptures and medial instability: valgus stress, anteromedial drawer, and Kleiger tests (Figs. 9.3, 9.4, and 9.5).

Radiographic signs, unless demonstrating a complete tibiotalar displacement, are not reliable for diagnostic confirmation [25, 26]. Medial clear space can change in accordance with ankle position (talar dome anatomy), and, although helpful, weight-bearing radiographs are not always possible to perform. Stress radiographs, as described in the literature, are vastly variable as they depend on patient conformity and perfect positioning [27, 28]. Ultrasound (US) is also a significant tool when analyzing these patients as it permits movement to the joint and allows dynamism to the assessment [23, 29].

When compared to syndesmosis or Lisfranc lesions, the dilemma among lesion and instability is also present in acute deltoid injuries. This is one of the main reasons magnetic resonance imaging (MRI) is not a definitive subsidiary exam when dealing with this type of lesion [22, 25]. A complete tear of the deep and superficial

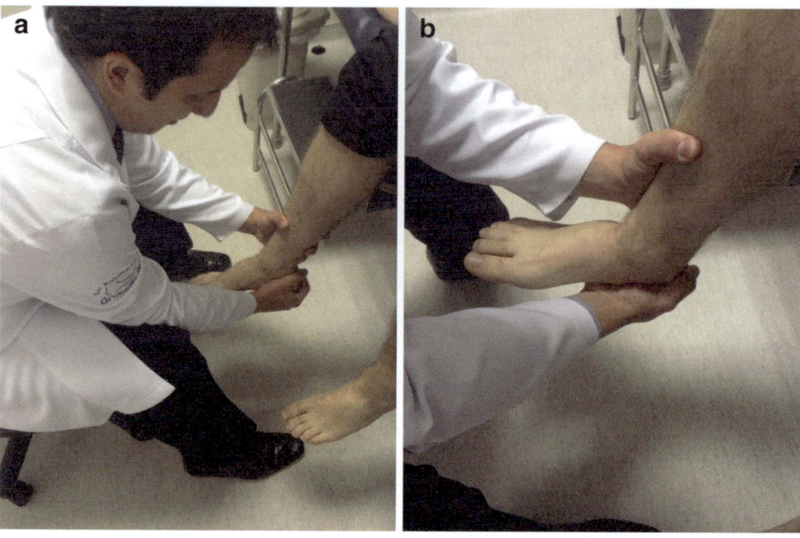

Fig. 9.3 (**a, b**) Valgus stress test. Patient is placed seated on stretcher with the legs dangling and the examiner sitting in front. With one hand, the leg is held at this distal and lateral region as the other hand embraces the calcaneus from its plantar aspect. The hindfoot is everted and compared to the contralateral side. Increase in valgus movement or pain at the deltoid area is considered positive

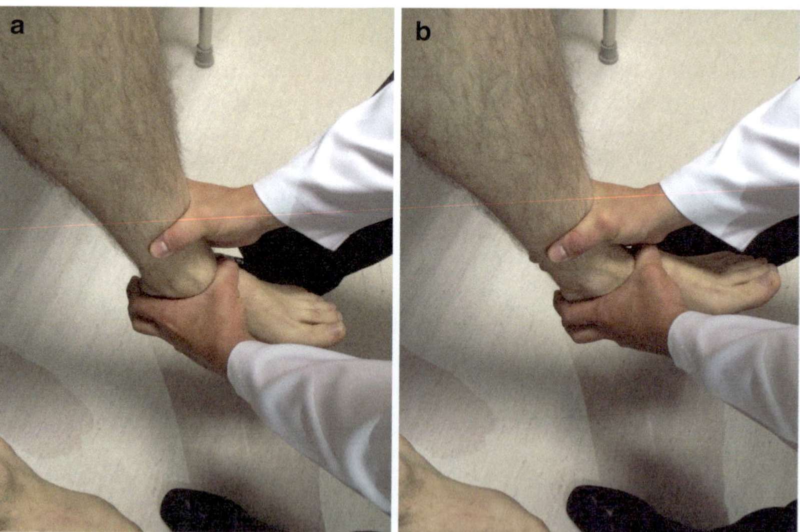

Fig. 9.4 (**a, b**) Anteromedial drawer test. Patient is placed seated on stretcher with the legs dangling and the examiner sitting in front. With one hand, the leg is held at this distal and lateral region as the other hand embraces the calcaneus from its posterior to anterior aspect, from its medial side, placing the index and middle fingers at the heel and the thumb at the talar neck region. Anterior translation of the hindfoot combined with external rotation is applied and compared with the contralateral side. Increase in translation or rotation is considered positive

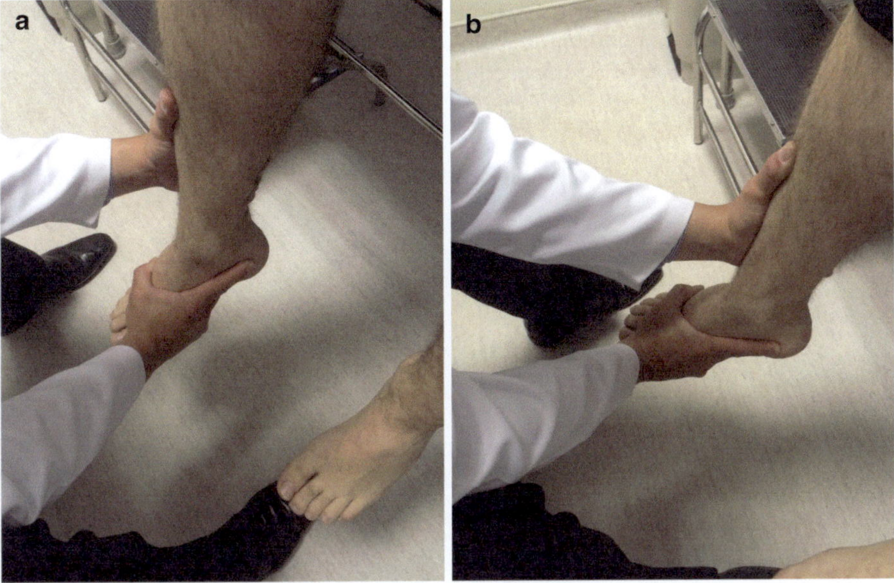

Fig. 9.5 (**a, b**) Kleiger test. Patient is placed seated on stretcher with the legs dangling and the examiner sitting in front. With one hand, the leg is held at this distal and lateral region as the other hand embraces the midfoot and forefoot from its medial side. With the ankle in plantarflexion, the foot is externally rotated. Pain at the deltoid topography is considered positive

layers is a strong indicator of acute medial instability. High-degree lesions should be evaluated under the unstable perspective, especially if associated lesions are present [30]. Partial ruptures have a trend for stability, although this is not a certainty [31]. Weight-bearing computed tomography (WBCT) and nano scope are new diagnostic options in determining medial instability outside the surgical ambient [32, 33].

The final diagnosis of a deltoid tear and for acute medial ankle instability still relies on the combination of clinical findings and imaging since no gold-standard and conclusive diagnostic method is established [23]. Nortunen et al. in 2014 were able to demonstrate that the MRI was not suitable for clinical decision-making regarding lesion and acute instability of this area. Correlation between medial clear space and rupture identification was reasonable. Ultrasound was found to have a high specificity and sensitivity although the tests were performed in sedated patients [34]. Arthroscopy, an invasive diagnostic method, still remains the standard for deltoid rupture confirmation [35].

Chronic

Complete and unstable deltoid injuries have unpredictable healing, especially if not properly treated [1, 12]. Poor deltoid ligament repair may lead to chronic pain and late-onset medial ankle instability [36]. Patients generally remember a previous acute ankle trauma and complain about achiness at the medial joint aspect [3, 9]. Instability or sensation of losing medial restraint could be evident, in addition to changes in footstep pattern [11].

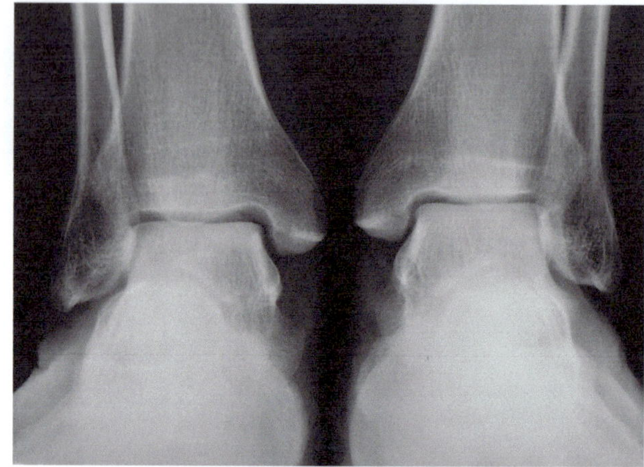

Fig. 9.6 Right talar tilt in a weight-bearing radiograph of a patient with chronic medial ankle instability

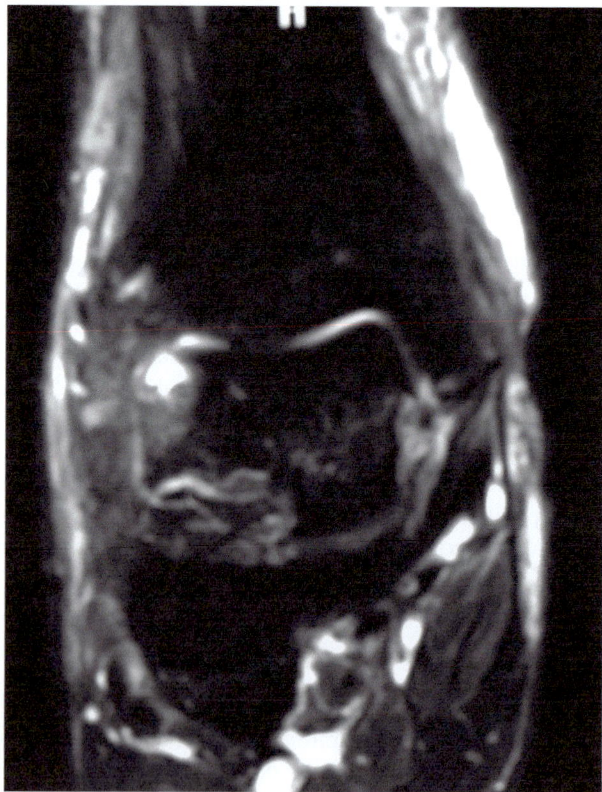

Fig. 9.7 Deltoid heterogenicity in a T2 coronal MR image

Physical inspection may reveal an asymmetric collapsed foot deformity (flatfoot) that can be corrected with posterior tibial tendon (PTT) activation [9, 37]. Pain when palpating the medial ankle gutter is a common and relevant finding in this condition. PTT may have signs of overuse, as well as other medial structures. The same maneuvers for the acute setting may be performed here, and if an established deformity is observed, flexibility evaluation should be performed.

Standing bilateral radiographs might demonstrate signs of previous deltoid injuries in the form of calcifications around ligament topography [38]. Valgus talar tilting (Fig. 9.6), even subtle, should be considered a primary indication of joint instability [9]. US might portrait the erratic ligament healing, structures in overload, and abnormal movement at the ankle.

MRI, as for the acute cases, is not able to diagnose instability but has a high capacity in showing signs of previous deltoid injuries such as areas of ligament disinsertion, tissue heterogenicity (Fig. 9.7), and calcification [1, 9, 39]. WBCT has the capability of confirming medial instability directly by displaying a valgus orientation of the talus as well as other common associated instabilities, such as syndesmosis and midtarsal instability. Baropodometry or gait analysis might suggest an asymmetric sagging and/or medial overload (Fig. 9.8).

Fig. 9.8 Baropodometry picturing the modification of the foot strike pattern

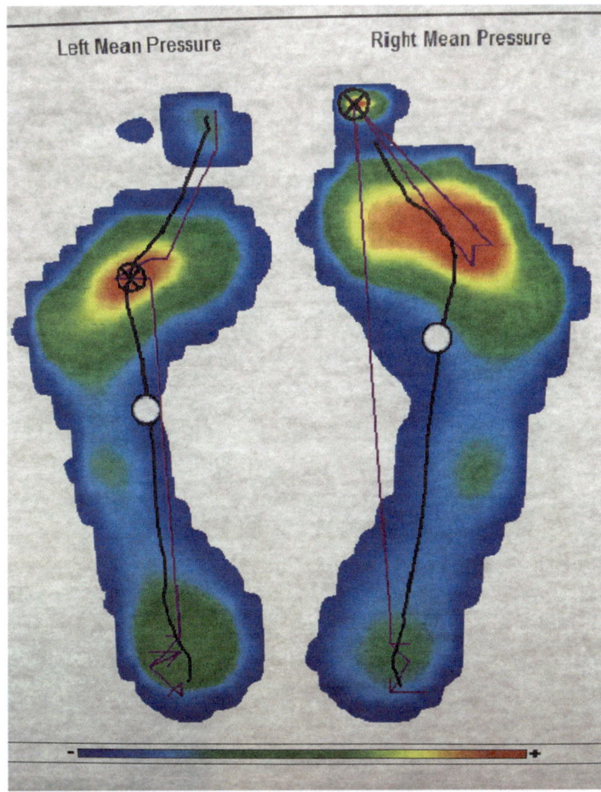

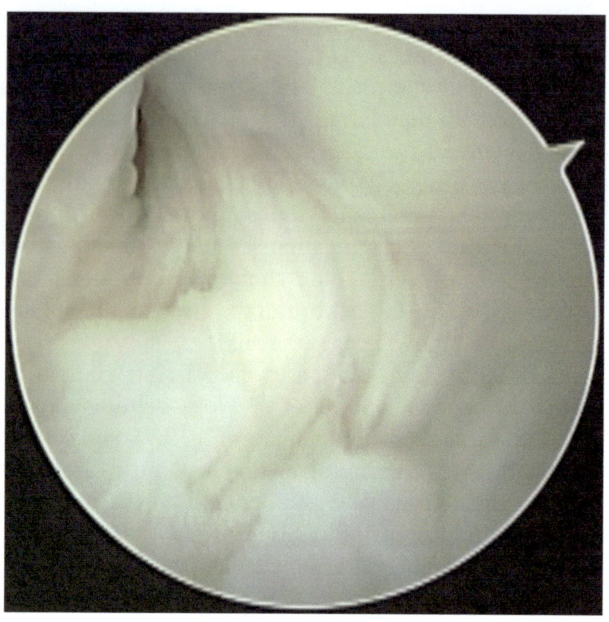

Fig. 9.9 Medial joint opening and deltoid degeneration visible during ankle arthroscopy

Differential diagnoses for medial ankle instability include primary progressive collapsing foot deformity (previously adult acquired flatfoot deformity), osteochondral talar lesions, PTT tendinopathy, isolated tibiospring injuries, and medial malleolus stress fractures [9, 40]. Arthroscopic assessment remains the standard in confirming chronic medial instability [11]. The ability of inserting a 5 mm probe into the medial gutter (or medial clear space) and the observation of indirect signs of poor deltoid healing support the diagnoses (Fig. 9.9).

Treatment

Acute

Management of an acute deltoid lesion is still based on poor evidence. No high-quality data that could guide clinicians on the decision regarding the necessity of repairing a deltoid lesion in an ankle fracture scenario was produced since the trial by Stromsoe et al. in 1995 [41]. This study supported many surgeons in defending a non-approach to this injury despite its methodological problems. Moderate comparative articles have shown conflicting results regarding functional and radiographic outcomes [42, 43]. Lack of long-term clinical data to back the non-approach and concerns regarding the late effects of poor deltoid healing are the main reasons for surgical attempts to repair the ligaments [36, 43].

This controversy could be extended to deltoid lesions that are isolated or associated with other ankle ligament injuries with literature that is even more scarce [22]. Choosing how to repair the medial complex is also debatable, with direct stump sutures, superficial reinsertion with an anchor, superficial and deep reinsertions with anchors, and arthroscopic techniques having been described over the last several years [8, 22]. No superiority of any method has been established.

Postoperative care of acute lesions usually requires a non-weight-bearing regimen (4 to 6 weeks) in order to unload the healing deltoid. Range of motion is started at 2 to 3 weeks, but eversion and external rotation are not allowed until the sixth week. Loading is initiated and progressively increased in a boot (2 weeks) and in an ankle brace thereafter (4 weeks).

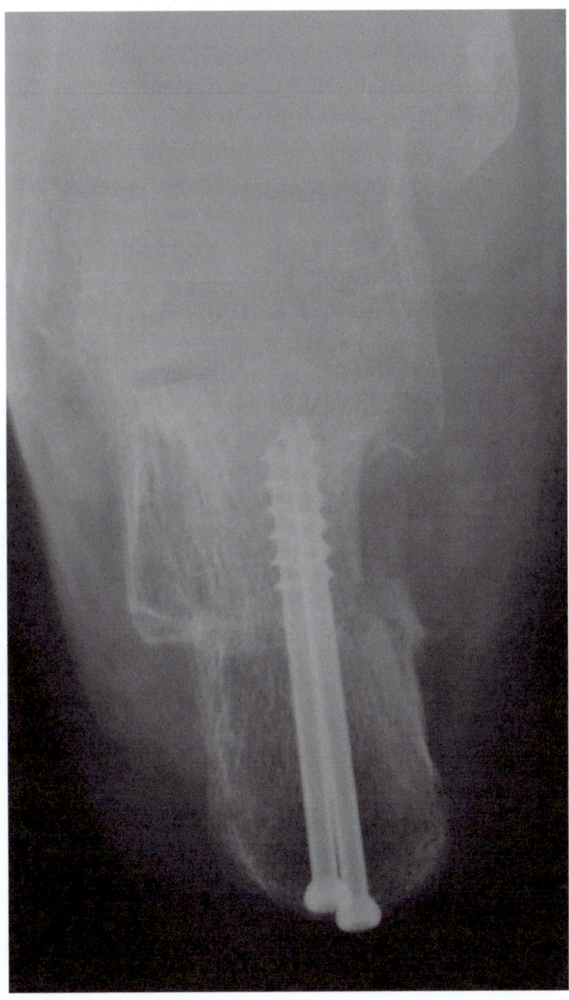

Fig. 9.10 Example of a calcaneal osteotomy, a procedure often necessary in chronic cases

Chronic

Different from the acute state, chronic medial ankle instabilities commonly receive surgical treatment due to its intrinsic deleterious feature [1, 10, 44]. Nonoperative approach is reserved only for extremely morbid patients. Tissue viability for retensioning or ligamentoplasty has been put into question over the last several years and has led authors to invest in reconstruction using grafts or synthetic materials [45]. When PCFD is evident, bone alignment procedures should be performed to properly treat the condition and protect the ligaments [46, 47].

Reconstruction techniques usually utilize allografts and autografts, although some authors still rely on the plication of the native ligament with the use of anchors. For reconstruction, one tunnel is performed at the tibia, another at the medial talar body, and the last at the calcaneus. Several implants might be used for fixation, and the tibiospring ligament may also be included in the reconstruction when necessary [48–51]. Osteotomies for ankle or foot realignment should always be considered in chronic patients (Fig. 9.10). Malleolar fracture sequelae must be assessed in conjunction with proper fibula and tibia correction. PCFD guidelines for the use of medializing calcaneus osteotomies (MCO), Evans, Cotton, Lapidus, Spring, and tendon transfer procedures need to be respected when this intra-articular deformity is present [52].

Evidence-Based/Critical Appraisal of the Literature

A comprehensive literature search was performed, with no time limit to maximize the pool of work available, conforming to the PRISMA statement. The databases used were PubMed, CINAHL, and EMBASE. The article abstracts were reviewed, and those that were not involving humans, the management of deltoid ligament injuries, nor had English translation if original articles were not in English were excluded. The search found a literature review of deltoid ligament injuries, which provided further articles that were available for analysis.

No systematic reviews (SR) of randomized controlled trials (RCTs) regarding acute and chronic deltoid injury were published in the indexed database. Dabash et al. conducted a SR for deltoid ligament repair in ankle fractures but was only able to include one RCT [41] and four retrospective cohorts [41, 53]. Although likely due to the quality of data analyzed, the study concluded there was an absence of a clear indication for reparation, even though some biomechanical advantages could occur.

A meta-analysis of comparative studies for deltoid repair was performed in the same year by Salameh et al. and found superior radiological reduction results for patients having the ligament sutured [54]. No functional differences were observed among the two groups.

Another SR about the subject was published in 2009 by van de Bekerom et al. that evaluated diagnostic methods for deltoid lesions [23]. The author found nine studies that concluded that Lauge-Hansen classification, radiographs, and clinical findings (swelling, ecchymoses, medial pain) were poor predictors of lesions and/or instability. External rotation stress radiographs showing more than 5 mm of medial space widening were noticed to be a reliable method to suspect the injury, although the review claimed that no definitive conclusion could be reached by using only one finding in clinical decision [55].

The presence of RCTs is also very scarce for both themes. Only Stromsoe et al. in 1995 tried to compare deltoid suture with a non-approach in ankle fracture patients ultimately finding no clinical difference among groups. Although it carries a myriad of methodological problems, it is still the only level one study published on acute deltoid treatment to this day [41].

Chronic deltoid injuries and medial ankle instabilities (MAI) have few strong supporting publications in the literature for diagnosis, decision-making, and treatment, likely due to its epidemiology. Most of the clinical judgment is based on case series and expert opinions [1, 10]. In the clinical setting, medial gutter pain and asymmetric valgus seem to be valuable findings during investigation. Subsidiary exams, with indirect discoveries, sustain the diagnosis, but, once again, are merely descriptions in articles regarding authors' experiences. The available procedures to address medial ankle instability are generally technical descriptions with some small case series.

Final Treatment Algorithm

Acute

Author's preference based on the literature for acute cases (regarding the deltoid approach) begins with the clinical decision constructed on a combination of physical exam (medial tenderness and deltoid provocative maneuvers) and subsidiary findings (valgus tilt, widening, ligament heterogenicity and detachment). The diagnosis threshold for active and young patients should be low in order to prevent mistreatment of an important lesion. Partial lesions with no signs of acute instability should be treated nonoperatively with a 2–3-week non-weight-bearing regimen followed by a brace for 3–4 weeks.

Complete ruptures and acute medial instabilities must receive surgical care. A medial longitudinal approach from the medial malleolus toward the navicular is pursued and the posterior tibial tendon sheath opened to allow access to the deltoid deep portion. An anchor is inserted at the medial talus body and sutures are passed through the deep deltoid. Another anchor is placed in the anterior colliculus of the medial malleolus, and sutures are passed through the tibionavicular and the tibiospring components of the superficial layer (Fig. 9.11). The constructed is then tightened with the ankle in mild inversion. Arthroscopic reinsertion is a less invasive possibility for select cases and is performed with anchor insertion at the quadrant described by Vega and arthroscopic sutures at the deltoid topography (Fig. 9.12) [8, 56].

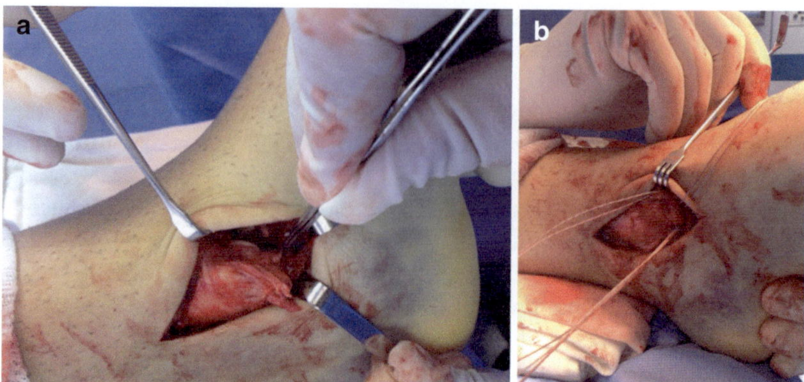

Fig. 9.11 Medial approach to an acute deltoid repair. Visualization of the superficial rupture at the medial malleolus and the deep rupture at the talus (**a**). After anchor insertion in these sites, sutures are passed through the ligaments. Tightening is completed (**b**) subsequently to finalization of other possible procedures (lateral ligaments, syndesmosis, malleolar fractures, etc.)

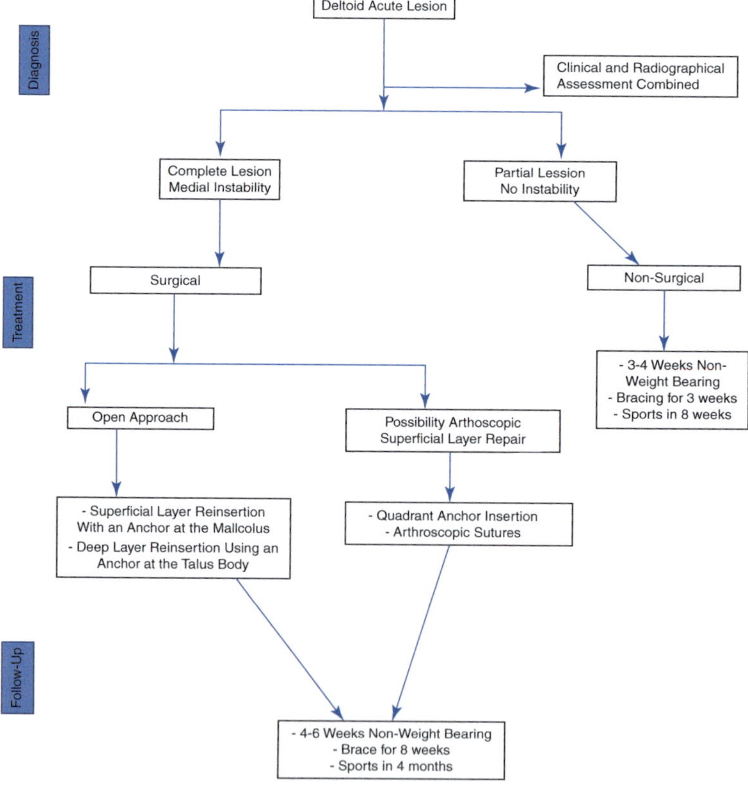

Fig. 9.12 Author's flowchart for deltoid acute lesions based on the strongest available evidence

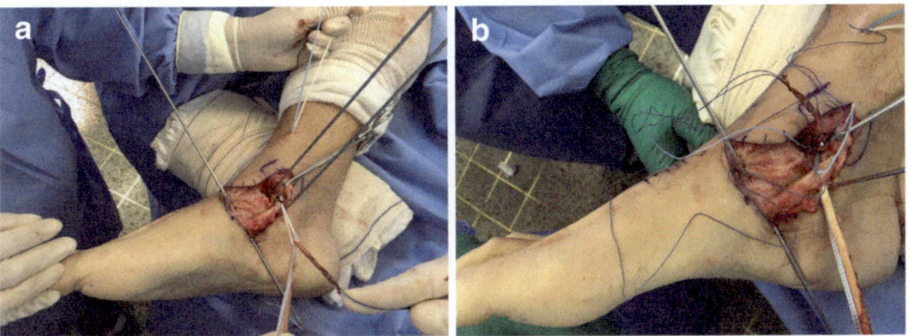

Fig. 9.13 Chronic medial instability reconstruction using a free graft. The malleolar tunnel is performed, and the folded semitendinosus graft passed and secured with a tibial button (**a**). After talus and calcaneus tunnels are completed, graft parts are inserted and stabilized with interference screws. If needed, the remaining graft may be used to reconstruct the spring ligament complex (**b**)

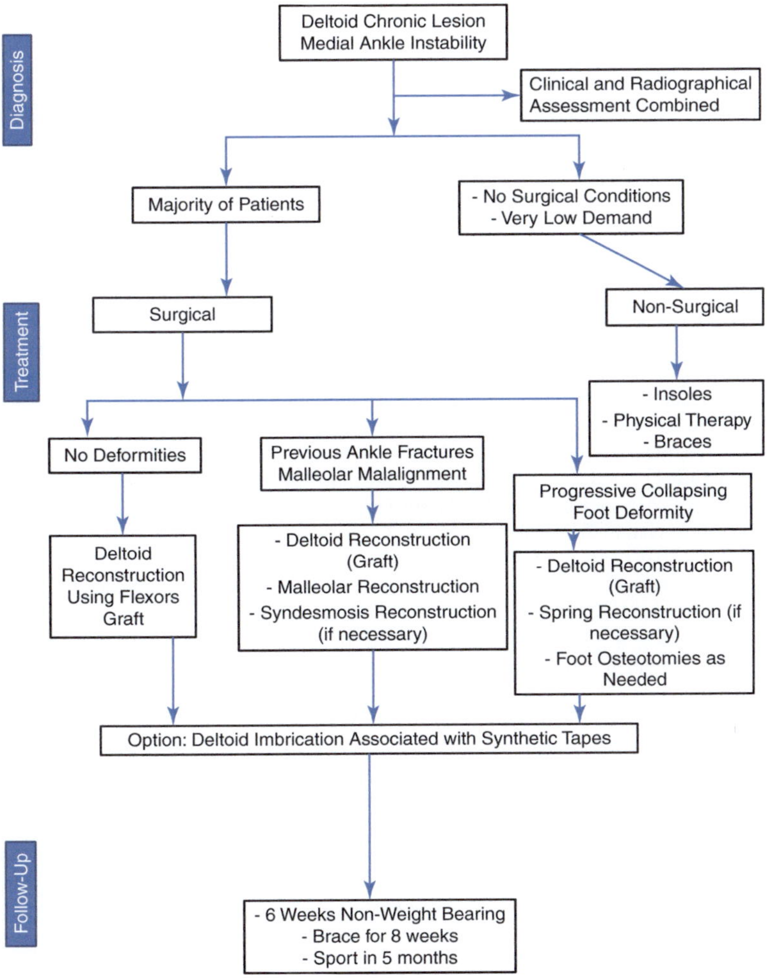

Fig. 9.14 Author's flowchart for deltoid chronic lesions based on the strongest available evidence

Chronic

Clinical findings for chronic deltoid lesions and medial ankle instabilities may be more challenging compared to acute injuries. The diagnosis in some cases may be obscure, but patients typically present with medial gutter pain and a mild change in walking stride. History of trauma should be considered, and indirect radiographic findings such as talar tilting, flattening, deltoid calcification, and ligament degeneration should support the investigation.

Only patients with nonsurgical conditions and extremely low demand should proceed with nonoperative treatment. Operative planning must consider the necessity for malleolar reconstructions and PCFD procedures [1]. Author's preferred technique for the deltoid uses a semitendinosus graft folded in two and then inserted in a medial malleolus tunnel and finally fixed with a button [48]. One bundle is inserted through a tunnel in the medial talar body and the other (after passing underneath the PTT), via another tunnel, below the medial calcaneal facet (Fig. 9.13). After positioning the ankle and foot in mild varus, the graft is secured with interference screws. Deltoid imbrication using anchors and augmented with synthetic tapes (using similar reconstruction tunnels) is a technical option (Fig. 9.14) [39, 45].

References

1. Alshalawi S, Galhoum AE, Alrashidi Y, Wiewiorski M, Herrera M, Barg A, et al. Medial ankle instability: the deltoid dilemma. Foot Ankle Clin. 2018;23(4):639–57.
2. Lee TH, Jang KS, Choi GW, Jeong CD, Hong SJ, Yoon MA, et al. The contribution of anterior deltoid ligament to ankle stability in isolated lateral malleolar fractures. Injury. 2016;47(7):1581–5.
3. Knupp M, Lang TH, Zwicky L, Lötscher P, Hintermann B. Chronic ankle instability (medial and lateral). Clin Sports Med. 2015;34(4):679–88.
4. Kopec TJ, Hibberd EE, Roos KG, Djoko A, Dompier TP, Kerr ZY. The epidemiology of deltoid ligament sprains in 25 National Collegiate Athletic Association Sports, 2009–2010 through 2014–2015 academic years. J Athl Train. 2017;52(4):350–9.
5. Lee S, Lin J, Hamid KS, Bohl DD. Deltoid ligament rupture in ankle fracture. J Am Acad Orthop Surg. 2019;27(14):e648–58.
6. Ortiz CA, Wagner P, Wagner E. State-of-the-art in ankle fracture Management in Chile. Foot Ankle Clin. 2016;21(2):367–89.
7. Hsu AR, Lareau CR, Anderson RB. Repair of acute superficial deltoid complex avulsion during ankle fracture fixation in National Football League Players. Foot Ankle Int. 2015;36(11):1272–8.
8. Acevedo JI, Kreulen C, Cedeno AA, Baumfeld D, Nery C, Mangone PG. Technique for arthroscopic deltoid ligament repair with description of safe zones. Foot Ankle Int. 2020;41(5):605–11.
9. Ribbans WJ, Garde A. Tibialis posterior tendon and deltoid and spring ligament injuries in the elite athlete. Foot Ankle Clin. 2013;18(2):255–91.
10. Alshalawi S, Galhoum AE, Alrashidi Y, Wiewiorski M, Herrera M, Barg A, et al. Medial ankle instability. Foot Ankle Clin. 2018;23(4):639–57.
11. Hintermann B. Medial ankle instability: an exploratory, prospective study of fifty-two cases. Am J Sports Med. 2004;32(1):183–90.

12. Jeng CL, Bluman EM, Myerson MS. Minimally Invasive Deltoid Ligament Reconstruction for Stage IV Flatfoot deformity. Foot Ankle Int. 2011;32(1):21–30.
13. Boss AP, Hintermann B. Anatomical study of the medial ankle ligament complex. Foot Ankle Int. 2002;23(6):547–53.
14. Cromeens BP, Kirchhoff CA, Patterson RM, Motley T, Stewart D, Fisher C, et al. An attachment-based description of the medial collateral and spring ligament complexes. Foot Ankle Int. 2015;36(6):710–21.
15. Panchani PN, Chappell TM, Moore GD, Tubbs RS, Shoja MM, Loukas M, et al. Anatomic study of the deltoid ligament of the ankle. Foot Ankle Int. 2014;35(9):916–21.
16. Campbell KJ, Michalski MP, Wilson KJ, Goldsmith MT, Wijdicks CA, Laprade RF, et al. The ligament anatomy of the deltoid complex of the ankle: a qualitative and quantitative anatomical study. J Bone Joint Surg Am. 2014;96(8):e62.
17. Yammine K. The morphology and prevalence of the deltoid complex ligament of the ankle. Foot Ankle Spec. 2017;10(1):55–62.
18. Debieux P, Wajnsztejn A, Mansur NSB. Epidemiology of injuries due to ankle sprain diagnosed in an orthopedic emergency room. Einstein (São Paulo). 2019;18:eAO4739.
19. Wei F, Villwock MR, Meyer EG, Powell JW, Haut RC. A biomechanical investigation of ankle injury under excessive external foot rotation in the human cadaver. J Biomech Eng. 2010;132(9):091001.
20. Bartoníček J, Rammelt S, Kašper Š, Malík J, Tuček M. Pathoanatomy of Maisonneuve fracture based on radiologic and CT examination. Arch Orthop Trauma Surg. 2019;139(4):497–506.
21. Wei F, Post JM, Braman JE, Meyer EG, Powell JW, Haut RC. Eversion during external rotation of the human cadaver foot produces high ankle sprains. J Orthop Res. 2012;30(9):1423–9.
22. Giza E, Wuellner J. Acute deltoid rupture: history, diagnosis, and a repair technique. Tech Foot Ankle Surg. 2014;13(2):73–80.
23. den Bekerom MPJ, Mutsaerts ELAR, Dijk CN. Evaluation of the integrity of the deltoid ligament in supination external rotation ankle fractures: a systematic review of the literature. Arch Orthop Trauma Surg. 2009;129(2):227–35.
24. Stenquist DS, Miller C, Velasco B, Cronin P, Kwon JY. Medial tenderness revisited: is medial ankle tenderness predictive of instability in isolated lateral malleolus fractures? Injury. 2020;51(6):1392–6.
25. Bäcker HC, Vosseller JT, Bonel H, Cullmann-Bastian J, Krause F, Attinger MC. Weightbearing radiography and MRI findings in ankle fractures. Foot Ankle Spec. 2021;14(6):489–95.
26. Nwosu K, Schneiderman BA, Shymon SJ, Harris T. A medial Malleolar "fleck sign" may predict ankle instability in ligamentous supination external rotation ankle fractures. Foot Ankle Spec. 2018;11(3):246–51.
27. van Leeuwen C, Haak T, Kop M, Weil N, Zijta F, Hoogendoorn J. The additional value of gravity stress radiographs in predicting deep deltoid ligament integrity in supination external rotation ankle fractures. Eur J Trauma Emerg Surg. 2019;45(4):727–35.
28. Baumfeld D, Baumfeld T, Cangussú J, Macedo B, Silva TAA, Raduan F, et al. Does foot position and location of measurement influence ankle medial clear space? Foot Ankle Spec. 2018;11(1):32–6.
29. Allen GM, Wilson DJ, Bullock SA, Watson M. Extremity CT and ultrasound in the assessment of ankle injuries: occult fractures and ligament injuries. Br J Radiol. 2020;93(1105):20180989.
30. Warner SJ, Garner MR, Fabricant PD, Schottel PC, Loftus ML, Hentel KD, et al. The diagnostic accuracy of radiographs and magnetic resonance imaging in predicting deltoid ligament ruptures in ankle fractures. HSS J. 2019;15(2):115–21.
31. Aiyer AA, Zachwieja EC, Lawrie CM, Kaplan JRM. Management of isolated lateral malleolus fractures. J Am Acad Orthop Surg. 2019;27(2):50–9.
32. Lepojärvi S, Niinimäki J, Pakarinen H, Leskelä H-V. Rotational dynamics of the normal distal tibiofibular joint with weight-bearing computed tomography. Foot Ankle Int. 2016;37(6):627–35.

33. Krähenbühl N, Bailey TL, Presson AP, Allen CM, Henninger HB, Saltzman CL, et al. Torque application helps to diagnose incomplete syndesmotic injuries using weight-bearing computed tomography images. Skelet Radiol. 2019;48(9):1367–76.
34. Henari S, Banks LN, Radiovanovic I, Queally J, Morris S. Ultrasonography as a diagnostic tool in assessing deltoid ligament injury in supination external rotation fractures of the ankle. Orthopedics. 2011;34(10):e639–43.
35. Chen X-Z, Chen Y, Liu C-G, Yang H, Xu X-D, Lin P. Arthroscopy-assisted surgery for acute ankle fractures: a systematic review. Arthroscopy. 2015;31(11):2224–31.
36. Jelinek JA, Porter DA. Management of unstable ankle fractures and syndesmosis injuries in athletes. Foot Ankle Clin. 2009;14(2):277–98.
37. Smith JT, Bluman EM. Update on stage IV acquired adult flatfoot disorder when the deltoid ligament becomes dysfunctional. Foot Ankle Clin. 2012;17(2):351–60.
38. Clanton TO, Williams BT, James EW, Campbell KJ, Rasmussen MT, Haytmanek CT, et al. Radiographic identification of the deltoid ligament complex of the medial ankle. Am J Sports Med. 2015;43(11):2753–62.
39. Pellegrini MJ, Torres N, Cuchacovich NR, Huertas P, Muñoz G, Carcuro GM. Chronic deltoid ligament insufficiency repair with internal brace™ augmentation. Foot Ankle Surg. 2019;25(6):812–8.
40. Bluman EM, Myerson MS. Stage IV posterior tibial tendon rupture. Foot Ankle Clin. 2007;12:341–62.
41. Strömsöe K, Höqevold HE, Skjeldal S, Alho A. The repair of a ruptured deltoid ligament is not necessary in ankle fractures. J Bone Joint Surg Br. 1995;77-B(6):920–1.
42. Zhao H-M, Lu J, Zhang F, Wen X-D, Li Y, Hao D-J, et al. Surgical treatment of ankle fracture with or without deltoid ligament repair: a comparative study. BMC Musculoskelet Disord. 2017;18(1):543.
43. Butler BA, Hempen EC, Barbosa M, Muriuki M, Havey RM, Nicolay RW, et al. Deltoid ligament repair reduces and stabilizes the talus in unstable ankle fractures. J Orthop. 2020;17:87–90.
44. Lack W, Phisitkul P, Femino JE. Anatomic deltoid ligament repair with anchor-to-post suture reinforcement: technique tip. Iowa Orthop J. 2012;32:227–30.
45. Nery C, Lemos AVKC, Raduan F, Mansur NSB, Baumfeld D. Combined spring and deltoid ligament repair in adult-acquired flatfoot. Foot Ankle Int. 2018;39(8):903–7.
46. Schon LC, de Cesar Netto C, Day J, Deland JT, Hintermann B, Johnson JE, et al. Consensus for the indication of a medializing displacement calcaneal osteotomy in the treatment of progressive collapsing foot deformity. Foot Ankle Int. 2020;41(10):1282–5.
47. Sangeorzan BJ, Hintermann B, Netto CDC, Day J, Deland JT, Ellis SJ, et al. Progressive collapsing foot deformity: consensus on goals for operative correction. Foot Ankle Int. 2020;41(10):1299–302.
48. Fonseca LF, Baumfeld D, Mansur N, Nery C. Deltoid insufficiency and flatfoot—oh gosh, I'm losing the ankle! What now? Tech Foot Ankle Surg. 2019;18(4):202–7.
49. Hayes B, Bluman EM. Augmented deltoid reconstruction techniques. Tech Foot Ankle Surg. 2014;13(2):81–8.
50. Deland JT, De Asla RJ, Segal A. Reconstruction of the chronically failed deltoid ligament: a new technique. Foot Ankle Int. 2004;25(11):795–9.
51. Acevedo J, Vora A. Anatomic reconstruction of the spring ligament complex: "internal brace" augmentation technique. Tech Foot Ankle Surg. 2014;13(2):89–93.
52. Deland JT, Ellis SJ, Day J, Netto CDC, Hintermann B, Myerson MS, et al. Indications for deltoid and spring ligament reconstruction in progressive collapsing foot deformity. Foot Ankle Int. 2020;41(10):1302–6.
53. Dabash S, Elabd A, Potter E, Fernandez I, Gerzina C, Thabet AM, et al. Adding deltoid ligament repair in ankle fracture treatment: is it necessary? A systematic review. Foot Ankle Surg. 2019;25(6):714–20.

54. Salameh M, Alhammoud A, Alkhatib N, Attia AK, Mekhaimar MM, D'Hooghe P, et al. Outcome of primary deltoid ligament repair in acute ankle fractures: a meta-analysis of comparative studies. Int Orthop. 2020;44(2):341–7.
55. Femino JE, Vaseenon T, Phistkul P, Tochigi Y, Anderson DD, Amendola A. Varus external rotation stress test for radiographic detection of deep deltoid ligament disruption with and without Syndesmotic disruption. Foot Ankle Int. 2013;34(2):251–60.
56. Vega J, Allmendinger J, Malagelada F, Guelfi M, Dalmau-Pastor M. Combined arthroscopic all-inside repair of lateral and medial ankle ligaments is an effective treatment for rotational ankle instability. Knee Surg Sports Traumatol Arthrosc. 2020;28(1):132–40.

Lateral Ankle Ligament Injuries

10

Matteo Guelfi [iD], Francesc Malagelada, Guillaume Cordier, Jordi Vega, and Miki Dalmau-Pastor [iD]

M. Guelfi
Foot and Ankle Unit, Casa di Cura Villa Montallegro, Genoa, Italy

Department of Orthopaedic Surgery "Gruppo Policlinico di Monza", Clinica Salus, Alessandria, Italy

GRECMIP-MIFAS (Groupe de Recherche et d'Etude en Chirurgie Mini-Invasive du Pied-Minimally Invasive Foot and Ankle Society), Mérignac, France

F. Malagelada
GRECMIP-MIFAS (Groupe de Recherche et d'Etude en Chirurgie Mini-Invasive du Pied-Minimally Invasive Foot and Ankle Society), Mérignac, France

Department of Trauma & Orthopaedics, The Royal London Hospital, Bart's Health NHS Trust, London, UK

G. Cordier
GRECMIP-MIFAS (Groupe de Recherche et d'Etude en Chirurgie Mini-Invasive du Pied-Minimally Invasive Foot and Ankle Society), Mérignac, France

Orthopaedic Department, Mérignac Sports Clinic, Mérignac, France

J. Vega
GRECMIP-MIFAS (Groupe de Recherche et d'Etude en Chirurgie Mini-Invasive du Pied-Minimally Invasive Foot and Ankle Society), Mérignac, France

Foot and Ankle Unit, iMove Traumatology- Clínica Tres Torres y Hospital Quirón Barcelona, Barcelona, Spain

Department of Pathology and Experimental Therapeutics, University of Barcelona, Barcelona, Spain

M. Dalmau-Pastor (✉)
GRECMIP-MIFAS (Groupe de Recherche et d'Etude en Chirurgie Mini-Invasive du Pied-Minimally Invasive Foot and Ankle Society), Mérignac, France

Department of Pathology and Experimental Therapeutics, University of Barcelona, Barcelona, Spain
e-mail: mikeldalmau@ub.edu

© Springer Nature Switzerland AG 2022
J. D. Cain, M. V. Hogan (eds.), *Tendon and Ligament Injuries of the Foot and Ankle*,
https://doi.org/10.1007/978-3-031-10490-9_10

Introduction

Ankle sprains are among the most prevalent injuries of the musculoskeletal system both in sports and in daily activities [1]. It has been calculated that approximately one ankle sprain occurs per 10,000 people every day worldwide. Most of these occur during athletic activity with some sports such as basketball, volleyball or soccer being more frequently associated with ankle sprains [1].

The vast majority of the ankle sprains occur following an inversion injury involving the lateral collateral ligaments (LCL).

Ankle sprains are usually treated conservatively according to the PRICE (Protection, Rest, Ice, Compression, Elevation) protocol. However, residual symptoms after ankle sprains are reported in 30–40% of cases [1], with patients complaining of chronic pain and subjective instability.

This chapter provides an overview of the most important aspects on the diagnosis and treatment of ankle lateral ligament injuries.

Ankle Lateral Ligaments Anatomy

A thorough knowledge of anatomy is paramount for the diagnosis and adequate management of ankle injuries. The ankle is a highly congruent synovial, hinge-type joint, in which the talus fits perfectly into the mortise formed by the tibial plateau, and the tibial and fibular malleoli. This allows movement across the bimalleolar axis, through which dorsiflexion and plantarflexion movements are produced. The congruency of the ankle mortise is stabilized by three main ligament complexes that can be identified based on their anatomical location, respectively: the lateral collateral ligament (LCL), the medial collateral ligament (MCL) and the distal tibiofibular ligaments.

The lateral collateral ligament (LCL) is the most commonly injured ligamentous structure of the lower limb, due to the highest frequency in inversion sprains [2]. The LCL has been classically described with three components, the anterior talofibular ligament (ATFL), the calcaneofibular ligament (CFL), and the posterior talofibular ligament (PTFL). Modern literature has shown that these ligaments are not completely independent, since some fibers and connections between the ATFL and the CFL or the PTFL are constantly present [3, 4]. As a result, the LCL's current description features three different components, the anterior talofibular ligament's superior fascicle (ATFLsf), the lateral fibulotalocalcaneal ligament complex (LFTCLC), and the posterior talofibular ligament (PTFL). This new description is based on the anatomical and functional relationship between these components which is described below.

Anterior Talofibular Ligament's Superior Fascicle (ATFLsf)

The anterior talofibular ligament's superior fascicle (ATFLsf) is the anterior component of the lateral collateral ligament. It originates in one single footprint just distal to the fibular attachment of the anterior tibiofibular ligament distal fascicle and runs toward the neck of the talus [5, 6]. The function of the ATFLsf is mainly to control talar internal rotation [5–7]. Tension of the ATFLsf occurs when the ankle is in plantarflexion while it is relaxed in ankle dorsiflexion (Fig. 10.1). It is the first ligament to be injured during an ankle sprain, thus being the most frequently injured ankle ligament of all [8–10]. The ATFLsf has been described as an intra-articular but extrasynovial structure [5, 11]. This fact could explain why chronic pain

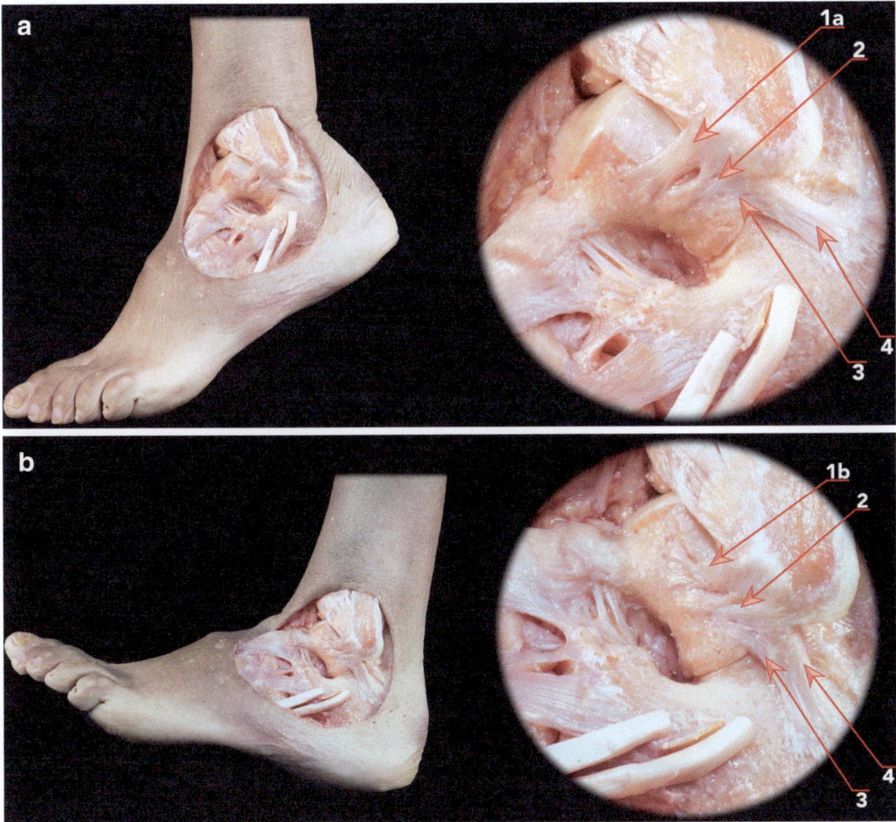

Fig. 10.1 Comparison of the morphology of the lateral ankle ligaments in plantarflexion (**a**) and dorsal flexion (**b**). Note how the structures forming the LFTCL complex maintain tension throughout the range of motion, while the ATFL superior fascicle does not. *1a*. Taut ATFL superior fascicle. *1b*. Lax ATFL superior fascicle. *2*. ATFL inferior fascicle. *3*. Arciform fibers of the LFTCL complex. *4*. CFL. Figure reproduced with permission from *Vega J, Malagelada F, Manzanares Céspedes MC, Dalmau-Pastor M. The lateral fibulotalocalcaneal ligament complex: an ankle stabilizing isometric structure. Knee Surg Sports Traumatol Arthrosc. 2020;28(1):8–17*

following an ankle sprain is still common after conservative treatment: the ATFLsf is unlikely to heal after tearing due to its intra-articular nature. Equally, its isolated injury can be difficult to detect with standard diagnostic tests or imaging.

Between the ATFLsf and the ATFL inferior fascicle (part of the lateral fibulota-localcaneal ligament complex), some branches pierce through from the perforating peroneal artery and its anastomosis with the lateral malleolar artery [12]. This explains the presence of the localized swelling, ecchymosis and hematoma that appear after an ankle sprain.

Lateral FibuloTaloCalcaneal Ligament Complex (LFTCLC)

The Lateral FibuloTaloCacaneal Ligament Complex, LFTCLC, is formed by the Anterior talofibular ligament's inferior fascicle, the calcaneofibular ligament and the connecting arc-shaped fibers between them (Fig. 10.2).

Originating from a common fibular attachment near the tip of the lateral malleolus (Fig. 10.3), the ATFL fascicle of the LFTCLC (ATFL's inferior fascicle) runs from the talar neck and inserts plantar to the ATFL superior fascicle, while the CFL inserts at the lateral side of the calcaneus and slightly posterior from its origin at the lateral malleolus [6]. In addition to the talocrural joint, the CFL component also crosses the subtalar joint, thereby stabilizing both joints.

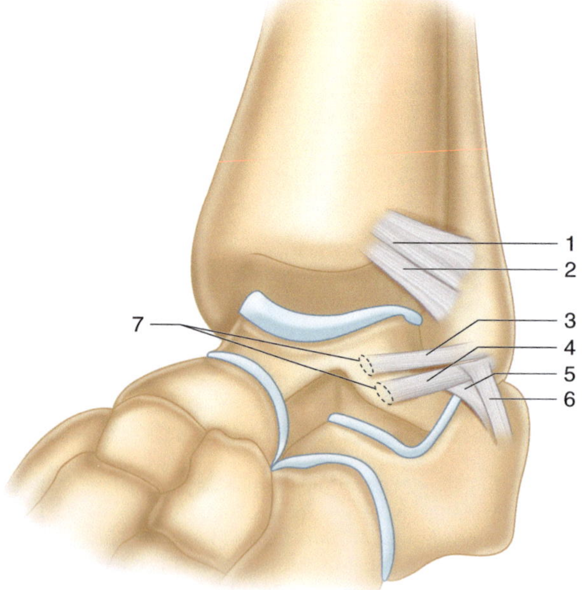

Fig. 10.2 Schematic drawing of the LFTCL complex. *1*. Anterior tibiofibular ligament. *2*. Distal fascicle of the anterior tibiofibular ligament. *3*. ATFL superior fascicle. *4*. ATFL inferior fascicle. *5*. Arciform fibers of the LFTCL complex. *6*. CFL. *7*. Note the different talar insertion points of ATFL fascicles

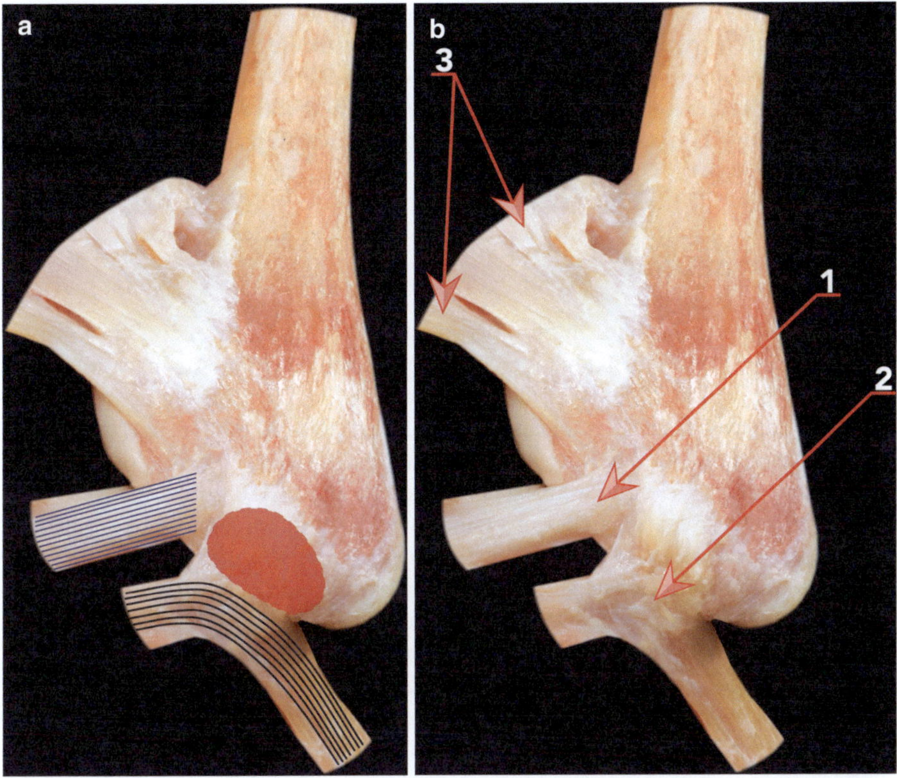

Fig. 10.3 Schematic view of the LFTCL complex with the lateral malleolus disarticulated from the ankle. (**a**) View with the lateral ankle ligaments highlighted: ATFL superior fascicle (blue lines), LFTCL complex (black lines), and area showing the common origin of the LFTCL complex (red area). (**b**) Classic view of the LFTCL complex. *1*. ATFL superior fascicle. *2*. LFTCL complex. *3*. Anterior tibiofibular ligament and distal fascicle. Figure reproduced with permission from *Vega J, Malagelada F, Manzanares Céspedes MC, Dalmau-Pastor M. The lateral fibulotalocalcaneal ligament complex: an ankle stabilizing isometric structure. Knee Surg Sports Traumatol Arthrosc. 2020;28(1):8–17*

The LFTCLC is an isometric structure that remains taut throughout the entire ankle arc of motion (Fig. 10.1) (neutral position, dorsiflexion and plantarflexion), possibly due to the presence of the connecting arc-shaped fibres. This ligamentous complex is injured in approximately 20% of all ankle sprains [9]. As an extra-articular structure, once torn it is likely to heal with adequate treatment.

Posterior Talofibular Ligament (PTFL)

The posterior talofibular ligament, PTFL, originates from the malleolar fossa in the medial posterior surface of the lateral malleolus and follows a horizontal course to insert along the lateral posterior surface of the talus [6]. It has a triangular shape with fibers inserting also into the talar posterolateral tubercle or *os trigonum*, when present. More recently, intra-articular connections to the rest of the lateral ankle ligaments have been described [4]. Tension of the PTFL occurs mainly when the ankle is in dorsiflexion. The PTFL is less frequently involved in ankle sprains and damage of the PTFL usually occurs in combination with other ligamentous ankle injuries.

Mechanism of Trauma

The most common mechanism of injury to the LCL is under inversion via a combination of supination and adduction of the plantarflexed foot. An inversion ankle sprain is observed in 75–90% of all ankle sprains [13–15], resulting in an injury to the ATFL superior fascicle in all cases [9, 16]. This is due to the fact that the ATFL's superior fascicle is the first ligament to be tensioned during inversion of the ankle, and that it appears to be the weakest component of the LCL complex [3, 6].

With the occurrence of higher inversion forces, the injury continues to propagate tearing the Lateral FibuloTaloCacaneal Ligament Complex [9, 17]. The PTFL is usually not injured, unless a lateral dislocation of the ankle joint occurs [18, 19]. An inversion mechanism can also damage posteromedial structures due to the kickback injury that affects the deep tibiotalar component of the medial collateral ligament, between the medial malleolus and the talus [20].

Ligamentous injuries of the medial collateral ligament (MCL) complex and the syndesmosis are much less common and are most likely associated with collision sports such as soccer, American football, or skiing. The trauma mechanism associated with ligamentous injuries of the MCL complex is excessive pronation and abduction (eversion), while the mechanism associated with syndesmotic injuries is forced dorsiflexion and external rotation. Both MCL and syndesmotic injuries rarely occur alone and are more often associated with other ligamentous injuries or fractures.

Diagnosis

Accurate diagnosis after ankle trauma is important in order to assess the severity of the injury and to exclude potential fractures or associated lesions. Ottawa ankle rules can be used to decide in which cases radiographs are recommended to exclude fractures [21]. When a fracture is excluded, the ankle should be examined further to rule out ligamentous damage. Because of pain, routine physical examination to assess ligament involvement is difficult and a full clinical exam should be delayed 5–7 days from the acute phase [22]. Hematoma, swelling, pain on palpation of the LCL and stress tests for ligament stability are all important aspects of physical examination following an ankle sprain.

Pain on palpation of the ATFL is one of the most common signs and suggests rupture of this ligament [23]. Pain is usually localized over the anterior border of the fibular malleolus as the ATFL usually tears at the fibular attachment. Two main clinical tests are performed to assess lateral ankle ligament injuries: the anterior drawer test and the inversion talar tilt test. The anterior drawer test is meant to assess the integrity of the ATFL, with a sensitivity of 73% and a specificity of 97% for rupture of the ATFL; and an increased sensitivity of 96% and a specificity of 84% when in combination with hematoma and pain on palpation of the ligaments [23].

Classically, the severity of the LCL injury after an acute ankle sprain was graded from I to III, based on increasing levels of ligamentous damage [24]. In this classification, grade I indicated mild stretching of the ATFL with some ligament fibers torn (the ankle might be stable or mildly unstable on physical examination); grade II indicated moderate injury with a complete tear of the ATFL and possibly a partial tear of the CFL (unstable ankle on physical examination with a positive anterior drawer and negative inversion tilt test); grade III indicated complete disruption of both the ATFL and CFL (severely unstable ankle on physical examination with positive anterior drawer and positive inversion talar tilt test). With the irruption of the recently described anatomical concepts, a new classification should be considered, with grade I indicating ATFL's superior fascicle injury, resulting in ankle microinstability; grade II indicating a complete tear of the ATFL's superior fascicle and partial injury of the LFTCLC; and grade III indicating a complete tear of ATFL's superior fascicle and LFTCLC.

Additional imaging studies such as ultrasound (US) and magnetic resonance imaging (MRI) are commonly used to diagnose associated injuries, while their use to evaluate ligament injuries is dependent on the radiologist or clinician interpreting the results, ideally in conjunction with proper physical examination. For this reason, imaging during the acute phase can be useful to rule out associated injuries or in case of severely unstable ankles or persistent symptoms [25]. Using these imaging tests to diagnose ATFLsf and ATFL inferior fascicle separately is probably the next step in order to improve ankle sprain diagnostics.

In cases of chronic ankle ligament injury, patients describe a subjective feeling of ankle instability, recurrent ankle sprains, chronic anterolateral pain, or a combination of them. The physical examination of chronic ankle instability (CAI) should include comparative assessment of both ankles including the anterior drawer test, the talar tilt test and ankle range of motion. An evaluation of generalized joint laxity should also be performed. The anterior drawer test compared to the contralateral side is the most specific test for CAI, while the talar tilt test is frequently difficult to assess and less reliable [23].

Imaging studies should include standard weight-bearing radiographs and MRI or US. Plain radiographs allow for the assessment of hindfoot alignment and may identify osteophytes and loose bodies. However, only 40% of the tibial and 32% of the talar osteophytes are detected by the standard lateral radiographs [26]. For this reason, in those cases with a suspect of anteromedial impingement an oblique anteromedial impingement view is suggested [26]. This view has shown a specificity of 93% and sensitivity of 67% for detecting anteromedial osteophytes. Other modalities like weight-bearing CT have shown more accurate measurement of deformities associated with lateral ankle injuries along with the ability to detect osteophytes or loose bodies [27]. Stress radiographs are not useful in the diagnosis of CAI and are no longer recommended because of the high percentage of false positive [25].

Ankle MRI is the most useful imaging study when investigating chronic ankle instability, especially to detect concomitant osteochondral lesions, tendon tears or other intra-articular pathologies in addition to LCL injury [28].

Treatment

When fracture is not present, acute ankle injuries are usually treated nonoperatively using a functional treatment with the goal of providing optimal healing capabilities by decreasing pain, swelling and hematoma and to prevent further damage. During the first few days, the RICE protocol is based on rest, ice, compression and elevation. Early weight-bearing and active range of motion exercises are encouraged as soon as tolerated. Once the acute phase treatment is implemented and function is restored, therapy will aim at improving ankle stability with neuromuscular coordination training and strengthening exercises on muscles and tendons [25, 29, 30]. Conservative treatments are successful in most patients; however, 30–40% of patients will have residual symptoms after an ankle sprain including chronic pain, recurrent giving way or instability [1]. In these patients for whom the conservative treatment failed, and depending on their activity level or sports involvement, surgical intervention is indicated to treat the ligament injury.

Several operative procedures have been described for the treatment of LCL injuries. They have been broadly divided into anatomic repair, nonanatomic reconstruction and anatomic reconstruction. The anatomic repair technique provides a reattachment of the native remnant restoring ankle stability and preserving physiological function. For this reason, it is preferred over the reconstruction procedures, representing the gold standard technique for CAI. Up to 93% of unstable ankles undergoing surgery present concomitant intra-articular pathologies such as soft-tissue or bony impingement, osteochondral defects, loose bodies or deltoid ligament injuries [31, 32]. For this reason, and although the recommended anatomical repair can be performed by an open or arthroscopic procedure, arthroscopic techniques are gaining popularity becoming probably the next gold standard procedure treating CAI [33, 34].

Arthroscopy allows concomitant treatment of the LCL injury and any intra-articular pathologies, through the same arthroscopic approach, providing the benefits of minimally invasive surgery and a faster recovery including return to sports activities.

From all ankle arthroscopic stabilizing techniques, the authors' preferred technique is the all-inside ligament repair. The all-inside arthroscopic repair, originally described by Vega et al. in 2013, is a fully arthroscopic technique that provides an anatomic repair of the LCL with a knotless suture anchor [35–38]. Supporting this technique, reports of excellent clinical results with a low complication rate are published in the literature [39, 40]. Compared to other arthroscopic techniques, such as

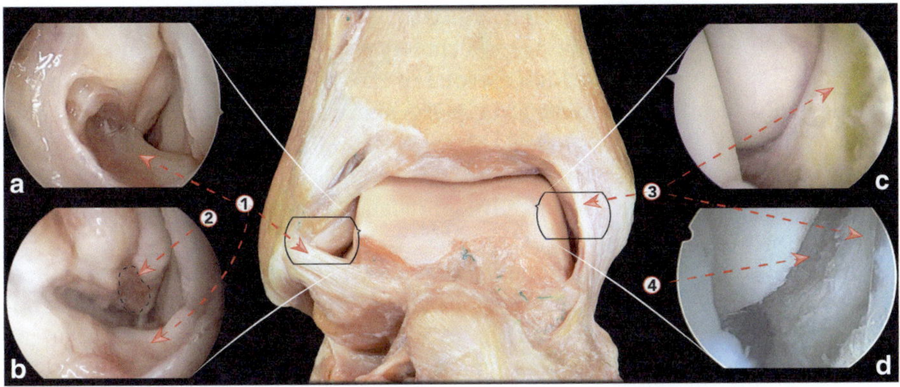

Fig. 10.4 Anatomical perspective of the ankle. Arthroscopic views of lateral and medial gutters showed to depict normal appearance (**a**, lateral gutter, and **c**, medial gutter) and pathological appearance with a ligament rupture (**b**, ATFL detachment, and **d**, deltoid ligament "open book" injury). (*1*) ATFL. (*2*) Fibular footprint of the ATFL (highlighted with black dotted line). (*3*) Anterior area of the deltoid ligament. (*4*) Deltoid ligament "open book" detachment. Figure reproduced with permission from Vega J, Allmendinger J, Malagelada F, Guelfi M, Dalmau-Pastor M. *Combined arthroscopic all-inside repair of lateral and medial ankle ligaments is an effective treatment for rotational ankle instability. Knee Surg Sports Traumatol Arthrosc. 2020;28(1):132–40*

the arthroscopic Broström, the all-inside provides better functional results with a lower complication rate [40]. The fact that both the medial and lateral ankle ligaments have an intra-articular portion [11] allows for its arthroscopic treatment, either isolated or in combination (Fig. 10.4) [35].

Literature Review

To date, a few systematic reviews are available in literature comparing open and arthroscopic ligament repair [41, 42]. The first systematic review by Guelfi et al. included 19 studies, 13 on open procedures [43–55] and 6 on arthroscopic procedures [35, 56–60]. Subjects of the selected studies were all patients with chronic ankle instability secondary to lateral ankle injuries that underwent an open or arthroscopic repair of the lateral ankle ligaments [41]. The meta-analysis of the AOFAS scores in patients treated with open procedures, performed in the 11 available studies, showed an overall score of 90.34 (95% CI [88.10; 92.58]), while a surgery-related complication occurred in 40 (7.92%) out of 505 treated ankles. Regarding the arthroscopic procedures, the meta-analysis of the AOFAS scores showed an overall score of 92.50 (95% CI [89.57; 95.43]), while a surgery-related complication was observed in 33/216 arthroscopically treated ankles (15.27%). The higher rate of complications was explained by the technique performed in five of the six arthroscopic studies included in the review, which was not an all-inside repair but an arthroscopically assisted repair with a percutaneous passage of the suture, which increases the risk for neurological complications.

The second systematic review performed by Brown et al. includes four comparative studies of arthroscopic and open techniques for lateral ankle ligament repair [42, 61–64]. In this review, including a total of 207 ankle ligament repair, there was a statistically significant difference in AOFAS score in favor of the arthroscopic repair (MD; 1.41, 95% CI 0.29–2.52, I2 = 0%, $p < 0.05$), and a not statistically significant difference in Karlsson score (MD; 0.00, 95% CI − 3.51 to 3.51, I2 = 0%, n.s.) [42]. In addition, a no statistically significant difference in total complications (nerve, or wound) was observed [42].

In conclusion the present literature provides consistent advantages, excellent results, and low rate of complication for the arthroscopic treatment of ankle instability. Although more studies with a high level of evidence and longer follow-up are required, the arthroscopic ligament repair is close to replace open surgery as the gold standard for CAI [34].

Treatment Algorithm

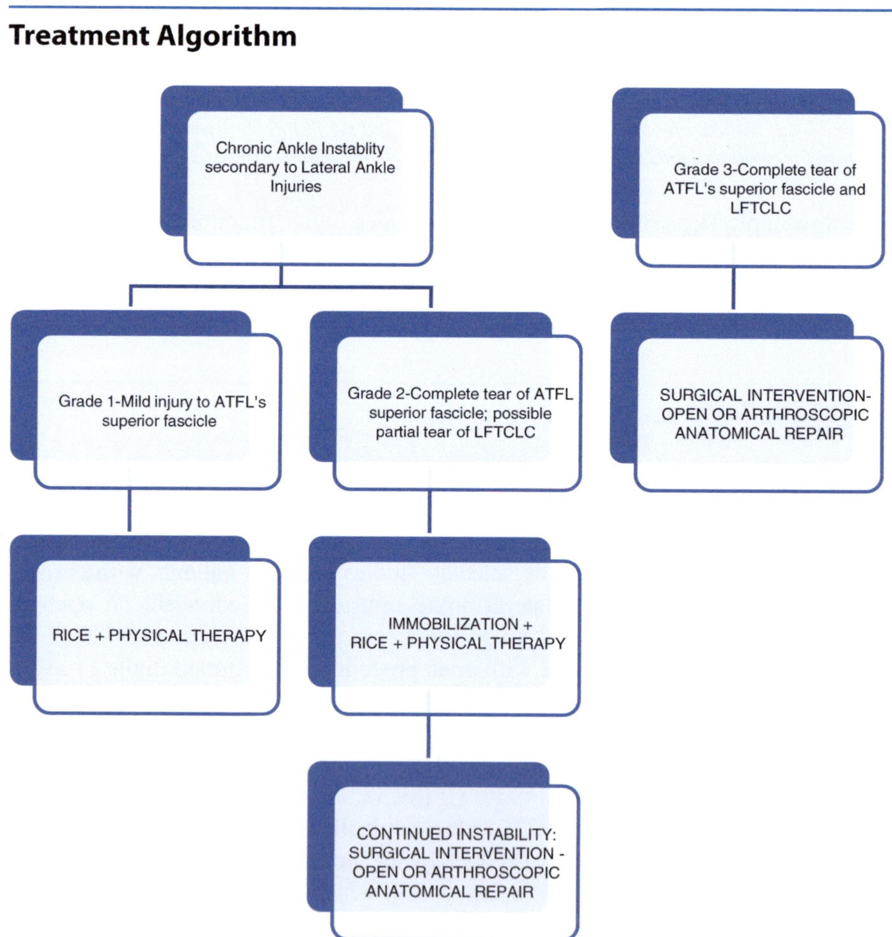

Postoperative Protocol

Postoperatively, immobilization with a removable walking boot is maintained for the first 3–4 weeks attempting weight bearing as tolerated with the aid of crutches. Once the walking boot is discontinued, physical therapy is initiated with range-of-motion exercises and gait training. Two weeks later, strengthening and balance exercises are initiated. Noncontact sports (swimming or bicycling) are allowed 2 months postoperatively, and sporting activities, including contact sports, can be expected at 3–6 months depending on muscle conditioning.

References

1. Ferran NA, Maffulli N. Epidemiology of sprains of the lateral ankle ligament complex. Foot Ankle Clin. 2006;11:659–62.
2. van Dijk CN. On diagnostic strategies in patient with severe ankle sprain. Thesis, University of Amsterdam, The Netherlands. 1994.
3. Golanó P, Dalmau-Pastor M, Vega J, et al. Anatomy of the ankle. In: d'Hooghe PPRN, Kerkhoffs GMMJ, editors. The ankle in football, sports and traumatology. Heidelberg: Springer; 2014. p. 1–24.
4. Dalmau-Pastor M, Malagelada F, Calder J, Manzanares MC, Vega J. The lateral ankle ligaments are interconnected: the medial connecting fibres between the anterior talofibular, calcaneofibular and posterior talofibular ligaments. Knee Surg Sports Traumatol Arthrosc. 2020;28(1):34–9.
5. Vega J, Malagelada F, Manzanares Céspedes MC, Dalmau-Pastor M. The lateral fibulotalocalcaneal ligament complex: an ankle stabilizing isometric structure. Knee Surg Sports Traumatol Arthrosc. 2020;28(1):8–17.
6. Golanó P, Vega J, de Leeuw PAJ, et al. Anatomy of the ankle ligaments: a pictorial essay. Knee Surg Sports Traumatol Arthrosc. 2010;18(5):557–69.
7. Caputo AM, Lee JY, Spritzer CE, et al. In vivo kinematics of the tibiotalar joint after lateral ankle instability. Am J Sports Med. 2009;37(11):2241–8.
8. Vega J, Malagelada F, Karlsson J, Kerkhoffs GMMJ, Guelfi M, Dalmau-Pastor M. A step-by-step arthroscopic examination of the anterior ankle compartment. Knee Surg Sports Traumatol Arthrosc. 2020;28(1):24–33.
9. Broström L. Sprained ankles. VI. Surgical treatment of "chronic" ligament ruptures. Acta Chir Scand. 1966;132:551–65.
10. Colville MR, Marder RA, Boyle JJ, et al. Strain measurement in lateral ankle ligaments. Am J Sports Med. 1990;18:196–200.
11. Dalmau-Pastor M, Malagelada F, Kerkhoffs GM, Karlsson J, Guelfi M, Vega J. Redefining anterior ankle arthroscopic anatomy: medial and lateral ankle collateral ligaments are visible through dorsiflexion and non-distraction anterior ankle arthroscopy. Knee Surg Sports Traumatol Arthrosc. 2020;28(1):18–23.
12. McKeon KE, Wright RW, Johnson JE, et al. Vascular anatomy of the tibiofibular syndesmosis. J Bone Joint Surg. 2012;94:931–8.
13. AFH R, Lynch SA. Acute injuries of the ankle. Foot Ankle Clin. 1999;4:697–711.
14. Balduini FC, Tetzlaff J. Historical perspectives on injuries of the ligaments of the ankle. Clin Sports Med. 1982;1(1):3–12.
15. Woods C, Hawkins R, Hulse M, Hodson A. The football association medical research Programme: an audit of injuries in professional football: an analysis of ankle sprains. Br J Sports Med. 2003;37(3):233–8.

16. Prins JG. Diagnosis and treatment of injury to the lateral ligament of the ankle. A comparative clinical study. Acta Chir Scand Suppl. 1978;486:3–149.
17. Baumhauer JF, O'Brien T. Surgical considerations in the treatment of ankle instability. J Athl Train. 2002;37:458–62.
18. Karlsson J, Andreasson GO. The effect of external ankle support in chronic lateral ankle joint instability. An electromyographic study. Am J Sports Med. 1992;20(3):257–61.
19. Karlsson J, Lansinger O. Lateral instability of the ankle joint. Clin Orthop Relat Res. 1992;276:253–61.
20. Paterson RS, Brown JN. The posteromedial impingement lesion of the ankle: a series of six cases. Am J Sports Med. 2001;29:550–7.
21. Bachmann LM, Kolb E, Koller MT, Steurer J, ter Riet G. Accuracy of Ottawa ankle rules to exclude fractures of the ankle and mid-foot: systematic review. BMJ. 2003;326(7386):417.
22. van den Bekerom MP, Kerkhoffs GM, McCollum GA, Calder J, van Dijk CN. Management of acute lateral ankle ligament injury in the athlete. Knee Surg Sports Traumatol Arthrosc. 2013;21(6):1390–5.
23. van Dijk CN, Lim S, Bossuyt PM, Marti RK. Physical examination is sufficient for the diagnosis of sprained ankles. J Bone Joint Surg Br. 1996;78(6):958–62.
24. Lynch SA, Renstrom PA. Treatment of acute lateral ankle ligament rupture in the athlete. Conservative versus surgical treatment. Sports Med. 1999;27(1):61–71.
25. Vuurberg G, Hoorntje A, Lm W, et al. Diagnosis, treatment and prevention of ankle sprains: update of an evidence-based clinical guideline. Br J Sports Med. 2018;52(15):956.
26. Tol JL, Van Dijk CN. Etiology of the anterior ankle impingement syndrome: a descriptive anatomical study. Foot Ankle Int. 2004;25:382–6.
27. Richter M, Seidl B, Zech S, Hahn S. PedCAT for 3D-imaging in standing position allows for more accurate bone position (angle) measurement than radiographs or CT. Foot Ankle Surg. 2014;20(3):201–7.
28. Verhagen RAW, Maas M, Dijkgraaf MGW, Tol JL, Krips R, van Dijk CN. Prospective study on diagnostic strategies in osteochondral lesions of the talus. J Bone Joint Surg Br. 2005;87(B-1):41–6.
29. Kerkhoffs GM, Rowe BH, Assendelft WJ, Kelly K, Struijs PA, Van Dijk CN. Immobilization and functional treatment for acute lateral ankle ligament injuries in adults (Cochrane review). Cochrane Database Syst Rev. 2002;(3):CD003762. https://doi.org/10.1002/14651858.
30. Kerkhoffs GM, Struijs PA, Marti RK, Blankevoort L, Assendelft WJ, Van Dijk CN. Functional treatments for acute ruptures of the lateral ankle ligament: a systematic review. Acta Orthop Scand. 2003;74(1):69–77.
31. Hintermann B, Boss A, Schäfer D. Arthroscopic findings in patients with chronic ankle instability. Am J Sports Med. 2002;30:402–9.
32. Komenda GA, Ferkel RD. Arthroscopic findings associated with the unstable ankle. Foot Ankle Int. 1999;20:708–13.
33. Vega J, Dalmau-Pastor M, Malagelada F, Fargues-Polo B, Peña F. Ankle arthroscopy: an update. J Bone Joint Surg Am. 2017;99:1395–407.
34. Vega J, Dalmau-Pastor M. Editorial commentary: arthroscopic treatment of ankle instability is the emerging gold standard. Art Ther. 2021;37(1):280–1.
35. Vega J, Golanó P, Pellegrino A, Rabat E, Peña F. All-inside arthroscopic lateral collateral ligament repair for ankle instability with a knotless suture anchor technique. Foot Ankle Int. 2013;34(12):1701–9.
36. Takao M, Matsui K, Stone JW, et al. Arthroscopic anterior talofibular ligament repair for lateral instability of the ankle. Knee Surg Sports Traumatol Arthrosc. 2015;24(4):1003–6.
37. Vega J, Allmendinger J, Malagelada F, Guelfi M, Dalmau-Pastor M. Combined arthroscopic all-inside repair of lateral and medial ankle ligaments is an effective treatment for rotational ankle instability. Knee Surg Sports Traumatol Arthrosc. 2020;28(1):132–40.
38. Vega J, Guelfi M, Malagelada F, Peña F, Dalmau-Pastor M. Arthroscopic all-inside anterior talofibular ligament repair through a three-portal and no-ankle-distraction technique. JBJS Essent Surg Tech. 2018;8(3):1–11.

39. Guelfi M, Vega J, Malagelada F, Dalmau-Pastor M. The arthroscopic all-inside ankle lateral collateral ligament repair is a safe and reproducible technique. Knee Surg Sports Traumatol Arthrosc. 2020;28(1):63–9.
40. Guelfi M, Nunes GA, Malagelada F, Cordier G, Dalmau-Pastor M, Vega J. Arthroscopic-assisted vs all-arthroscopic ankle stabilization technique. A comparative clinical study. Foot Ankle Int. 2020;41(11):1360–7.
41. Guelfi M, Zamperetti M, Pantalone A, et al. Open and arthroscopic lateral ligament repair for treatment of chronic ankle instability: a systematic review. Foot Ankle Surg. 2018;24(1):11–8.
42. Brown A, Shimozono Y, Hurley ET, Kennedy JG. Arthroscopic repair of lateral ankle ligament for chronic lateral ankle instability: a systematic review. Knee Surg Sports Traumatol Arthrosc. 2018;34(8):2497–503.
43. Buerer Y, Winkler M, Burn A, Chopra S, Crevoisier X. Evaluation of a modified Broström–Gould procedure for treatment of chronic lateral ankle instability: a retrospective study with critical analysis of outcome scoring. Foot Ankle Surg. 2013;19:36–41.
44. Ferkel RD, Chams RN. Chronic lateral instability: arthroscopic findings and long-term results. Foot Ankle Int. 2007;28:24–31.
45. Maffulli N, Del Buono A, Maffulli GD, Oliva F, Testa V, Capasso G, et al. Isolated anterior talofibular ligament brostrom repair for chronic lateral ankle instability: 9-year follow-up. Am J Sports Med. 2013;41:858–64.
46. Brodsky AR, O'Malley MJ, Bohne WH, Deland JA, Kennedy JG. An analysis of outcome measures following the Broström–Gould procedure for chronic lateral ankle instability. Foot Ankle Int. 2005;26:816–9.
47. Porter M, Shadbolt B, Stuart R. Primary ankle ligament augmentation versus modified Brostrom–Gould procedure: a 2-year randomized controlled trial. ANZ J Surg. 2015;85:44–8.
48. Messer TM, Cummins CA, Ahn J, Kelikian AS. Outcome of the modified brostrom procedure for chronic lateral ankle instability using suture anchors. Foot Ankle Int. 2000;21:996–1003.
49. Chen CY, Huang PJ, Kao KF, Chen JC, Cheng YM, Chiang HC, et al. Surgical reconstruction for chronic lateral instability of the ankle. Injury. 2004;35:809–13.
50. Schmidt R, Benesch S, Friemert B, Herbst A, Claes L, Gerngroß H. Anatomical repair of lateral ligaments in patients with chronic ankle instability. Knee Surg Sports Traumatol Arthrosc. 2005;13:231–7.
51. Bell SJ, Mologne TS, Sitler DF, Cox JS. Twenty-six-year results after Broström procedure for chronic lateral ankle instability. Am J Sports Med. 2006;34:975–8.
52. Li X, Killie H, Guerrero P, Busconi BD. Anatomical reconstruction for chronic lateral ankle instability in the high-demand athlete: functional outcomes after the modified Broström repair using suture anchors. Am J Sports Med. 2009;37:488–94.
53. Hua Y, Chen S, Li Y, Chen J, Li H. Combination of modified Broström procedure with ankle arthroscopy for chronic ankle instability accompanied by intra-articular symptoms. Art Ther. 2010;26:524–8.
54. Lee KT, Park YU, Kim JS, Kim JB, Kim KC, Kang SK. Long-term results after modified Brostrom procedure without calcaneofibular ligament reconstruction. Foot Ankle Int. 2011;32:153–7.
55. Molloy AP, Ajis A, Kazi H. The modified Broström-Gould procedure – early results using a newly described surgical technique. Foot Ankle Surg. 2014;20:224–8.
56. Nery C, Raduan F, Del Buono A, Asaumi ID, Cohen M, Maffulli N. Arthroscopic-assisted brostrom-gould for chronic ankle instability: a long-term follow-up. Am J Sports Med. 2011;39:2381–8.
57. Kim ES, Lee KT, Park JS, Lee YK. Arthroscopic anterior talofibular ligament repair for chronic ankle instability with a suture anchor technique. Orthopedics. 2011;34:1–9.
58. Cottom JM, Rigby RB. The "all inside" arthroscopic brostrom procedure: a prospective study of 40 consecutive patients. J Foot Ankle Surg. 2013;52:568–74.
59. Corte-real NM, Moreira RM. Arthroscopic repair of chronic lateral ankle instability. Foot Ankle Int. 2015;5:213–7.
60. Acevedo JI, Mangone P. Arthroscopic Brostrom technique. Foot Ankle Int. 2015;36:465–73.

61. Li H, Hua Y, Li H, Ma K, Li S, Chen S. Activity level and function 2 years after anterior talofibular ligament repair: a comparison between arthroscopic repair and open repair procedures. Am J Sports Med. 2017;45:2044–51.
62. Matsui K, Takao M, Miyamoto W, Matsushita T. Early recovery after arthroscopic repair compared to open repair of the anterior talofibular ligament for lateral instability of the ankle. Arch Orthop Trauma Surg. 2016;136:93–100.
63. Rigby RB, Cottom JM. A comparison of the "all-inside" arthroscopic Broström procedure with the traditional open modified Broström–Gould technique: a review of 62 patients. Foot Ankle Surg. 2019;25(1):31–6.
64. Yeo ED, Lee KT, Sung IH, Lee SG, Lee YK. Comparison of all-inside arthroscopic and open techniques for the modified Broström procedure for ankle instability. Foot Ankle Int. 2016;37:1037–45.

Syndesmotic Injuries

11

François Lintz, Céline Fernando, Alessio Bernasconi, Ronny Lopes, Giovany Padiolleau, and Renaud Guiu

Introduction

The distal tibiotalar syndesmosis has been a long-standing clinical challenge and scientific puzzle for foot and ankle surgeons and researchers. Its complex ligamentous anatomy is a strong contributor to this matter of fact, and conversely, its relatively simple bony shape (two close-to-flat articular surfaces facing each other) has made it very difficult to evaluate using conventional imaging solutions such as two-dimensional radiography. Furthermore, obvious acute injuries associated with ankle fractures are rather rare. The most frequent situations are subtle injuries either associated with an ankle fracture, an ankle sprain, or misdiagnosed as such. This leads to delayed management, rendering diagnosis and treatment even more challenging. In this small and constrained joint, with small range of motion, and little or no reliable surface landmarks, clinical examination remains very subjective and poorly reproducible. The same is true of the reproducibility and reliability of conventional, two-dimensional radiography. However, recent advances in imaging technics are

Supplementary Information The online version contains supplementary material available at [https://doi.org/10.1007/978-3-031-10490-9_11].

F. Lintz (✉) · C. Fernando
Department of Orthopedics, Foot and Ankle Center, Ramsay Healthcare, Clinique de l'Union, Saint Jean, France

A. Bernasconi
Foot and Ankle, Orthopaedics and Trauma Department, University of Naples Federico II, Naples, Italy

R. Lopes · G. Padiolleau
Department of Orthopedics, Atlantic Nantes Foot and Ankle Centre, Atlantic Health, Saint Herblain, France

R. Guiu
Sports Medicine, Paris, France

© Springer Nature Switzerland AG 2022
J. D. Cain, M. V. Hogan (eds.), *Tendon and Ligament Injuries of the Foot and Ankle*,
https://doi.org/10.1007/978-3-031-10490-9_11

shedding a new light on syndesmotic lesions. In this chapter, we will focus on dynamic ultrasound scanning which could be the next step in early diagnosis and cone beam weight-bearing CT, which has the potential to immediately and at a later stage provide precise three-dimensional evaluation of this challenging joint. The consequences in terms of health improvement could be very significant because of the potential adverse effects of a misdiagnosed syndesmotic lesion. While classically described as a rare injury, more modern research based on arthroscopic findings during sprain and fracture treatment has shown that up to 15% of syndesmotic lesions could be associated with ankle sprains [1] and 90% in ankle fractures [2], while going underseen in a majority of cases. In those cases, chronic syndesmotic lesions lead to longer healing time and secondary ankle arthritis [3]. While new opportunities are arising in terms of diagnosis, new treatment algorithms are also being investigated, taking advantage in particular of the recent advances in arthroscopic ligament repairs in the foot and ankle, which allow for excellent intra-articular visualization of the anterior distal syndesmosis, as well as new opportunities for intraoperative clinical testing.

In this chapter, we will investigate the following points and report on the latest advances based on an up-to-date review of the literature.

Anatomy

The distal tibiofibular syndesmosis is a small, constrained, fibrous joint [4]. Its role is to ensure stability for the talo-tibiofibular mortise especially with regard to the valgus constraints which are physiologically applied during gait. Its shape is triangular, with an apex situated 6–8 cm above the level of the tibiotalar joint [5]. The tibial side is concave (fibular incisura) and the fibular side is convex. The anterior and posterior borders are defined by the anterior tubercule (Chaput's tubercule) and the posterior tubercule which is the pivot point for external rotation of the fibula during ankle dorsiflexion. The base of the triangle is situated just above the cartilage of the fibular facet of the talofibular joint. This corresponds to a tibiofibular contact area which is very small and inconsistently present [5]. The literature usually describes four main strong ligaments which ensure the stability of the joint: the anterior inferior tibiofibular ligament (AITFL), the posterior (or posterior inferior) tibiofibular ligament or PTFL/PITFL, the interosseous membrane or tibiofibular interosseous ligament, and the transverse tibiofibular ligament or posterior inter-malleolar ligament. The anatomy of the syndesmosis, especially the posterior aspect, is variable, and not all publications agree on the number and denominations of all fibrous and ligamentous structures (Fig. 11.1).

In terms of functional anatomy, the syndesmosis ensures stability of the ankle joint during dorsiflexion and external rotation. Ankle dorsiflexion happens passively during the third stage of gait at every step, while external rotation happens mainly under load during physical activity such as pivot and contact sports. The

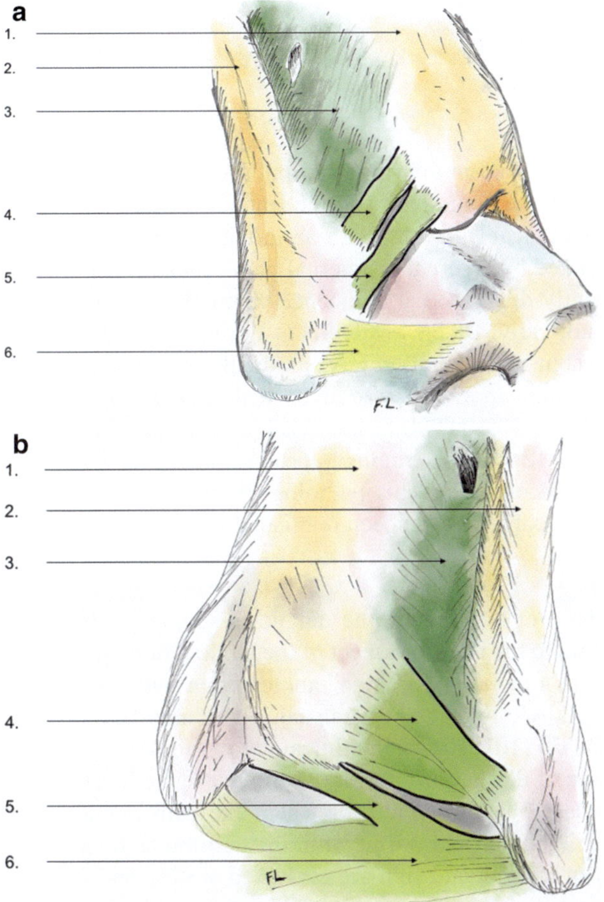

Fig. 11.1 (**a**) Anterior view of the tibiofibular syndesmosis [1]. Tibia [2]. Fibula [3]. Interosseous membrane [4]. Anterior inferior tibiofibular ligament, superior bundle [5]. Anterior inferior tibiofibular ligament, inferior bundle [6]. Anterior talofibular ligament. (**b**) Posterior view of the tibiofibular syndesmosis [1]. Tibia [2]. Fibula [3]. Interosseous membrane [4]. Posterior (inferior) tibiofibular ligament [5]. Posterior inter-malleolar or transverse tibiofibular ligament [6]. Posterior talofibular ligament

syndesmosis demonstrates an increased diastasis of 1–2 mm as the talus moves into dorsiflexion, while the fibula undergoes 3–5° external rotation. On plantarflexion, the process is reversed [6].

The role of the medial collateral ligaments (deep and superficial or deltoid) should not be understated because, even though they are not anatomically part of the syndesmosis, they are functionally part of the same complex, ensuring resistance to excessive dorsiflexion, external rotation, and valgus constraints [7]. This explains the large number of associated lesions in a traumatic context.

Diagnosis

Clinical Evaluation

Background

The clinical diagnosis of an inferior tibiofibular syndesmosis (DTFS) lesion is considered difficult in the acute phase of the trauma. In fact, during the ankle sprain mechanism, the clinical signs on DTFS are often in the background, and the symptoms are dominated by external or internal pain. These lesions are therefore unfortunately frequently diagnosed at a distance when chronic and irreversible damage has set in. Historically, DTFS involvement during an ankle sprain mechanism is considered rare, but several authors have gradually questioned this dogma. For Hunt [8], one in five ankle sprains is associated with a DTFS lesion. Other authors [9] report a rate of over 50% DTFS lesions visible on MRI. Mulcahay [9] studied this in a population of 1216 ankle sprains in professional footballers and found 53% of DTFS involvement on MRI. This pathology is therefore largely underestimated, while reliable clinical tests have been published to make the diagnosis.

Clinical Tests

In the acute phase of the trauma, the diagnosis should be made when the patient complains of pain to the anterior aspect of the ankle radiating into the leg. The clinician is faced with a picture of a "high" ankle sprain with painful symptoms on the outside of the ankle less marked than usual. There may be a bruise on the anterior aspect of the DTFS [10]. The main clinical sign to look for in this acute context is pain on palpation of the antero-inferior tibiofibular ligament (AiTFL) [10]. This differs from the classic lateral sprain for which the pain is mainly localized on the calcaneofibular ligament and on the anterior talofibular ligament. The sensitivity and specificity of this clinical sign are evaluated at 92% and 79%, respectively, for Sman [11]. This difference in painful localization should give rise to suspicion of an impaired DTFS and therefore requires seeing the patient again a few days later to perform dynamic tests. Indeed, pain in the acute phase of the sprain can make it difficult to interpret the clinical maneuvers described below. When the pain allows it, clinical maneuvers can therefore be performed to confirm DTFS involvement. Six main clinical tests have been described: the squeeze test, the Frick test, the cross-leg test, the Cotton test, the fibular translation test, and the stabilization test. They can be combined in the event of doubt.

The squeeze test [12] was published in 1990 by Hopkinson and consists of performing a lateral compression of the leg. The examiner places his dominant hand just above the upper half of the patient's leg. The thumb is placed on the tibia and the lateral fingers on the fibula. The examiner performs a squeezing movement between his thumb and lateral fingers and looks for pain caused by this maneuver in the DTFS (photo 1). Different authors [11, 13, 14] report a good specificity of 88% to 93% but a low sensitivity estimated at 30% (Fig. 11.2).

Kiter [15] offers a self-test performed by the patient himself: the cross-leg test. The patient is seated on the edge of the examination table. He positions the leg to be tested on the opposite knee. The point of support of the leg on the knee should be

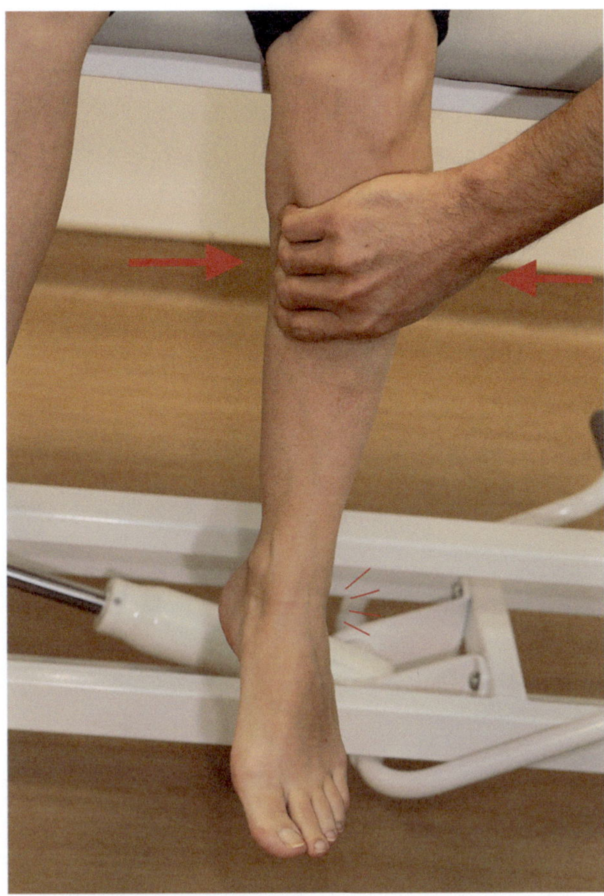

Fig. 11.2 The squeeze test

located at the junction 1/3 lower-2/3 upper of the calf. Pressure is applied by the patient on his knee and pain in the DTFS is sought (Fig. 11.3).

The Frick test [16], also called the forced lateral rotation test, is performed on a patient in a seated position with the knee bent at 90°. The ankle is initially in a neutral position. The examiner's upper hand is resting on the knee and his lower hand grasps the heel. The medial aspect of the foot is positioned resting on the forearm, and then a lateral rotation movement of the ankle is applied. The test is positive if it produces pain in the DTFS (Fig. 11.4). The sensitivity of this test is evaluated between 30% and 71% and the specificity at 85% [14, 17, 18].

In severe cases, anteroposterior mobility between the tibia and the fibula may be found. The examiner grasps the fibula between his fingers and looks for an anteroposterior piston movement (Fig. 11.5): the fibular translation test [19].

Cotton [20] described an increase in mediolateral translation of the talus below the tibia in the presence of DTFS.

Ward [21] performs a compression/dorsiflexion test while standing. He positions himself behind the patient and asks him to perform a dorsiflexion movement with

Fig. 11.3 The cross-leg test

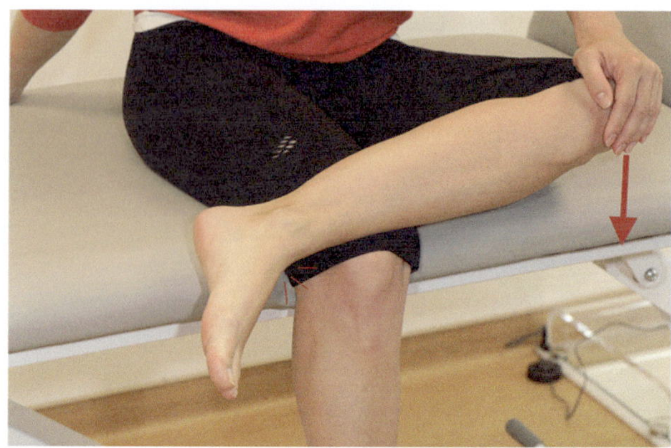

Fig. 11.4 The Frick test

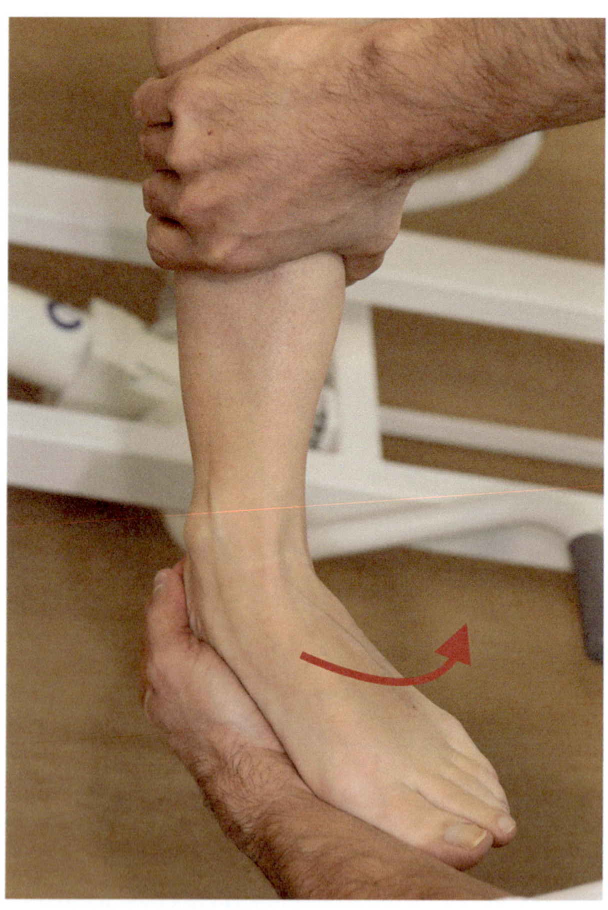

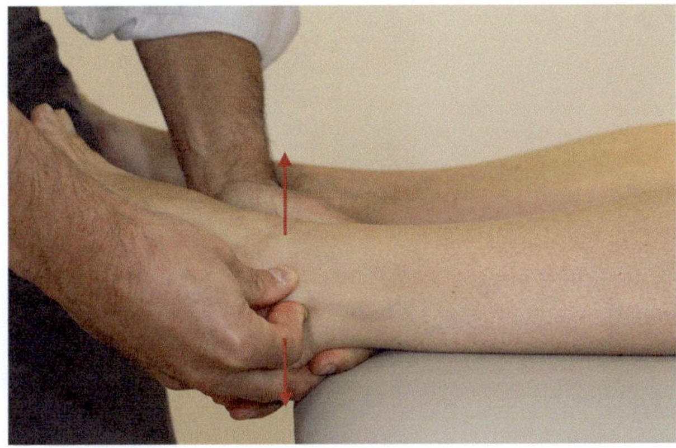

Fig. 11.5 The fibular translation test

the ankle under load. In a second step, the examiner performs a compression movement in the supramalleolar region. The test is positive if this compression maneuver relieves the patient (Fig. 11.6). A variant of this test exists by replacing manual compression by strapping.

In conclusion, the clinical picture reported by the patient and the positivity of these different tests make it possible to highlight a painful symptomatology on DTFS in the event of acute, subacute, or chronic lesions. By increasing the number of tests, the overall sensitivity of the clinical examination is increased. However, clinical diagnosis alone is insufficient to make a therapeutic decision. It should be supplemented by a suitable iconographic assessment confirming the diagnosis of DTFS instability and which will allow the surgical strategy to be defined.

Imaging

If a syndesmosis injury is suspected, imaging should be considered in addition to the clinical history and physical examination with stress tests to confirm the diagnosis. Conventional imaging (radiography and CT) are widely used, but suffer from lack of reproducibility and diagnostic power. Advanced modalities including MRI and weight-bearing CT (WBCT) offer new perspectives and opportunities to diagnose syndesmotic lesions earlier in order to apply adapted treatment algorithms before secondary onset degenerative evolution of the ankle joint occurs.

Radiography

Anteroposterior (AP) and mortise views are generally employed for assessment of the distal tibiofibular syndesmosis. Syndesmotic injuries can happen in isolation or in association with fractures. The most common are pronation-external rotation and

Fig. 11.6 The Ward test

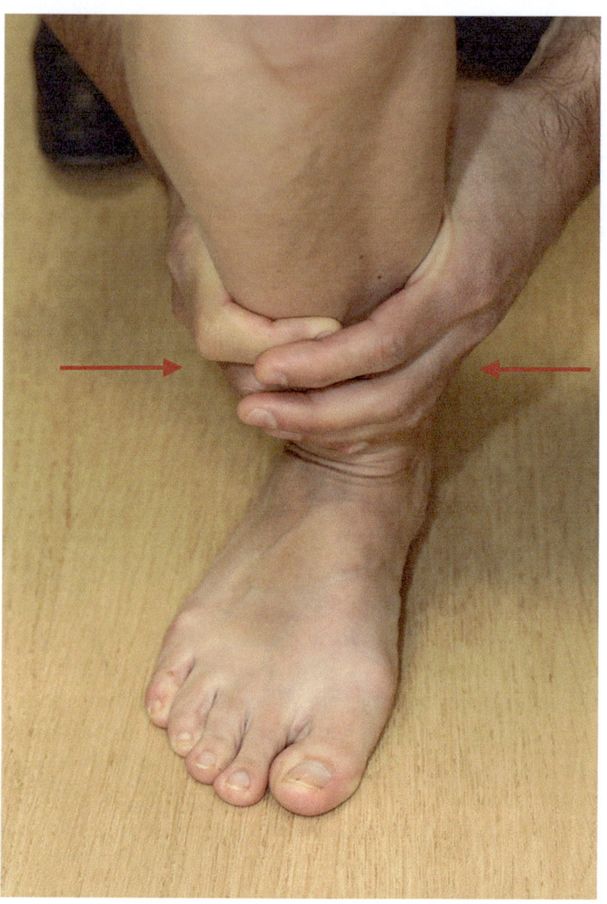

supination-external rotational (SER) fractures, Weber type C (Fig. 11.7), and proximal fibular fractures (Maisonneuve type). A lateral view is required to see an avulsion fracture at the posterior tibial tubercle, or a view of the proximal tibia and fibula when a Maisonneuve fracture is suspected.

The most common measurements used for detecting syndesmosis lesions on plain radiographs are the tibiofibular clear space (TFCS, the distance between the medial border of the fibula and the floor of the incisura at a level 1 cm proximal to the tibial plafond), the tibiofibular overlap (TFO, the distance between medial border of the fibula and the anterior tubercle of the tibia), and the medial clear space that can be increased with lateral shift of the talus (MCS, the distance between the medial border of the talar dome and the lateral border of the medial malleolus on mortise view) (Fig. 11.8).

In a cadaveric study, Harper and Keller first described these measurements in normal situation: the TFCS on the AP and mortise views should normally be less than 6 mm and seem to be the most reliable measurements, the TFO should be greater than 6 mm on the AP view or 42% of fibular width and greater than

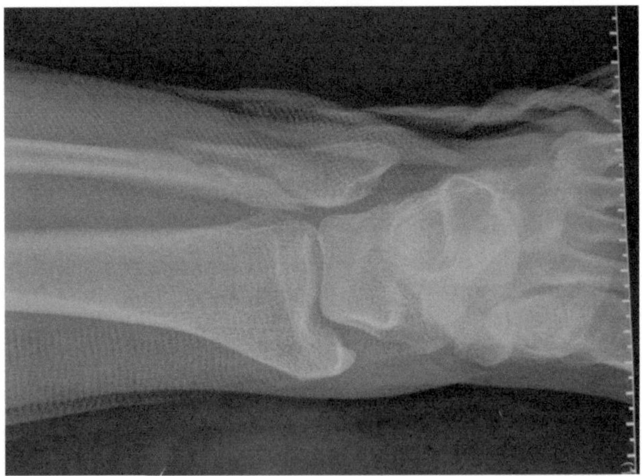

Fig. 11.7 Typical Weber type C fracture pattern with disruption of the distal syndesmosis, increased TFCS and MCS, and negative TFO

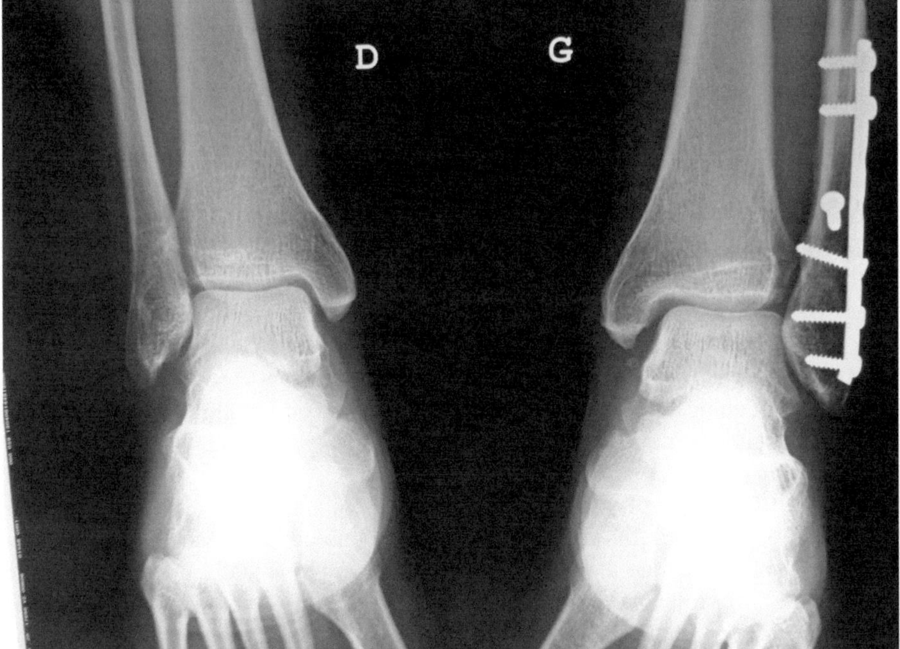

Fig. 11.8 Postoperative aspect with persisting increased TFCS and MCS

1 mm on the mortise view, and the MCS should be less than or equal to the superior joint space [22]. A more recent study showed that variability exists in these measurements among normal individuals and that a lack of overlap on the mortise view can be visualized in some normal cases [23]. Based on these observations, obtaining contralateral views for comparison in equivocal cases may be helpful.

Several studies were carried out to predict syndesmotic disruption based on malleolar fracture patterns [24, 25]. Hermans et al. demonstrated that by combining radiographic measurement with the Lauge-Hansen fracture classification, the accuracy of syndesmotic injury prediction was increased [26].

Rotation stress or gravity stress views may be used to confirm latent diastasis [27, 28]. Radiographic measurements of the distal tibiofibular syndesmosis can be modified by rotation of the ankle/limb, which makes standardization of radiographic measurements more difficult [29, 30]. As mentioned above, the TFCS on the AP view seems to be the most reliable parameter for diagnosing syndesmosis lesions: the reason for this is that it doesn't change with rotation [31]. Similarly, in a study in patients without ankle fractures evaluating the sensitivity of RX measurement comparing to MRI diagnosis of syndesmotic injury, Schoennagel et al. similarly found that TFCS is the best parameter [32].

Moreover, Jenkinson et al. demonstrated that intraoperative fluoroscopy stress examination detected more undiagnosed unstable syndesmotic injuries than preoperative radiography alone [33]. They compared intraoperative mortise views of Weber type C fractures with syndesmosis injury to the contralateral uninjured ankle. Assessment of contour changes in lateral malleolar shape, and the appearance of the lateral malleolar fossa cortex, proved to be a reliable method to detect distal fibula rotational malreduction [34].

In a diagnostic meta-analysis study, Chun et al. found that the pooled sensitivity for radiography to diagnose syndesmosis injury was 0.528 and 0.984 for the pooled specificity which is dependent on the presence of ankle fractures [35].

To conclude, conventional radiographs are mainly useful to assess gross syndesmotic injuries often associated with Weber type C fractures, but it is largely an insensitive test in more subtle lesions. It results that treatment decisions based only on RX may result in either failure to treat or overtreatment. The diagnosis of incomplete syndesmotic injuries remains difficult, particularly in cases when there is no fracture (high ankle sprain), and requires more advanced imaging for confirmation of syndesmosis disruption.

Computed Tomography (CT)

Computed tomography by providing excellent bone contrast and high-resolution imaging is more accurate than conventional radiography, mostly in cases of subtle syndesmotic injuries, low diastasis, and nondisplaced or subtle fractures such as Wagstaffe-LeFort fractures that can be missed or undetected on plain radiographs [36]. It has been used in subtle or complex cases over the past 20 years. However, with the advent of cone beam weight-bearing CT which provides similar quality but much less radiation dose, things may evolve rapidly in the future in favor of a more widespread use of the latter, toward a standard utilization in A&E, trauma, and specialized foot and ankle centers.

Elgafy et al. noticed variations in the anatomy of the incisura fibularis on CT. Nevertheless, using same reference points in normal patients, they found a mean of 2 mm for the width of the anterior tibiofibular syndesmosis (between the tip of the anterior tibial tubercle and the nearest point of the fibula) and a mean of 4 mm for the posterior tibiofibular syndesmosis (between the nearest point of the lateral border of the posterior tibial tubercle and the medial border of the fibula) [37].

Taser et al. used 3D reconstruction of axial CT images to calculate the volume of tibiofibular joint space, with the aim of detecting tibiofibular diastasis. They found that a 1-mm diastasis increases approximately 43% of the joint space volume, while from 1 to 3 mm, there is about a 20% increase for each 1-mm increase [38].

As for plain radiographs, given anatomic variability between individuals [39–41], bilateral CT is very useful and strongly recommended for the evaluation of syndesmotic injuries or malreduction [39, 42, 43]. However, this represents a high radiation dose compared to what a modern, bilateral weight-bearing cone beam CT offers, which questions the legitimacy of such an investigation today.

In case of chronic syndesmotic injuries, CT is used to assess fibular length, degenerative changes within the syndesmosis or tibiotalar joint, osteochondral lesions, the presence of a synostosis, or fracture malreduction.

In a cadaveric study with simulated malreduction models, Schon et al. found that the most reliable measurements for detecting the magnitude and direction of the malreduction are the clear space for lateral translation, the anterior tibiofibular distance for posterior translation, and the talar dome angle for external rotation of the fibula [44]. According to Knops et al., the most reliable and accurate method for the difficult assessment of fibular rotational malreduction is the measurement of the angle between the tangent of the anterior tibial surface and the bisection of the vertical midline of the fibula at the level of the incisura [45].

A study evaluated syndesmotic measurements during active motion of the ankle using four-dimensional computed tomography (4DCT) in asymptomatic ankles [46]. They found no change for all the syndesmotic measurements except for the syndesmotic translation (defined by the distance between the anterior margins of the tibia and the line tangential to the anterolateral surface of the fibula) which has a propensity to decrease during plantarflexion, so the authors propose that changes of syndesmotic measurements during dorsiflexion or plantarflexion in symptomatic ankles could indicate syndesmosis-related instability. In contrast, a recent cadaveric study showed that ankle plantarflexion (from 0° to 30°) doesn't affect CT measurements of the syndesmosis [47].

To conclude, although more expensive than radiographs, CT is a useful tool for accurate assessment of the tibiofibular anatomy and subtle fractures and also to guide surgical planning and fixation strategies [48] and to analyze malreduction intraoperatively [49–52] or postoperatively. However, with recent endeavors such as the development of stress CT (with external rotation and dorsiflexion) and cone beam, the ongoing trend is clearly in favor of weight-bearing CT, which offers similar or better spatial definition at a much lower cost and radiation dose.

Cone Beam Weight-Bearing CT (WBCT)

Although some studies tried to analyze the syndesmosis during stance prior to the emergence of this technology in the 2010's such as by 3D/2D registration technique or stereophotogrammetric analysis [53, 54], it was the emergence of cone beam weight-bearing CT (WBCT) that allowed for the first time the analysis of syndesmosis on axial views during true weight bearing [55]. Weight-bearing CT is more accurate than radiographs by preventing inaccuracies of projections and/or foot orientation and allows studying bone positions in standing position in contrast to conventional radiography and CT [56] (Fig. 11.9).

The influence of weight bearing on 2D measurements performed on CT scans is still debated. However, this must not overshadow the advantages of cone beam CT, which offers CT images at a much lower cost and radiation dose. The weight-bearing aspect is a bonus of WBCT, not its nature. Indeed, Shakoor et al. didn't find significant differences in syndesmotic measurements, except for the MCS (medial

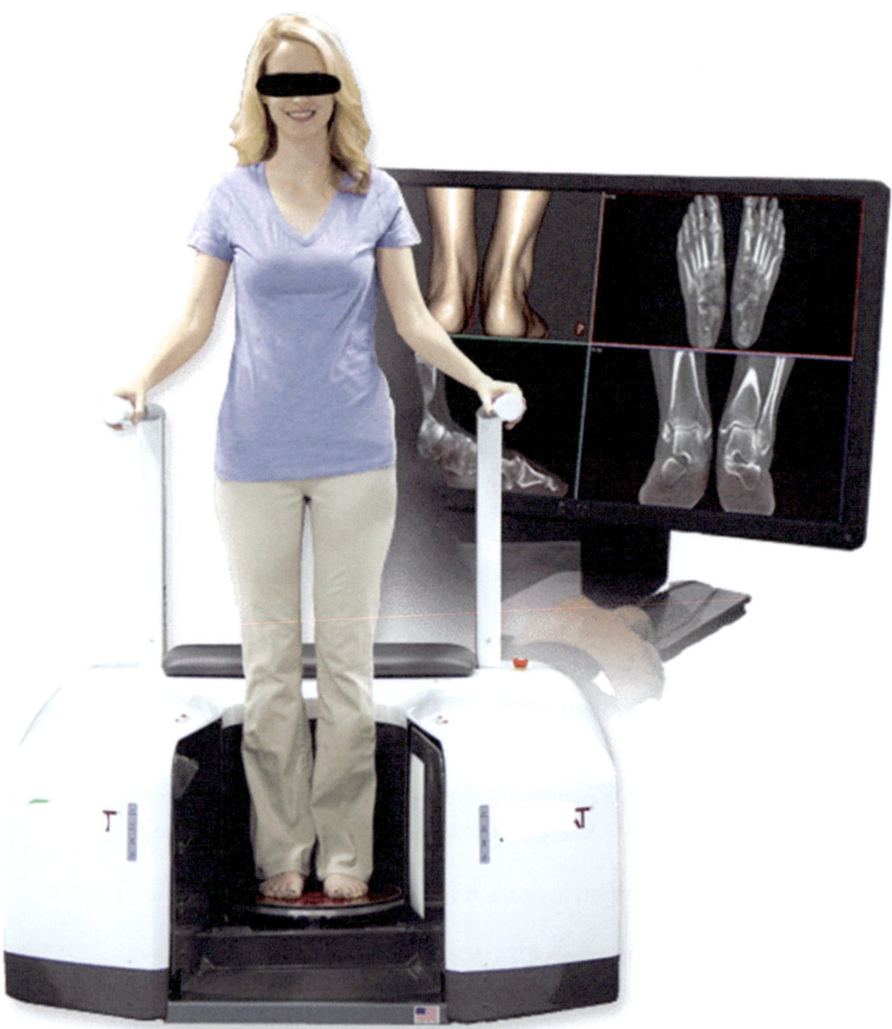

Fig. 11.9 Example of a cone beam WBCT scan (courtesy of Curvebeam, LLC)

clear space), when weight bearing is applied during cone beam CT acquisition of asymptomatic uninjured ankles [57]. Similarly a cadaveric study showed no difference between measurements of the distal tibiofibular syndesmosis in incomplete and more complete syndesmotic injuries with and without load application, and only more complete injuries of the distal tibiofibular syndesmosis could be identified using axial WBCT images [58]. In contrast, in a study comparing WBCT with conventional CT, it has been demonstrated that weight bearing is a reproducible method for assessing the syndesmosis with the following changes observed in WBCT: lateral and posterior translation and external rotation of the fibula in relation to the incisura [59]. In patients with a history of ankle injury, it has been shown that weight bearing changes significantly some angular measurements and increases posterior tibiofibular distance and diastasis [60].

In a cadaver study, when using WBCT, Krähenbühl and colleagues demonstrated on digitally reconstructed radiographs (DRR) and axial images that torque application helps to diagnose incomplete syndesmotic injuries: the tibiofibular overlap (TFO) was useful to differentiate isolated AITFL transection from native ankles. The medial clear space (MCS) and the tibiofibular clear space (TFCS) were useful predictors for more complete injuries by identifying an additional deltoid ligament transection or PITFL transection, respectively [61, 62].

In a retrospective comparative study, Burssens et al. proposed a method to quantify the displacement of a syndesmotic lesion. They used the 3D-mirrored healthy ankle as template on bilateral WBCT scans in case of a high ankle sprains and on bilateral non-weight-bearing CT in case of a fracture-associated syndesmotic lesion (Fig. 11.10) [63]. Patel et al. did not find any significant syndesmotic differences between right and left legs in patients' healthy ankles [64]. So, as in conventional radiographs or CT, for the diagnosis of syndesmosis and to determine if syndesmotic measurements are normal or abnormal, the uninjured side as an internal

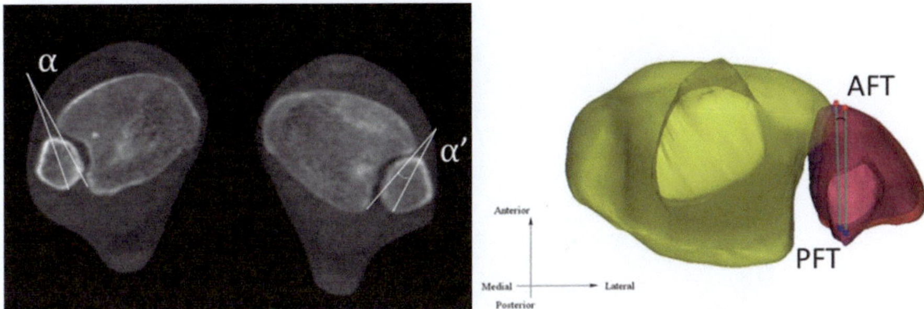

Fig. 11.10 Right-sided chronic syndesmotic ankle lesion in a 32-year-old male. Clinical examination demonstrated a positive squeeze and external rotation test. Weight-bearing CT images revealed an increased posterior translation of the fibula (posterior sagging), and external rotation demonstrated a reduced angle α compared to angle α' (left). A 3D reconstruction of the same patient was obtained after mirroring and matching the right on the left side based on the geometry of the tibia. Computed anatomical landmarks allowed to quantify this lesion according to the 6 degrees of freedom. Images provided by Dr. Kristian Buedts and analyzed by Dr. Arne Burssens (Ghent University, Belgium)

control seemed to be a better reference than population-based ranges of normal values since there is significant variation between sex and individuals [55, 65, 66]. Nevertheless, it has been shown that the intra- and interobserver reliability of syndesmotic reduction assessment with WBCT was low. However, this may be due to the fact that 2D techniques (angles and distances) were applied in a 3D environment [67]. The introduction of cone beam WBCT as a mainstream examination requires the development of new, computerized tools such as semiautomatic 3D biometric software [68]. Syndesmotic area calculation, followed by fibular rotation, has already demonstrated high reliability [69]. Pushing this concept further, Bhimani et al. have recently published on the use of volumetric measurements in a case-control study of patients who were evaluated using a bilateral WBCT [70]. They found significant increase in comparison with contralateral syndesmotic volume in the case group, with the volumetric measurement being more sensitive than their 2D counterparts.

Furthermore, in another very recent study, Del Rio et al. demonstrated that WBCT allows visualizing greater diastasis in unstable ankles than with conventional non-weight-bearing CT and that dynamic change in syndesmotic area from NWB to WB and WB comparison with the contralateral uninjured ankle are two parameters that may be useful for evaluating syndesmotic instability in the future [71].

To conclude, WBCT presents the advantage of standardizing the position of the foot and to perform bilateral full 3D standing scans of the foot and ankle complex (Fig. 11.11). More studies will be performed in the very near future to standardize syndesmotic area and volume measurements. In particular, the development of bone segmentation has recently paved the way to new techniques such as distance mapping, which registers pixel per pixel (rather voxel per voxel since WBCT is in a 3D

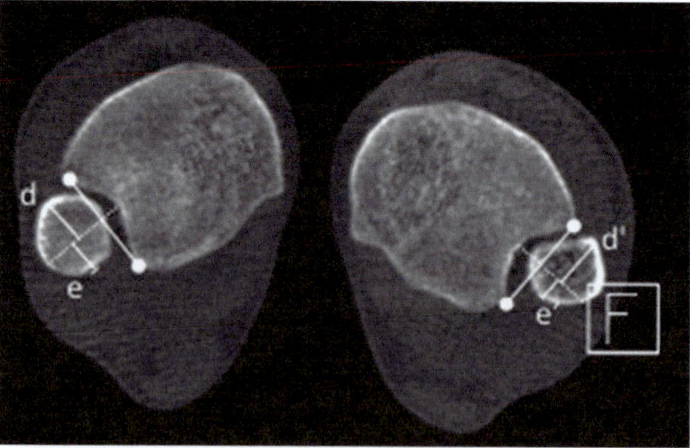

Fig. 11.11 Left-sided syndesmotic ankle sprain in a 21-year-old male hockey player. Clinical examination demonstrated gross instability during the fibular translation test. Weight-bearing CT images reveal an increased anterior fibular translation (increased distance d' and reduced distance e' relative to distance d and e). Images provided by Dr. Kristian Buedts and analyzed by Dr. Arne Burssens (Ghent University, Belgium)

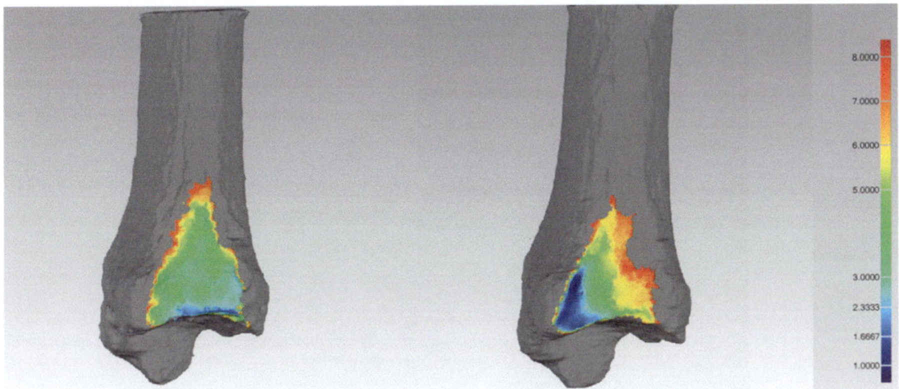

Fig. 11.12 Distance mapping of the tibial incisura, comparative of a normal (left) versus injured side (right). Image provided by Dr. Francois Lintz, analysis by Pr Sorin Sigler (Drexel University, Philadelphia, USA)

environment) a joint surface interactions map [72] (Fig. 11.12). In parallel, the development of automatic measurement software which has arisen from the growing use of cone beam WBCT as standard of care in orthopedic practices will help to identify more precisely syndesmotic pathology, particularly in patients with occult syndesmotic instability or to assess postoperative reduction.

Magnetic Resonance Imaging (MRI)

Magnetic resonance imaging (MRI) of the syndesmotic complex is a useful diagnostic tool to evaluate the integrity of syndesmotic ligaments often misdiagnosed by conventional imaging. Thereby, it helps to evaluate the grade of injury by determining which ligament(s) are torn (grades I to IV) [10, 73]. Using standard 3.0 T protocol, especially the T1 and T2 axial images, an abnormal course, a wavy irregular appearance (fuzzy contours), discontinuity, and abnormal signal intensity (enhancement or non-visualization) are signs of a ligament injury (Fig. 11.13).

MRI is a highly sensitive and specific tool for pretherapeutic evaluation of both acute and chronic syndesmotic injuries [74]. In comparison with arthroscopy as a definitive diagnostic standard, it has been demonstrated that MRI diagnosis was 100% sensitive for both anterior inferior tibiofibular ligament (AITFL) and posterior inferior tibiofibular ligament (PITFL) disruptions, 70–94% specific for AITFL injury and 100% specific for PITFL rupture [75, 76]. In similar studies, Han et al. and Clanton et al. also reported high sensitivity, specificity, and accuracy for MRI in detecting syndesmotic injury [77, 78].

Based on this knowledge, several studies have demonstrated that there is no correlation between the tibiofibular clear space (TFCS) and tibiofibular overlap (TFO) on radiographs with anterior or posterior syndesmotic ligament injury on MRI scans [26, 79].

It has also been shown that the presence of the lambda sign (Fig. 11.14) noted as a high-intensity signal on coronal MRI that resembles the Greek letter lambda with

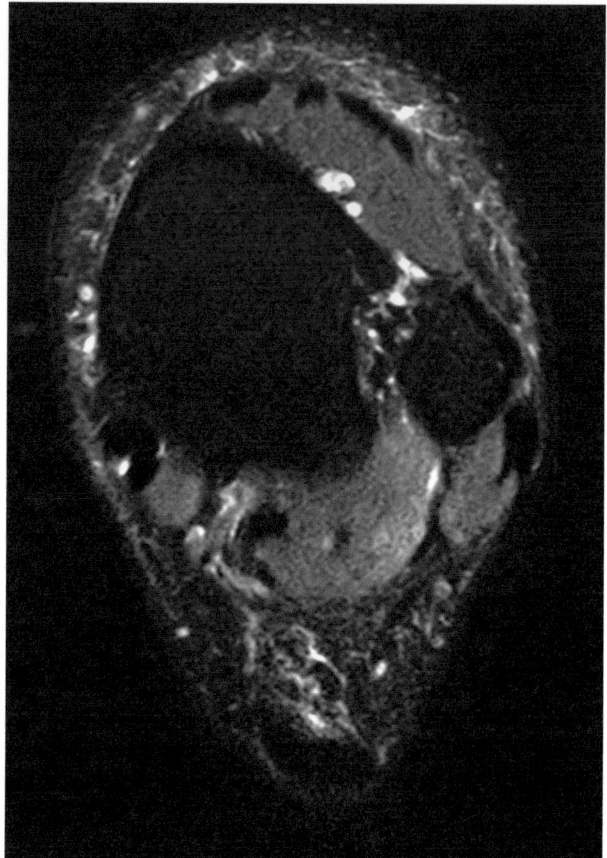

Fig. 11.13 Example of AITFL rupture in a 40-year-old football player

physical exam findings suggestive of syndesmotic pain was sensitive (75%) and specific (85%) for injuries involving greater than 2 mm of diastasis on arthroscopic stress examination [51].

It appears that MRI may be helpful in planning surgical approaches by revealing syndesmotic injury patterns less predictable on the radiographs. Indeed, some ankle fractures are quite frequently unclassifiable under the Lauge-Hansen system, and MRI demonstrated that this classification has limitations as a predictor of the mechanism of injury and the presence of ligamentous disruption associated with ankle fractures [80].

In addition, secondary findings can be concurrently assessed by MRI such as bone contusions, tibiofibular joint incongruity, height of the tibiofibular recess, osteochondral lesions, tendinous structures, and subtle bony injuries [81, 82].

Despite its good sensitivity and specificity in detecting a syndesmotic lesion, there remains controversy about the ability of MRI to diagnose whether the latter is the

Fig. 11.14 Localization of the "lambda sign," from the Greek letter λ, between the superior aspect of the talar dome, the talofibular facet, and the syndesmosis, where the most proximal extremity of the λ corresponds to the inferior aspect of the syndesmosis, where an AITFL rupture corresponds to a low T1 signal and a hyper T2 signal. Image Courtesy of Pr Cesar de Cesar Netto (University of Iowa, Iowa City, USA)

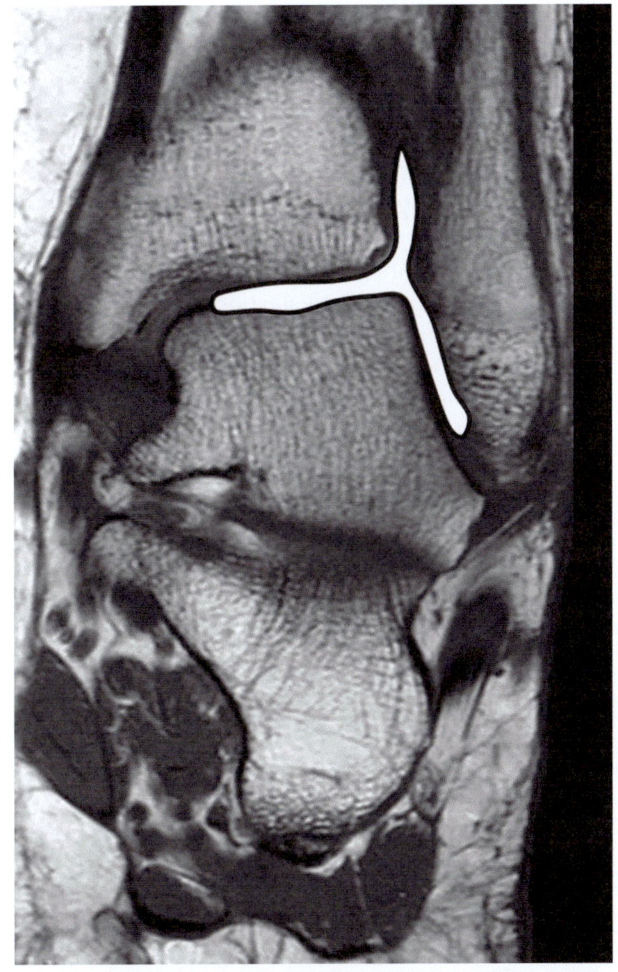

cause for instability as it's not a dynamic test. Several pitfalls in the MRI diagnosis of syndesmotic ligament injury should be avoided. Firstly, the AITFL, PITFL, and the anterior, posterior talofibular ligaments are close and have similar obliquity on axial views: they can therefore easily be confused. Secondly, a ligament disruption should not be confused with the striated appearance of the AITFL resulting from interspersed areas of fat between the multiple bands of the ligament [83]. Finally, syndesmotic ligaments obliqueness can lead to false positive as compared to intraoperative findings since they might appear interrupted when the MRI slice is not parallel to the ligament, resulting also in false positives. Hermans et al. described the advantage of MRI scanning not in the orthogonal axial plane but in an oblique plane of about 45°, parallel to the AITFL and PITFL to improve visualization and to decrease the risk of false-positive diagnosis of partial or complete ligament ruptures [84].

To conclude, MRI is a very helpful tool to assess the presence or absence of syndesmotic lesions and potential concurrently associated lesions, but has to be balanced with knowledge of anatomy and imaging pitfalls. However, being a non-weight-bearing, static imaging, it does not permit to conclude that any lesion is the cause for instability.

Ultrasonography

Ultrasound (US) is an easy and reliable but underused tool in the assessment of the syndesmosis. Research on syndesmotic injuries is more interested in complex, invasive, and often expensive evaluation methods. A specific US protocol, both static and dynamic, could however be effective in the future to help with the diagnosis of the majority of acute and chronic lesions. The first articles describing the use of US for syndesmosis assessment are more than 20 years old [85]. Despite this, US does not seem to be considered as a reliable tool to assess the syndesmotic joint [35, 86]. The two main limitations of US are its operator dependence and the fact that US scan is not able to visualize intra-articular injuries. However, it is a low-cost, noninvasive, quick, and effective exam which allows both static and dynamic evaluation. Ligamentous US dynamic assessment can be effective by showing enlargement of the space between the ends of a ligament, elongation or rupture, or modification of joint biomechanics, but this method still requires standardization and reproducibility criteria [87, 88] to be effective in clinical practice.

Syndesmosis Static Assessment

Syndesmotic sprains always start with antero-inferior tibiofibular ligament (AITFL) rupture, which is the anterior lock of the joint. Then the severity of the injury increases with interosseous membrane (IOM) tear and finally postero-inferior tibiofibular ligament (PITFL) lesion. The deltoid ligament (DL) can be injured during the trauma and must also be systematically investigated.

Antero-Inferior Tibiofibular Ligament (AITFL)

On an anterior-posterior view [89–91], it runs obliquely downward and laterally from the anterior tibial tubercle to the anterior border of lateral malleolus. It is composed of several fascicles.

Normal AITFL thickness ranges from 2.6 to 4 mm. It appears as an echogenic fibrillary structure like any other ligament (Fig. 11.15). The US beam should be as perpendicular as possible to the ligament to avoid anisotropy artifacts.

Acute ruptures will show ligament discontinuity or hypoechoic, thickened, and heterogeneous areas in the ligament with loss of fibrillary aspect (Fig. 11.16). Chronic injury may have similar appearances, but the clinical context and dynamic maneuvers will help with the diagnosis.

Interosseous Membrane (IOM)

After AITFL visualization, the interosseous membrane can be assessed by putting the probe in a horizontal plane and by moving slowly upward. It appears as

Fig. 11.15 AITFL, normal

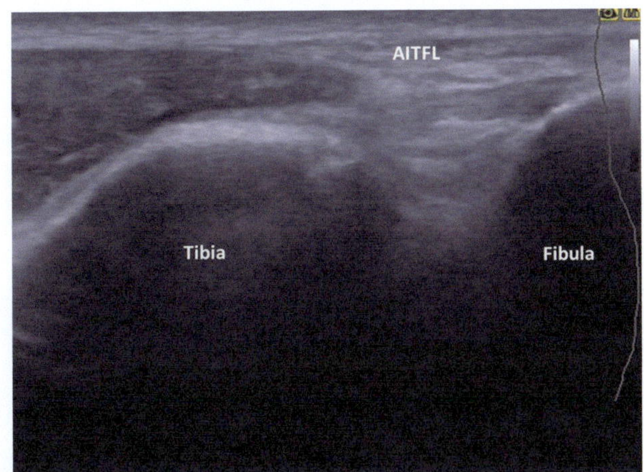

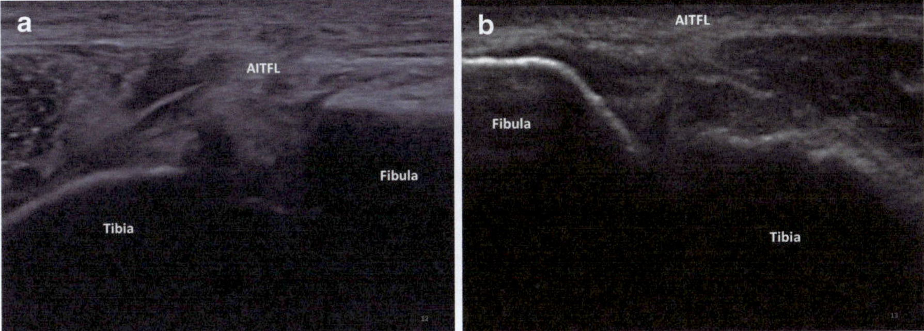

Fig. 11.16 (a, b) AITFL acute tears

a thin hyperechoic and continuous line between the tibia and fibula (Fig. 11.17). The injured IOM is poorly defined and hypoechoic and can be discontinuous [92].

Posterior Inferior Tibiofibular Ligament (PITFL)

As recently described, it is possible to visualize the PITFL directly (Fig. 11.18). This requires the patient to lie in prone position, ideally with the foot hanging off the end of the table.

The ligament runs obliquely upward and medially from the posterior tip of the distal fibula to the lateral process of the tibia. The superficial component of PITFL appears as a tense and fibrillar structure, whereas its deep component, the transverse ligament, is more difficult to visualize [93].

PITFL injuries (Fig. 11.19) always occur in the same area near its tibial insertion with visualization of a thickened and hypoechoic ligament or small bony avulsions [94–96].

Fig. 11.17 Normal IOM

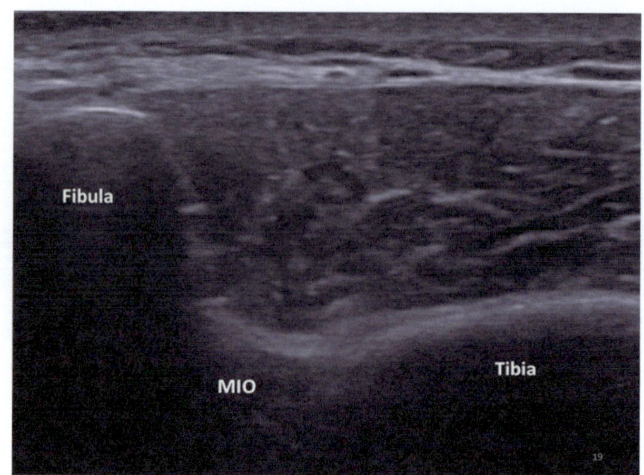

Fig. 11.18 Normal PITFL

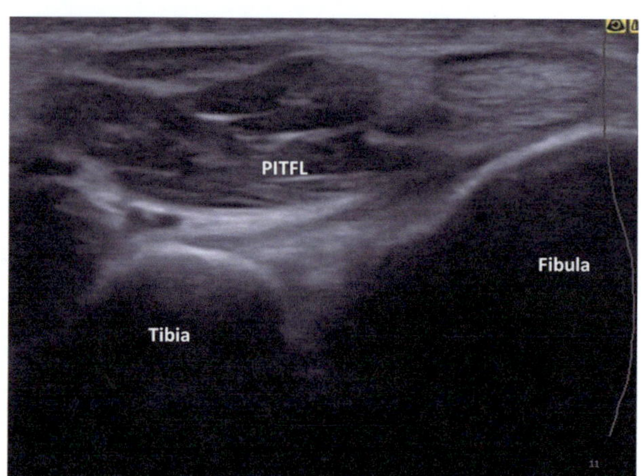

Fig. 11.19 PITFL acute injury

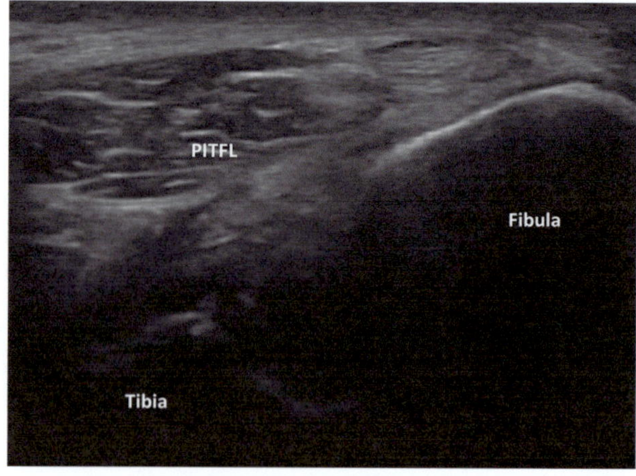

Deltoid Ligament (DL)

Due to its biomechanical role in limiting ankle abduction, external rotation, and dorsal flexion, the examination of the DL must be systematic.

We are used to describing an anterior superficial deltoid and a posterior deep deltoid. But its anatomy is much more complex, and DL injury assessment can be challenging, ranging from the identification of hypoechoic areas, and swelling without frank disruption, and involving several bundles [97–99].

MRI studies have shown that superficial deltoid injuries are the most frequent and are always superficial tibial avulsion, whereas lesions of the posterior deltoid concern the posterior tibiotalar ligament and are mostly found at the level of its talar insertion.

Syndesmosis Dynamic Assessment

The dynamic maneuvers to assess the normal (Fig. 11.20; Videos 11.1, 11.2, 11.3, and 11.4), acute (Fig. 11.21; Videos 11.5 and 11.6), and chronic (Fig. 11.22) syndesmosis already published consist, on a subject in supine position with knee flexed at 90° and ankle in ankle dorsiflexion, in causing external and internal rotation on the ankle and measuring clear space between the tibia and fibula. This clear space increases in external rotation, especially when the AITFL is injured, and decreases in internal rotation [100–102].

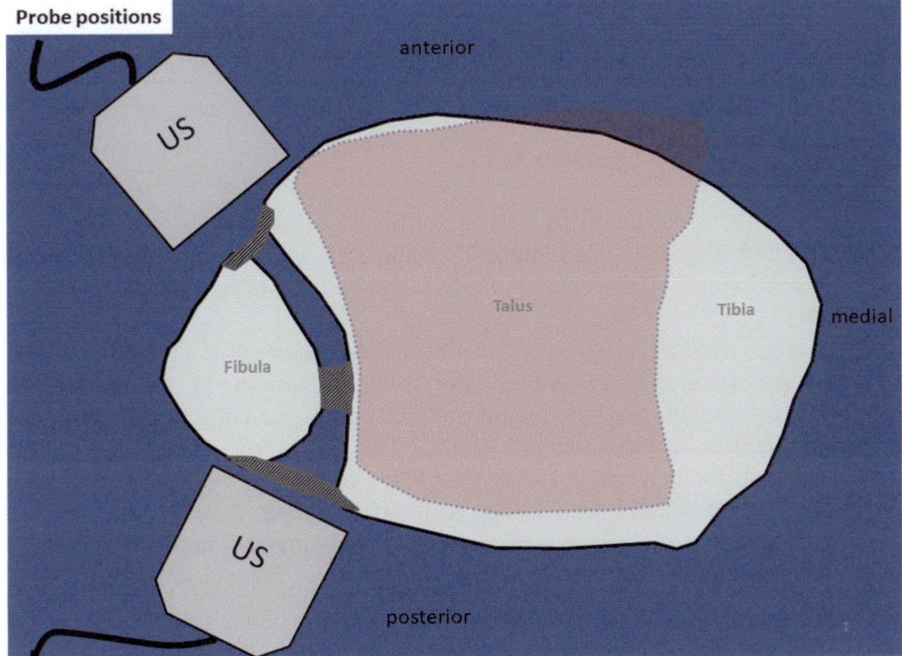

Fig. 11.20 Dynamic US protocol of normal syndesmosis assessment

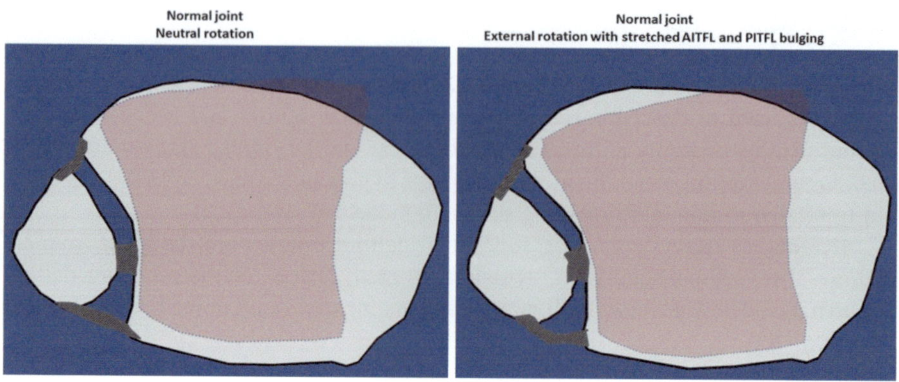

Fig. 11.21 Acute syndesmosis injury assessment

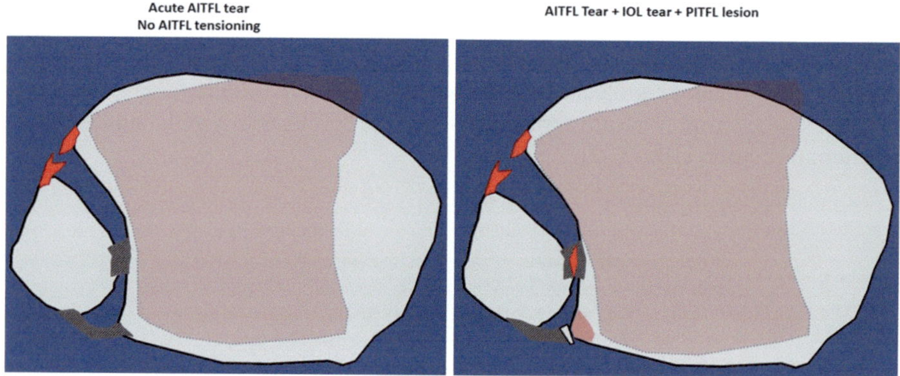

Fig. 11.22 Chronic syndesmosis injury assessment

However, the reproducibility and reliability of clear space measurement in 2D ultrasound scan are questionable. Furthermore, we have identified significant interindividual differences in physiological mobility of syndesmosis [103, 104].

We prefer a dynamic analysis of the associated mobility of the tibia and fibula. For this it is possible to assess not only the AITFL but also the PITFL on a patient in prone position with the foot hanging off the end of the table by applying soft external rotation on a relaxed ankle.

The external rotation and posterior translation of the fibula [55, 105] and ligaments tensioning [106, 107] can thus be perfectly visualized.

Furthermore, ultrasonography also enables the assessment of the deep and superficial components of the medial collateral ligament (Fig. 11.23; Videos 11.7 and 11.8).

Normal Syndesmosis Assessment
Anterior view (Video 11.3)

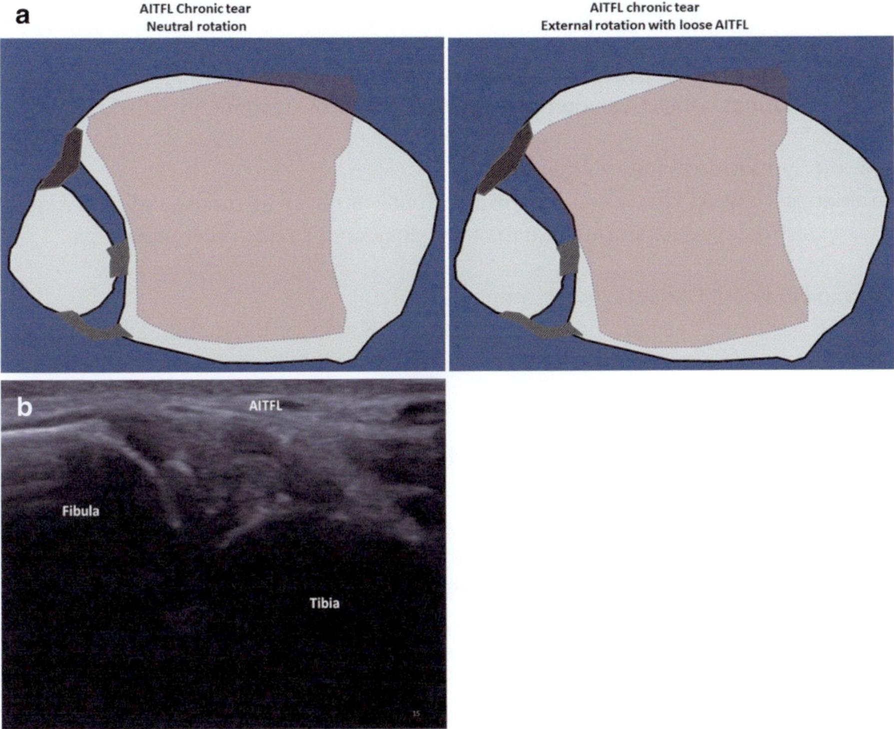

Fig. 11.23 (**a, b**) Deltoid ligament dynamic assessment

1. Posterior translation (1–3 mm) and external rotation of the fibula in relation to the tibia
2. Tensioning of the AITFL
3. Associated mobilization of the fibula and tibia in external rotation

   Posterior view (Video 11.4)
   Approximation in a mediolateral axis of the tibia and fibula with bulging (posterior convexity) of the PITFL.

Acute Syndesmosis Injury Assessment
Anterior view (Video 11.5)

1. Posterior translation and external rotation of the fibula
2. No tensioning of the AITFL
3. Increased motion of the fibula without transmission to the tibia - > complete dissociation (acute lesion) of tibiofibular mobility

Posterior view (Video 11.6)

1. Alteration of tibial posterior malleolar, bone, or periosteal avulsion
2. No additional objective contribution from posterior dynamic visualization

Chronic Syndesmosis Injury Assessment

In anterior view, AITFL is most of the time loose or rarely disrupted and tibia mobility appears delayed. Posterior visualization does not provide other elements.

Deltoid Ligament Dynamic Assessment

The DL has never been the subject of dynamic US studies, but mobilization in external rotation, eversion, or dorsal flexion makes it possible to put in tension the different bundles.

Syndesmosis Standardized Ultrasound Scan

This examination should not be limited to a quick AITFL view in supine position.

IOM must be assessed too because its injury would confirm serious AITFL damage. Then, the DL, with its two components, superficial and deep, should be checked.

Then the patient should be placed in a prone position to allow the dynamic assessment of AITFL and PITFL. In this position it is easy to test at the same time ATFL, CFL, and DL.

In acute injuries and associated with a radiological examination (to not miss a fracture or a frank diastasis), this US standardized scan allows a sufficient assessment of the syndesmosis enabling a therapeutic decision.

In chronic cases and according to the experience of the operator, it is an extremely effective method to diagnose chronic lesions (AITFL, PITFL, IOM, deltoid) but also to evaluate, in a comparative manner with the other ankle, physiological or pathological joint laxity and thus to highlight a potential instability of the syndesmosis.

Evidence-Based Critical Appraisal of the Literature Conforming to PRISMA Statement

Dynamic or Static Stabilization to Fix Syndesmotic Injuries: What Does the Literature Say?

Over the last years, a few randomized trials have compared dynamic and static stabilization methods to fix ankle syndesmotic injuries (Fig. 11.24). Multiple meta-analyses have been published [108–113], with particular attention toward the suture-button technique. In 2020, a biomechanical comparison on cadaveric specimens by Lee et al. demonstrated how the dynamic fixation performed using suture button led to less rigidity as compared to metal or bioabsorbable screws, with a final construct much more similar to the physiological syndesmosis in terms of micromotion.

Among the clinical meta-analyses, the larger and most recent one has been conducted by Grassi et al. and published in March 2020 on the *American Journal of*

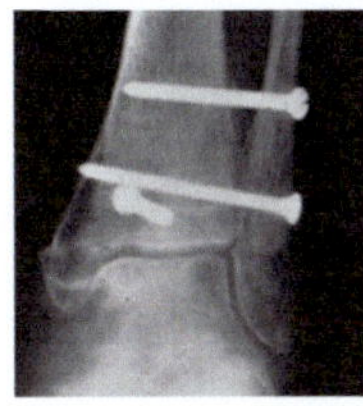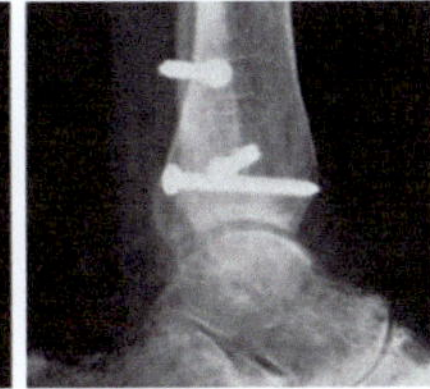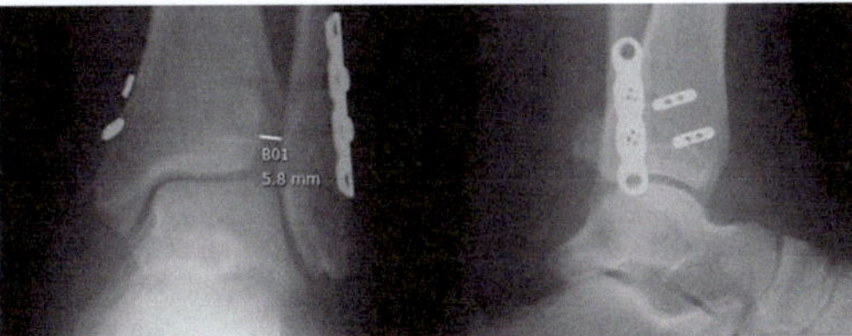

Fig. 11.24 Examples of rigid (left) and dynamic (right) fixation systems. Images courtesy of Dr. Cesar de Cesar Netto (University of Iowa, Iowa City, USA)

Sports Medicine. In this study, performed according to the Preferred Reporting Items for Systematic Reviews and Meta-Analyses (PRISMA) guidelines, seven randomized controlled trials (level I of evidence) were included, for a total of 168 patients treated with dynamic fixation (in five studies the suture button was used, in one cerclages and in one elastic hook plate) and 167 with static fixation (transsyndesmotic screws). Follow-up in primary studies was between 12 and 24 months.

For what concerns the complications related to surgery, dynamic fixation was associated with a reduced risk of inadequate reduction at final follow-up, recurrent diastasis or instability, implant breakage, and implant loosening. This finding was confirmed regardless of the type of device used, the decision to retain or remove the screw, and the length of follow-up (shorter or longer than 12 months). Interestingly, in a subgroup analysis where authors considered only "clinically relevant complications" (i.e., all but implant breakage and loosening), there was no difference between the dynamic and the static stabilization group.

Although the reoperation rate was similar between the two groups, the authors found a reduced risk of being reoperated after dynamic fixation if compared with static stabilization with permanent screws. The use of different devices and the length of follow-up didn't seem to affect the result in this case either.

In terms of clinical outcome, the analysis of the Olerud-Molander score did not reveal any significant difference between the two methods of treatment. Conversely, the American Orthopaedic Foot & Ankle Society (AOFAS) score was higher (therefore better) by six points at 3 months, by five points at 12 months, and by eight points at 24 months for patients who have undergone dynamic stabilization when compared to the static fixation. The Visual Analog Scale (VAS) also revealed a better control of pain for the dynamic fixation group, with mean values being lower by −0.7 and −0.5 points by 6 and 12 months. It should be emphasized that, although these differences resulted statistically significant, the minimally clinical important difference of these parameters in ankle fractures has not been established yet. This means that it's difficult to translate the advantages shown through these scores into daily practice, and a clear conclusion about the superiority of one technique versus one other in clinical terms cannot be drawn.

Finally, the time to return to work and to sport (which are important parameters from a patient perspective) were evaluated only in two and one study, respectively; therefore further analyses are warranted to verify whether dynamic fixation allows a quicker recovery or not.

The Ultimate Treatment Algorithm

Based on the evidence in the literature and the author's experience.

Introduction

The treatment of syndesmotic injuries is a challenge for sports physicians and surgeons.

This report only presents isolated syndesmotic lesions.

We present a simple algorithm to help determine the management of these injuries based on the most recent data in the literature and our personal experience.

In the decisional algorithms that have already been proposed in the literature [114, 115], management is determined according to the delay before surgery (acute, subacute, chronic). Certain notions in these treatment algorithms are highly theoretical (latent or clear instability, possibility of ligament repair, etc.) and difficult to apply.

Our goal is to present a final treatment algorithm that is reproducible in clinical practice.

Because of the severe and rapid consequences of poorly treated syndesmotic lesions, we advise being extremely cautious and even overtreating these injuries.

There are two stages of management, chronic and acute. The acute stage is defined as 6 weeks after injury in clinical practice [115].

Acute Phase

"One can only treat what one finds, find what one looks for, and look for what one knows." This saying is particularly true for syndesmotic lesions, which often go unrecognized.

Making a Diagnosis

Before the lesion can be treated, a diagnosis must be made. To prevent a misdiagnosis, syndesmotic lesions should be suspected in the presence of any ankle injury.

The mechanism of injury (rotational force on a foot that is planted on the ground) and the cause (contact sport, rugby, judo, American football, sports on artificial grass surface) should prompt the physician to systematically perform a squeeze test of AITFL and a forced lateral rotation test.

Determine Disease Severity

X-rays are standard practice, and an MRI should be performed in case of clinical signs to determine the severity of ligament damage. The treatment strategy will depend on the grade of severity and the number of damaged ligaments. Sikka [73] et al. have proposed a four-grade classification:

- Anterior inferior talofibular (AITFL)
- IOL (interosseous ligament)
- Posterior talofibular ligament (PTFL)
- Medial collateral ligament (MCL)
- Grade 1: Isolated AITFL injury
- Grade 2: AITFL + IOL (± interosseous membrane)
- Grade 3: AITFL + IOL + PTFL
- Grade 4: AITFL + IOL + PTFL + MCL

Treatment

Once the diagnosis has been made and the severity of the injuries has been identified, treatment can be determined based on these elements.

There is a consensus in the literature on the management of stages 1, 3, and 4.

Grade 1: Conservative Orthopedic Treatment

There is no consensus on the amount of time weight should be kept off the foot for orthopedic treatment or on the type and duration of immobilization [114, 116, 117]. Flexible, removable splints such as the Aircast device do not sufficiently control flexion and extension of the ankle and are contraindicated in our practice. We prefer strict non-weight bearing and immobilization with an orthopedic boot for 21 days. The patient will only place weight on the foot when the ankle is completely pain-free. Non-weight bearing can be extended to 6 weeks. The walking boot makes it possible to begin physical rehabilitation immediately and limit loss of muscle tone. There are three phases to rehabilitation described in the literature [117–120]. The initial goal is to relieve pain with manual lymphatic drainage and compressive cryotherapy. Compression socks are used as soon as possible. Preventive anticoagulation is associated with the non-weight-bearing phase.

The goal of the second phase of rehabilitation is to recover complete joint range of motion and strengthen the active stabilizers in the foot. Special attention is paid to the intrinsic foot muscles, in particular the medial plantar muscle, and the primary muscles of ankle inversion (common flexor muscles of the toes, the extensor hallucis longus, the tibialis posterior). Finally, proprioceptive neuromuscular facilitation work is begun.

The third phase involves physical training to allow the patient to return to all his/her activities. This can never begin before week 6.

Grades 3 and 4: They Are Treated Surgically

Numerous studies have been performed to evaluate the type (static or dynamic), number of fixation, their influence on the quality of reduction, and the medico-economic impact of these options [5, 6, 10, 13, 17, 114–116, 121–134]. There seems to be an advantage to a double dynamic fixation [55, 109, 134–138]. In our practice anterior arthroscopy of the ankle is systematically performed first to confirm inferior tibiofibular instability [41–44], to directly repair the AITFL injury if the quality of remaining tissue is good, and to search for and treat associated injuries such as detachment of the deep fibers of the medial collateral ligament.

Although certain authors [123, 139] prefer direct repair of ligament damage, this has not been shown to be better than isolated fixation.

Rehabilitation following surgical treatment is similar to that with orthopedic management.

Grade 2

This is the only grade of severity that is a subject of debate. For numerous authors management depends on the patient, his/her age, and activity. It has been shown that 1 mm of lateral talar shift under the tibia results in a reduction in contact area of 42% [140]. In our practice, surgical treatment is systematic, because of the significant risk of rapid deterioration and morbidity. As described above treatment begins with arthroscopy to confirm the instability of the lesion by hook palpation. If the hook can be inserted into the syndesmosis, the test is positive, and the joint is considered to be unstable [141]. Stabilization is obtained with two cortical suture endobuttons.

The Case of Chronic Lesions

Like acute disease, the diagnosis is mainly based on a clinical examination and questioning of the patient. The patient usually mentions pain, a feeling of instability, swelling, and an inability to perform his/her usual activities. Additional tests confirm the suspected clinical diagnosis.

Surgical treatment will depend on the presence of degenerative changes in the inferior tibiofibular joint and/or the tibiotalar joint.

Although certain authors propose different treatment options depending on the function of the remaining ligaments [114, 115], we find this approach difficult to apply in clinical practice.

Lesions without Degenerative Changes

Although numerous treatments have been tested to manage these cases, only two options are now considered: arthroscopic debridement and anatomical reconstruction. These two treatment options are generally protected by static or dynamic stabilization.

Reconstruction by open surgery is proposed by Grambart et al. [142] for up to a year after injury, based on empirical evidence alone.

To our knowledge there are no studies comparing the results of simple debridement to ligament reconstruction.

Most articles on ligament reconstruction are technical notes [143–147] except for the report by Yasui et al. [148] who evaluated six patients and described excellent results after a mean 38 months of follow-up for isolated reconstruction of the AITFL.

Simple debridement with stabilization is less invasive. This is the approach taken in our practice, even if a study by Han [77] did not find any statistically significant

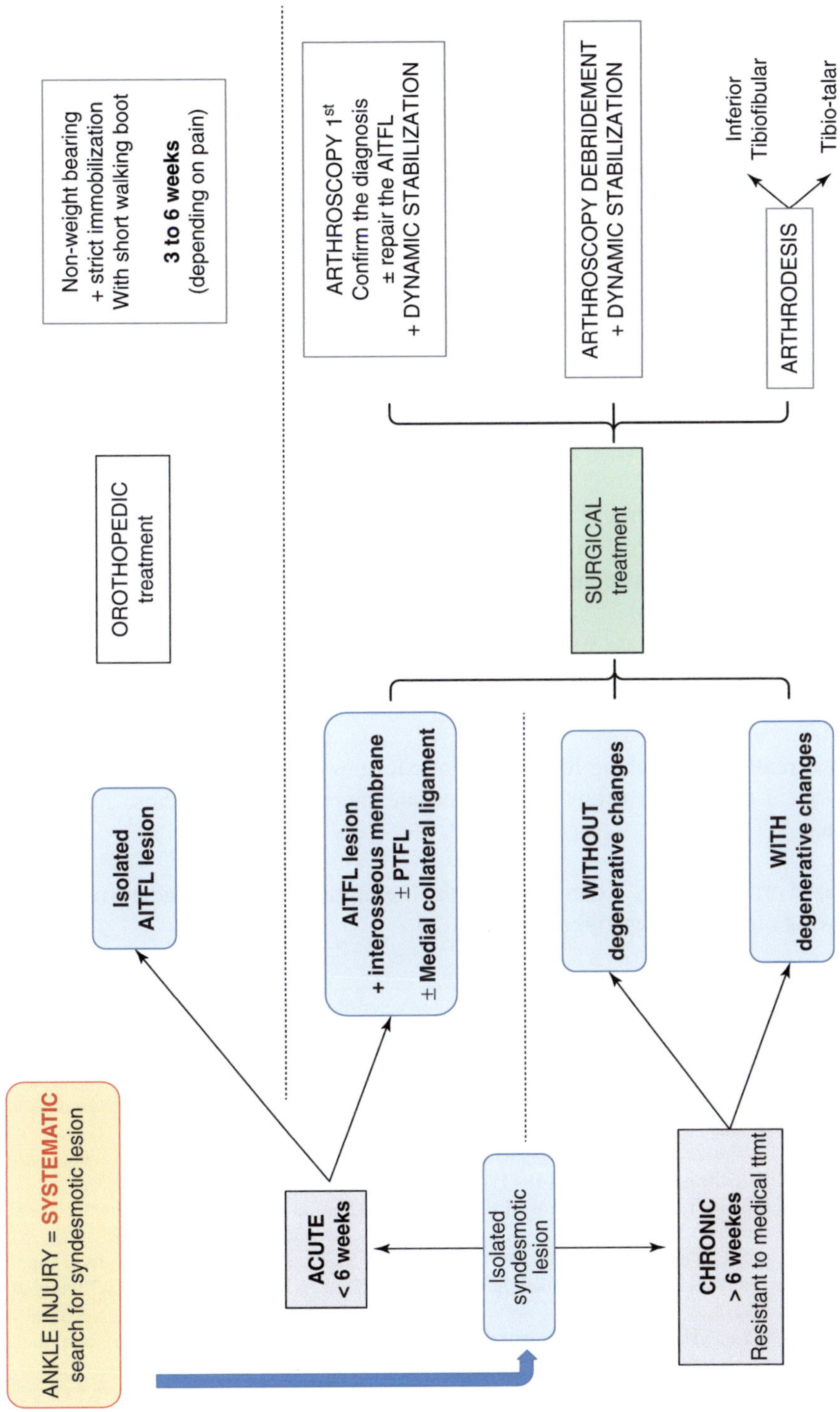

ANKLE INJURY = **SYSTEMATIC**
search for syndesmotic lesion

OROTHOPEDIC treatment

Non-weight bearing
+ strict immobilization
With short walking boot
3 to 6 weeks
(depending on pain)

Isolated
AITFL lesion

ACUTE
< 6 weeks

Isolated syndesmotic lesion

AITFL lesion
+ interosseous membrane
± PTFL
± Medial collateral ligament

ARTHROSCOPY 1st
Confirm the diagnosis
± repair the AITFL
+ DYNAMIC STABILIZATION

SURGICAL treatment

CHRONIC
> 6 weekes
Resistant to medical ttmt

WITHOUT
degenerative changes

WITH
degenerative changes

ARTHROSCOPY DEBRIDEMENT
+ DYNAMIC STABILIZATION

ARTHRODESIS

Inferior
Tibiofibular

Tibio-talar

Fig. 11.25 Ultimate treatment algorithm

difference between debridement with and without stabilization. That study emphasized the role of soft tissue impingement as the origin of pain.

In the Presence of Degenerative Changes

If the degenerative changes are localized in the tibiofibular joint, arthrodesis of the inferior tibiofibular joint is performed [132, 149, 150] especially since this does not seem to limit dorsal or plantarflexion of the ankle [58, 151].

In case of talar degeneration, most authors propose ankle arthrodesis alone. On the other hand, others consider total ankle arthroplasty to be a feasible option [125].

Algorithm

Certain concepts in existing algorithms [114, 115] are abstract and difficult to evaluate in clinical practice when determining the appropriate therapeutic option:

- The stability of the injury
- The possibility of repairing the remaining ligament
- Whether the injury is considered subacute (between 6 weeks and 6 months) or chronic (> 6 months)

Because of the risk of morbidity in chronic lesions of the syndesmosis [152], we recommend:

- Systematically searching for syndesmotic lesions in all ankle injuries
- Surgical treatment for any lesions that are more severe than those in an isolated AITFL

Based on the authors' experience and the literature, we recommend the use of the following algorithm, described in Fig. 11.25.

References

1. Großterlinden LG, Hartel M, Yamamura J, Schoennagel B, Bürger N, Krause M, et al. Isolated syndesmotic injuries in acute ankle sprains: diagnostic significance of clinical examination and MRI. Knee Surg Sports Traumatol Arthrosc. 2016;24(4):1180–6.
2. Loren GJ, Ferkel RD. Arthroscopic assessment of occult intra-articular injury in acute ankle fractures. Arthroscopy. 2002;18(4):412–21.
3. Hunt KJ, Goeb Y, Behn AW, Criswell B, Chou L. Ankle joint contact loads and displacement with progressive Syndesmotic injury. Foot Ankle Int. 2015;36(9):1095–103.
4. Sarrafian SK, Kelikian AS. Sarrafian's anatomy of the foot and ankle: descriptive, topographic, functional. 3rd ed. Philadelphia: Wolters Kluwer Health, Lippincott Williams & Wilkins; 2011.
5. Yuen CP, Lui TH. Distal tibiofibular syndesmosis: anatomy, biomechanics, injury and management. Open Orthop J. 2017;11:670–7.

6. Tourné Y, Molinier F, Andrieu M, Porta J, Barbier G. Diagnosis and treatment of tibiofibular syndesmosis lesions. Orthop Traumatol Surg Res. 2019;105(8S):S275–86.
7. Massri-Pugin J, Lubberts B, Vopat BG, Wolf JC, DiGiovanni CW, Guss D. Role of the deltoid ligament in Syndesmotic instability. Foot Ankle Int. 2018;39(5):598–603.
8. Hunt KJ, Hurwit D, Robell K, Gatewood C, Botser IB, Matheson G. Incidence and epidemiology of foot and ankle injuries in elite collegiate athletes. Am J Sports Med. 2017;45(2):426–33.
9. Mulcahey MK, Bernhardson AS, Murphy CP, Chang A, Zajac T, Sanchez G, et al. The epidemiology of ankle injuries identified at the National Football League Combine, 2009–2015. Orthop J Sports Med. 2018;6(7):2325967118786227.
10. Switaj PJ, Mendoza M, Kadakia AR. Acute and chronic injuries to the syndesmosis. Clin Sports Med. 2015;34(4):643–77.
11. Sman AD, Hiller CE, Rae K, Linklater J, Black DA, Nicholson LL, et al. Diagnostic accuracy of clinical tests for ankle syndesmosis injury. Br J Sports Med. 2015;49(5):323–9.
12. Hopkinson WJ, St Pierre P, Ryan JB, Wheeler JH. Syndesmosis sprains of the ankle. Foot Ankle. 1990;10(6):325–30.
13. Vopat ML, Vopat BG, Lubberts B, DiGiovanni CW. Current trends in the diagnosis and management of syndesmotic injury. Curr Rev Musculoskelet Med. 2017;10(1):94–103.
14. van Dijk CN, Longo UG, Loppini M, Florio P, Maltese L, Ciuffreda M, et al. Classification and diagnosis of acute isolated syndesmotic injuries: ESSKA-AFAS consensus and guidelines. Knee Surg Sports Traumatol Arthrosc. 2016;24(4):1200–16.
15. Kiter E, Bozkurt M. The crossed-leg test for examination of ankle syndesmosis injuries. Foot Ankle Int. 2005;26(2):187–8.
16. Boytim MJ, Fischer DA, Neumann L. Syndesmotic ankle sprains. Am J Sports Med. 1991;19(3):294–8.
17. Rammelt S, Obruba P. An update on the evaluation and treatment of syndesmotic injuries. Eur J Trauma Emerg Surg. 2015;41(6):601–14.
18. Knapik DM, Trem A, Sheehan J, Salata MJ, Voos JE. Conservative management for stable high ankle injuries in professional football players. Sports Health. 2018;10(1):80–4.
19. Ogilvie-Harris DJ, Reed SC. Disruption of the ankle syndesmosis: diagnosis and treatment by arthroscopic surgery. Arthroscopy. 1994;10(5):561–8.
20. Cotton F. Dislocations and joint-fractures. Philadelphia: W. B. Saunders; 1910.
21. Ward DW. Syndesmotic ankle sprain in a recreational hockey player. J Manip Physiol Ther. 1994;17(6):385–94.
22. Harper MC, Keller TS. A radiographic evaluation of the tibiofibular syndesmosis. Foot Ankle. 1989;10(3):156–60.
23. Shah AS, Kadakia AR, Tan GJ, Karadsheh MS, Wolter TD, Sabb B. Radiographic evaluation of the normal distal tibiofibular syndesmosis. Foot Ankle Int. 2012;33(10):870–6.
24. Ebraheim NA, Weston JT, Ludwig T, Moral MZ, Carroll T, Liu J. The association between medial malleolar fracture geometry, injury mechanism, and syndesmotic disruption. Foot Ankle Surg. 2014;20(4):276–80.
25. Choi Y, Kwon S-S, Chung CY, Park MS, Lee SY, Lee KM. Preoperative radiographic and CT findings predicting syndesmotic injuries in supination-external rotation-type ankle fractures. J Bone Joint Surg Am. 2014;96(14):1161–7.
26. Hermans JJ, Wentink N, Beumer A, Hop WCJ, Heijboer MP, Moonen AFCM, et al. Correlation between radiological assessment of acute ankle fractures and syndesmotic injury on MRI. Skelet Radiol. 2012;41(7):787–801.
27. Xenos JS, Hopkinson WJ, Mulligan ME, Olson EJ, Popovic NA. The tibiofibular syndesmosis. Evaluation of the ligamentous structures, methods of fixation, and radiographic assessment. J Bone Joint Surg Am. 1995;77(6):847–56.
28. Schock HJ, Pinzur M, Manion L, Stover M. The use of gravity or manual-stress radiographs in the assessment of supination-external rotation fractures of the ankle. J Bone Joint Surg Br. 2007;89(8):1055–9.

29. Beumer A, Swierstra BA. The influence of ankle positioning on the radiography of the distal tibial tubercles. Surg Radiol Anat. 2003;25(5–6):446–50.

30. Beumer A, van Hemert WLW, Niesing R, Entius CAC, Ginai AZ, PGH M, et al. Radiographic measurement of the distal tibiofibular syndesmosis has limited use. Clin Orthop Relat Res. 2004;423:227–34.

31. Pneumaticos SG, Noble PC, Chatziioannou SN, Trevino SG. The effects of rotation on radiographic evaluation of the tibiofibular syndesmosis. Foot Ankle Int. 2002;23(2):107–11.

32. Schoennagel BP, Karul M, Avanesov M, Bannas P, Gold G, Großterlinden LG, et al. Isolated syndesmotic injury in acute ankle trauma: comparison of plain film radiography with 3T MRI. Eur J Radiol. 2014;83(10):1856–61.

33. Jenkinson RJ, Sanders DW, Macleod MD, Domonkos A, Lydestadt J. Intraoperative diagnosis of syndesmosis injuries in external rotation ankle fractures. J Orthop Trauma. 2005;19(9):604–9.

34. Chang S-M, Li H-F, Hu S-J, Du S-C, Zhang L-Z, Xiong W-F. A reliable method for intraoperative detection of lateral malleolar malrotation using conventional fluoroscopy. Injury. 2019;50(11):2108–12.

35. Chun D-I, Cho J-H, Min T-H, Park SY, Kim K-H, Kim JH, et al. Diagnostic accuracy of radiologic methods for ankle syndesmosis injury: a systematic review and meta-analysis. J Clin Med. 2019;8(7):968.

36. Ebraheim NA, Lu J, Yang H, Mekhail AO, Yeasting RA. Radiographic and CT evaluation of tibiofibular syndesmotic diastasis: a cadaver study. Foot Ankle Int. 1997;18(11):693–8.

37. Elgafy H, Semaan HB, Blessinger B, Wassef A, Ebraheim NA. Computed tomography of normal distal tibiofibular syndesmosis. Skelet Radiol. 2010;39(6):559–64.

38. Taser F, Shafiq Q, Ebraheim NA. Three-dimensional volume rendering of tibiofibular joint space and quantitative analysis of change in volume due to tibiofibular syndesmosis diastases. Skelet Radiol. 2006;35(12):935–41.

39. Mukhopadhyay S, Metcalfe A, Guha AR, Mohanty K, Hemmadi S, Lyons K, et al. Malreduction of syndesmosis—are we considering the anatomical variation? Injury. 2011;42(10):1073–6.

40. Nault M-L, Hébert-Davies J, Laflamme G-Y, Leduc S. CT scan assessment of the syndesmosis: a new reproducible method. J Orthop Trauma. 2013;27(11):638–41.

41. Liu GT, Ryan E, Gustafson E, VanPelt MD, Raspovic KM, Lalli T, et al. Three-dimensional computed tomographic characterization of normal anatomic morphology and variations of the distal tibiofibular syndesmosis. J Foot Ankle Surg. 2018;57(6):1130–6.

42. Malhotra G, Cameron J, Toolan BC. Diagnosing chronic diastasis of the syndesmosis: a novel measurement using computed tomography. Foot Ankle Int. 2014;35(5):483–8.

43. Ahrberg AB, Hennings R, von Dercks N, Hepp P, Josten C, Spiegl UJ. Validation of a new method for evaluation of syndesmotic injuries of the ankle. Int Orthop. 2020;44(10):2095–100.

44. Schon JM, Brady AW, Krob JJ, Lockard CA, Marchetti DC, Dornan GJ, et al. Defining the three most responsive and specific CT measurements of ankle syndesmotic malreduction. Knee Surg Sports Traumatol Arthrosc. 2019;27(9):2863–76.

45. Knops SP, Kohn MA, Hansen EN, Matityahu A, Marmor M. Rotational malreduction of the syndesmosis: reliability and accuracy of computed tomography measurement methods. Foot Ankle Int. 2013;34(10):1403–10.

46. Mousavian A, Shakoor D, Hafezi-Nejad N, Haj-Mirzaian A, de Cesar NC, Orapin J, et al. Tibiofibular syndesmosis in asymptomatic ankles: initial kinematic analysis using four-dimensional CT. Clin Radiol. 2019;74(7):571.e1–8.

47. Levack AE, Dvorzhinskiy A, Gausden EB, Garner MR, Warner SJ, Fabricant PD, et al. Sagittal ankle position does not affect axial CT measurements of the syndesmosis in a cadaveric model. Arch Orthop Trauma Surg. 2020;140(1):25–31.

48. Black EM, Antoci V, Lee JT, Weaver MJ, Johnson AH, Susarla SM, et al. Role of preoperative computed tomography scans in operative planning for malleolar ankle fractures. Foot Ankle Int. 2013;34(5):697–704.

49. Franke J, von Recum J, Suda AJ, Grützner PA, Wendl K. Intraoperative three-dimensional imaging in the treatment of acute unstable syndesmotic injuries. J Bone Joint Surg Am. 2012;94(15):1386–90.
50. Davidovitch RI, Weil Y, Karia R, Forman J, Looze C, Liebergall M, et al. Intraoperative syndesmotic reduction: three-dimensional versus standard fluoroscopic imaging. J Bone Joint Surg Am. 2013;95(20):1838–43.
51. Moon SW, Kim JW. Usefulness of intraoperative three-dimensional imaging in fracture surgery: a prospective study. J Orthop Sci. 2014;19(1):125–31.
52. Vetter SY, Euler J, Beisemann N, Swartman B, Keil H, Grützner PA, et al. Validation of radiological reduction criteria with intraoperative cone beam CT in unstable syndesmotic injuries. Eur J Trauma Emerg Surg. 2021;47(4):897–903.
53. Lundberg A. Kinematics of the ankle and foot. In vivo roentgen stereophotogrammetry. Acta Orthop Scand Suppl. 1989;233:1–24.
54. Wang C, Yang J, Wang S, Ma X, Wang X, Huang J, et al. Three-dimensional motions of distal syndesmosis during walking. J Orthop Surg Res. 2015;10:166.
55. Lepojärvi S, Niinimäki J, Pakarinen H, Leskelä H-V. Rotational dynamics of the Normal distal Tibiofibular joint with weight-bearing computed tomography. Foot Ankle Int. 2016;37(6):627–35.
56. Richter M, Seidl B, Zech S, Hahn S. PedCAT for 3D-imaging in standing position allows for more accurate bone position (angle) measurement than radiographs or CT. Foot Ankle Surg. 2014;20(3):201–7.
57. Shakoor D, Osgood GM, Brehler M, Zbijewski WB, de Cesar NC, Shafiq B, et al. Cone-beam CT measurements of distal tibio-fibular syndesmosis in asymptomatic uninjured ankles: does weight-bearing matter? Skelet Radiol. 2019;48(4):583–94.
58. Krähenbühl N, Bailey TL, Weinberg MW, Davidson NP, Hintermann B, Presson AP, et al. Is load application necessary when using computed tomography scans to diagnose syndesmotic injuries? A cadaver study. Foot Ankle Surg. 2020;26(2):198–204.
59. Malhotra K, Welck M, Cullen N, Singh D, Goldberg AJ. The effects of weight bearing on the distal tibiofibular syndesmosis: a study comparing weight bearing-CT with conventional CT. Foot Ankle Surg. 2019;25(4):511–6.
60. Osgood GM, Shakoor D, Orapin J, Qin J, Khodarahmi I, Thawait GK, et al. Reliability of distal tibio-fibular syndesmotic instability measurements using weightbearing and non-weightbearing cone-beam CT. Foot Ankle Surg. 2019;25(6):771–81.
61. Krähenbühl N, Bailey TL, Presson AP, Allen CM, Henninger HB, Saltzman CL, et al. Torque application helps to diagnose incomplete syndesmotic injuries using weight-bearing computed tomography images. Skelet Radiol. 2019;48(9):1367–76.
62. Krähenbühl N, Bailey TL, Weinberg MW, Davidson NP, Hintermann B, Presson AP, et al. Impact of torque on assessment of syndesmotic injuries using weightbearing computed tomography scans. Foot Ankle Int. 2019;40(6):710–9.
63. Burssens A, Vermue H, Barg A, Krähenbühl N, Victor J, Buedts K. Templating of syndesmotic ankle lesions by use of 3D analysis in weightbearing and nonweightbearing CT. Foot Ankle Int. 2018;39(12):1487–96.
64. Patel S, Malhotra K, Cullen NP, Singh D, Goldberg AJ, Welck MJ. Defining reference values for the normal tibiofibular syndesmosis in adults using weight-bearing CT. Bone Joint J. 2019;101-B(3):348–52.
65. Dikos GD, Heisler J, Choplin RH, Weber TG. Normal tibiofibular relationships at the syndesmosis on axial CT imaging. J Orthop Trauma. 2012;26(7):433–8.
66. Hagemeijer NC, Chang SH, Abdelaziz ME, Casey JC, Waryasz GR, Guss D, et al. Range of normal and abnormal syndesmotic measurements using weightbearing CT. Foot Ankle Int. 2019;40(12):1430–7.
67. Lintz F, de Cesar NC, Barg A, Burssens A, Richter M. Weight-bearing cone beam CT scans in the foot and ankle. EFORT Open Rev. 2018;3(5):278–86.
68. Lintz F, Welck M, Bernasconi A, Thornton J, Cullen NP, Singh D, et al. 3D biometrics for hindfoot alignment using weightbearing CT. Foot Ankle Int. 2017;38(6):684–9.

69. Abdelaziz ME, Hagemeijer N, Guss D, El-Hawary A, El-Mowafi H, DiGiovanni CW. Evaluation of syndesmosis reduction on CT scan. Foot Ankle Int. 2019;40(9):1087–93.
70. Bhimani R, Ashkani-Esfahani S, Lubberts B, Guss D, Hagemeijer NC, Waryasz G, et al. Utility of volumetric measurement via weight-bearing computed tomography scan to diagnose syndesmotic instability. Foot Ankle Int. 2020;41(7):859–65.
71. Del Rio A, Bewsher SM, Roshan-Zamir S, Tate J, Eden M, Gotmaker R, et al. Weightbearing cone-beam computed tomography of acute ankle syndesmosis injuries. J Foot Ankle Surg. 2020;59(2):258–63.
72. Lintz F, Jepsen M, De Cesar NC, Bernasconi A, Ruiz M, Siegler S. Distance mapping of the foot and ankle joints using weightbearing CT: the cavovarus configuration. Foot Ankle Surg. 2021;27(4):412–20.
73. Sikka RS, Fetzer GB, Sugarman E, Wright RW, Fritts H, Boyd JL, et al. Correlating MRI findings with disability in syndesmotic sprains of NFL players. Foot Ankle Int. 2012;33(5):371–8.
74. Vogl TJ, Hochmuth K, Diebold T, Lubrich J, Hofmann R, Stöckle U, et al. Magnetic resonance imaging in the diagnosis of acute injured distal tibiofibular syndesmosis. Investig Radiol. 1997;32(7):401–9.
75. Takao M, Ochi M, Oae K, Naito K, Uchio Y. Diagnosis of a tear of the tibiofibular syndesmosis. The role of arthroscopy of the ankle. J Bone Joint Surg Br. 2003;85(3):324–9.
76. Oae K, Takao M, Naito K, Uchio Y, Kono T, Ishida J, et al. Injury of the tibiofibular syndesmosis: value of MR imaging for diagnosis. Radiology. 2003;227(1):155–61.
77. Han SH, Lee JW, Kim S, Suh J-S, Choi YR. Chronic tibiofibular syndesmosis injury: the diagnostic efficiency of magnetic resonance imaging and comparative analysis of operative treatment. Foot Ankle Int. 2007;28(3):336–42.
78. Clanton TO, Ho CP, Williams BT, Surowiec RK, Gatlin CC, Haytmanek CT, et al. Magnetic resonance imaging characterization of individual ankle syndesmosis structures in asymptomatic and surgically treated cohorts. Knee Surg Sports Traumatol Arthrosc. 2016;24(7):2089–102.
79. Nielson JH, Gardner MJ, Peterson MGE, Sallis JG, Potter HG, Helfet DL, et al. Radiographic measurements do not predict syndesmotic injury in ankle fractures: an MRI study. Clin Orthop Relat Res. 2005;436:216–21.
80. Gardner MJ, Demetrakopoulos D, Briggs SM, Helfet DL, Lorich DG. The ability of the Lauge-Hansen classification to predict ligament injury and mechanism in ankle fractures: an MRI study. J Orthop Trauma. 2006;20(4):267–72.
81. Brown KW, Morrison WB, Schweitzer ME, Parellada JA, Nothnagel H. MRI findings associated with distal tibiofibular syndesmosis injury. AJR Am J Roentgenol. 2004;182(1):131–6.
82. Campbell SE, Warner M. MR imaging of ankle inversion injuries. Magn Reson Imaging Clin N Am. 2008;16(1):1–18. v
83. Perrich KD, Goodwin DW, Hecht PJ, Cheung Y. Ankle ligaments on MRI: appearance of normal and injured ligaments. AJR Am J Roentgenol. 2009;193(3):687–95.
84. Hermans JJ, Ginai AZ, Wentink N, Hop WCJ, Beumer A. The additional value of an oblique image plane for MRI of the anterior and posterior distal tibiofibular syndesmosis. Skelet Radiol. 2011;40(1):75–83.
85. Milz P, Milz S, Steinborn M, Mittlmeier T, Putz R, Reiser M. Lateral ankle ligaments and tibiofibular syndesmosis. 13-MHz high-frequency sonography and MRI compared in 20 patients. Acta Orthop Scand. 1998;69(1):51–5.
86. Krähenbühl N, Weinberg MW, Davidson NP, Mills MK, Hintermann B, Saltzman CL, et al. Imaging in syndesmotic injury: a systematic literature review. Skelet Radiol. 2018;47(5):631–48.
87. Oae K, Takao M, Uchio Y, Ochi M. Evaluation of anterior talofibular ligament injury with stress radiography, ultrasonography and MR imaging. Skelet Radiol. 2010;39(1):41–7.
88. Lee KT, Park YU, Jegal H, Park JW, Choi JP, Kim JS. New method of diagnosis for chronic ankle instability: comparison of manual anterior drawer test, stress radiography and stress ultrasound. Knee Surg Sports Traumatol Arthrosc. 2014;22(7):1701–7.

89. De Maeseneer M, Marcelis S, Jager T, Shahabpour M, Van Roy P, Weaver J, et al. Sonography of the normal ankle: a target approach using skeletal reference points. Am J Roentgenol. 2009;192(2):487–95.

90. Döring S, Provyn S, Marcelis S, Shahabpour M, Boulet C, de Mey J, et al. Ankle and midfoot ligaments: ultrasound with anatomical correlation: a review. Eur J Radiol. 2018;107:216–26.

91. Alves T, Dong Q, Jacobson J, Yablon C, Gandikota G. Normal and injured ankle ligaments on ultrasonography with magnetic resonance imaging correlation: normal and injured ankle ligaments. J Ultrasound Med. 2019;38(2):513–28.

92. Durkee NJ, Jacobson JA, Jamadar DA, Femino JE, Karunakar MA, Hayes CW. Sonographic evaluation of lower extremity interosseous membrane injuries: retrospective review in 3 patients. J Ultrasound Med. 2003;22(12):1369–75.

93. Stella SM, Ciampi B, Del Chiaro A, Vallone G, Miccoli M, Gulisano M, et al. Sonographic visibility of the main posterior ankle ligaments and para-ligamentous structures in 15 healthy subjects. J Ultrasound. 2021;24(1):23–33.

94. Becciolini M, Bonacchi G, Stella SM, Galletti S, Ricci V. High ankle sprain: sonographic demonstration of a posterior inferior tibiofibular ligament avulsion. J Ultrasound. 2020;23(3):431–3.

95. Warner SJ, Garner MR, Schottel PC, Hinds RM, Loftus ML, Lorich DG. Analysis of PITFL injuries in rotationally unstable ankle fractures. Foot Ankle Int. 2015;36(4):377–82.

96. Randell M, Marsland D, Ballard E, Forster B, Lutz M. MRI for high ankle sprains with an unstable syndesmosis: posterior malleolus bone oedema is common and time to scan matters. Knee Surg Sports Traumatol Arthrosc. 2019;27(9):2890–7.

97. Crim J, Longenecker LG. MRI and surgical findings in deltoid ligament tears. Am J Roentgenol. 2015;204(1):W63–9.

98. Chun K-Y, Choi YS, Lee SH, Kim JS, Young KW, Jeong M-S, et al. Deltoid ligament and tibiofibular syndesmosis injury in chronic lateral ankle instability: magnetic resonance imaging evaluation at 3T and comparison with arthroscopy. Korean J Radiol. 2015;16(5):1096.

99. Jeong MS, Choi YS, Kim YJ, Kim JS, Young KW, Jung YY. Deltoid ligament in acute ankle injury: MR imaging analysis. Skelet Radiol. 2014;43(5):655–63.

100. Mei-Dan O, Kots E, Barchilon V, Massarwe S, Nyska M, Mann G. A dynamic ultrasound examination for the diagnosis of ankle syndesmotic injury in professional athletes: a preliminary study. Am J Sports Med. 2009;37(5):1009–16.

101. Mei-Dan O, Carmont M, Laver L, Nyska M, Kammar H, Mann G, et al. Standardization of the functional syndesmosis widening by dynamic U.S examination. BMC Sports Sci Med Rehabil. 2013;5(1):9.

102. van Niekerk C, van Dyk B. Dynamic ultrasound evaluation of the syndesmosis ligamentous complex and clear space in acute ankle injury, compared to magnetic resonance imaging and surgical findings. S Afr J Radiol. 2017;21(1):8.

103. Anand PA. Syndesmotic stability: is there a radiological normal?—a systematic review. Foot Ankle Surg. 2018;24(3):174–84.

104. Cha SW, Bae KJ, Chai JW, Park J, Choi Y-H, Kim DH. Reliable measurements of physiologic ankle syndesmosis widening using dynamic 3D ultrasonography: a preliminary study. Ultrasonography. 2019;38(3):236–45.

105. Clanton TO, Williams BT, Backus JD, Dornan GJ, Liechti DJ, Whitlow SR, et al. Biomechanical analysis of the individual ligament contributions to syndesmotic stability. Foot Ankle Int. 2017;38(1):66–75.

106. Colville MR, Marder RA, Boyle JJ, Zarins B. Strain measurement in lateral ankle ligaments. Am J Sports Med. 1990;18(2):196–200.

107. Xu D, Wang Y, Jiang C, Fu M, Li S, Qian L, et al. Strain distribution in the anterior inferior tibiofibular ligament, posterior inferior tibiofibular ligament, and interosseous membrane using digital image correlation. Foot Ankle Int. 2018;39(5):618–28.

108. Shimozono Y, Hurley ET, Myerson CL, Murawski CD, Kennedy JG. Suture button versus syndesmotic screw for syndesmosis injuries: a meta-analysis of randomized controlled trials. Am J Sports Med. 2019;47(11):2764–71.

109. McKenzie AC, Hesselholt KE, Larsen MS, Schmal H. A systematic review and meta-analysis on treatment of ankle fractures with syndesmotic rupture: suture-button fixation versus cortical screw fixation. J Foot Ankle Surg. 2019;58(5):946–53.
110. Xie L, Xie H, Wang J, Chen C, Zhang C, Chen H, et al. Comparison of suture button fixation and syndesmotic screw fixation in the treatment of distal tibiofibular syndesmosis injury: a systematic review and meta-analysis. Int J Surg. 2018;60:120–31.
111. Chen B, Chen C, Yang Z, Huang P, Dong H, Zeng Z. To compare the efficacy between fixation with tightrope and screw in the treatment of syndesmotic injuries: a meta-analysis. Foot Ankle Surg. 2019;25(1):63–70.
112. Fan X, Zheng P, Zhang Y-Y, Hou Z-T. Dynamic fixation versus static fixation in treatment effectiveness and safety for distal tibiofibular syndesmosis injuries: a systematic review and meta-analysis. Orthop Surg. 2019;11(6):923–31.
113. Onggo JR, Nambiar M, Phan K, Hickey B, Ambikaipalan A, Hau R, et al. Suture button versus syndesmosis screw constructs for acute ankle diastasis injuries: a meta-analysis and systematic review of randomised controlled trials. Foot Ankle Surg. 2020;26(1):54–60.
114. de-Las-Heras Romero J, AML A, Sanchez FM, Garcia AP, Porcel PAG, Sarabia RV, et al. Management of syndesmotic injuries of the ankle. EFORT Open Rev. 2017;2(9):403–9.
115. van den Bekerom MP, de Leeuw PA, van Dijk CN. Delayed operative treatment of syndesmotic instability. Current concepts review. Injury. 2009;40(11):1137–42.
116. Press CM, Gupta A, Hutchinson MR. Management of ankle syndesmosis injuries in the athlete. Curr Sports Med Rep. 2009;8(5):228–33.
117. Williams GN, Jones MH, Amendola A. Syndesmotic ankle sprains in athletes. Am J Sports Med. 2007;35(7):1197–207.
118. Brosky T, Nyland J, Nitz A, Caborn DN. The ankle ligaments: consideration of syndesmotic injury and implications for rehabilitation. J Orthop Sports Phys Ther. 1995;21(4):197–205.
119. Gerber JP, Williams GN, Scoville CR, Arciero RA, Taylor DC. Persistent disability associated with ankle sprains: a prospective examination of an athletic population. Foot Ankle Int. 1998;19(10):653–60.
120. Nussbaum ED, Hosea TM, Sieler SD, Incremona BR, Kessler DE. Prospective evaluation of syndesmotic ankle sprains without diastasis. Am J Sports Med. 2001;29(1):31–5.
121. Yu GS, Lin YB, Xiong GS, Xu HB, Liu YY. Diagnosis and treatment of ankle syndesmosis injuries with associated interosseous membrane injury: a current concept review. Int Orthop. 2019;43(11):2539–47.
122. Liu G, Chen L, Gong M, Xing F, Xiang Z. Clinical evidence for treatment of distal tibiofibular syndesmosis injury: a systematic review of clinical studies. J Foot Ankle Surg. 2019;58(6):1245–50.
123. Akoh CC, Phisitkul P. Anatomic ligament repairs of syndesmotic injuries. Orthop Clin North Am. 2019;50(3):401–14.
124. Wu ZP, Chen PT, He JS, Wang JC. Classification and treatment of syndesmotic injury. Zhongguo Gu Shang. 2018;31(2):190–4.
125. Swords M, Brilhault J, Sands A. Acute and chronic syndesmotic injury: the authors' approach to treatment. Foot Ankle Clin. 2018;23(4):625–37.
126. Fort NM, Aiyer AA, Kaplan JR, Smyth NA, Kadakia AR. Management of acute injuries of the tibiofibular syndesmosis. Eur J Orthop Surg Traumatol. 2017;27(4):449–59.
127. Hunt KJ, Phisitkul P, Pirolo J, Amendola A. High ankle sprains and syndesmotic injuries in athletes. J Am Acad Orthop Surg. 2015;23(11):661–73.
128. Porter DA, Jaggers RR, Barnes AF, Rund AM. Optimal management of ankle syndesmosis injuries. Open Access J Sports Med. 2014;5:173–82.
129. Miller TL, Skalak T. Evaluation and treatment recommendations for acute injuries to the ankle syndesmosis without associated fracture. Sports Med. 2014;44(2):179–88.
130. Magan A, Golano P, Maffulli N, Khanduja V. Evaluation and management of injuries of the tibiofibular syndesmosis. Br Med Bull. 2014;111(1):101–15.

131. Lin CF, Gross ML, Weinhold P. Ankle syndesmosis injuries: anatomy, biomechanics, mechanism of injury, and clinical guidelines for diagnosis and intervention. J Orthop Sports Phys Ther. 2006;36(6):372–84.
132. Espinosa N, Smerek JP, Myerson MS. Acute and chronic syndesmosis injuries: pathomechanisms, diagnosis and management. Foot Ankle Clin. 2006;11(3):639–57.
133. Amendola A, Williams G, Foster D. Evidence-based approach to treatment of acute traumatic syndesmosis (high ankle) sprains. Sports Med Arthrosc Rev. 2006;14(4):232–6.
134. Amendola A. Controversies in diagnosis and management of syndesmosis injuries of the ankle. Foot Ankle. 1992;13(1):44–50.
135. Zhang P, Liang Y, He J, Fang Y, Chen P, Wang J. A systematic review of suture-button versus syndesmotic screw in the treatment of distal tibiofibular syndesmosis injury. BMC Musculoskelet Disord. 2017;18(1):286.
136. Clanton TO, Whitlow SR, Williams BT, Liechti DJ, Backus JD, Dornan GJ, et al. Biomechanical comparison of 3 current ankle syndesmosis repair techniques. Foot Ankle Int. 2017;38(2):200–7.
137. LaMothe JM, Baxter JR, Murphy C, Gilbert S, DeSandis B, Drakos MC. Three-dimensional analysis of fibular motion after fixation of syndesmotic injuries with a screw or suture-button construct. Foot Ankle Int. 2016;37(12):1350–6.
138. Schepers T. Acute distal tibiofibular syndesmosis injury: a systematic review of suture-button versus syndesmotic screw repair. Int Orthop. 2012;36(6):1199–206.
139. Zhan Y, Yan X, Xia R, Cheng T, Luo C. Anterior-inferior tibiofibular ligament anatomical repair and augmentation versus trans-syndesmosis screw fixation for the syndesmotic instability in external-rotation type ankle fracture with posterior malleolus involvement: a prospective and comparative study. Injury. 2016;47(7):1574–80.
140. Ramsey PL, Hamilton W. Changes in tibiotalar area of contact caused by lateral talar shift. J Bone Joint Surg Am. 1976;58(3):356–7.
141. Lubberts B, Guss D, Vopat BG, Johnson AH, van Dijk CN, Lee H, et al. The arthroscopic syndesmotic assessment tool can differentiate between stable and unstable ankle syndesmoses. Knee Surg Sports Traumatol Arthrosc. 2020;28(1):193–201.
142. Grambart ST, Prusa RD, Ternent KM. Revision of the chronic syndesmotic injury. Clin Podiatr Med Surg. 2020;37(3):577–92.
143. Vilá-Rico J, Sánchez-Morata E, Vacas-Sánchez E, Ojeda-Thies C. Anatomical arthroscopic graft reconstruction of the anterior tibiofibular ligament for chronic disruption of the distal syndesmosis. Arthrosc Tech. 2018;7(2):e165–9.
144. Morris MW, Rice P, Schneider TE. Distal tibiofibular syndesmosis reconstruction using a free hamstring autograft. Foot Ankle Int. 2009;30(6):506–11.
145. Lui TH. Tri-ligamentous reconstruction of the distal tibiofibular syndesmosis: a minimally invasive approach. J Foot Ankle Surg. 2010;49(5):495–500.
146. Grass R, Rammelt S, Biewener A, Zwipp H. Peroneus longus ligamentoplasty for chronic instability of the distal tibiofibular syndesmosis. Foot Ankle Int. 2003;24(5):392–7.
147. Che J, Li C, Gao Z, Qi W, Ji B, Liu Y, et al. Novel anatomical reconstruction of distal tibiofibular ligaments restores syndesmotic biomechanics. Knee Surg Sports Traumatol Arthrosc. 2017;25(6):1866–72.
148. Yasui Y, Takao M, Miyamoto W, Innami K, Matsushita T. Anatomical reconstruction of the anterior inferior tibiofibular ligament for chronic disruption of the distal tibiofibular syndesmosis. Knee Surg Sports Traumatol Arthrosc. 2011;19(4):691–5.
149. Katznelson A, Lin E, Militiano J. Ruptures of the ligaments about the tibio-fibular syndesmosis. Injury. 1983;15(3):170–2.
150. Peña FA, Coetzee JC. Ankle syndesmosis injuries. Foot Ankle Clin. 2006;11(1):35–50. viii
151. Albers GH, de Kort AF, Middendorf PR, van Dijk CN. Distal tibiofibular synostosis after ankle fracture. A 14-year follow-up study. J Bone Joint Surg Br. 1996;78(2):250–2.
152. Sagi HC, Shah AR, Sanders RW. The functional consequence of syndesmotic joint malreduction at a minimum 2-year follow-up. J Orthop Trauma. 2012;26(7):439–43.

Achilles Tendon Injuries

12

J. Randy Clements

Anatomy

The Achilles tendon is the tendinous convergence of the gastrocnemius-soleus muscular complex. It is the largest tendon in the human body [1] and a main contributor to propulsive force during walking, jumping, and running through a concentric contraction. Forces have been approximated to transmit up to almost 10 times the body weight through the Achilles tendon with running [2–4]. Due to these high forces and unique anatomy, traumatic, inflammatory, and degenerative disorders may result.

The Achilles tendon crosses both the ankle and subtalar joints inserting into the posterior calcaneus. Just before its insertion, the fibers of the Achilles tendon turn with the medial tendinous fibers inserting posteriorly with the contribution of the soleus portion being inserting medially and the contribution of the gastrocnemius muscle inserting laterally. Between the calcaneus and the Achilles tendon is the location of the retrocalcaneal bursa.

The Achilles tendon does not have a true synovial sheath, but rather a layer of paratenon. This paratenon is a single layer of cells composed of vascularized areolar tissue that is responsible for a significant portion of the blood supply to the Achilles tendon. Additionally, the tendon receives blood supply from the posterior tibial and peroneal arteries, proximally from the muscle belly, and distally from the calcaneus. Studies have shown a hypovascular area 2 to 6 cm proximal to the insertion on the calcaneus that is considered a watershed zone that is prone to injury and impaired healing [5].

J. R. Clements (✉)
Department of Orthopaedic Surgery, Carillon Clinic Orthopaedic Surgery, Viriginia Tech Carilion School of Medicine, Roanoke, VA, USA
e-mail: jrclements@carilonclinic.org

© Springer Nature Switzerland AG 2022
J. D. Cain, M. V. Hogan (eds.), *Tendon and Ligament Injuries of the Foot and Ankle*,
https://doi.org/10.1007/978-3-031-10490-9_12

Paratenonitis

Paratenonitis is an overuse injury commonly seen in athletes, particularly distance runners, who may have increased or changed their training regimen. On physical examination, swelling and tenderness along the course of the inflamed paratenon can be appreciated. The tenderness and thickness will remain fixed with ankle motion in isolated paratenonitis [6].

Diagnosis of paratenonitis is made clinically; however, MRI or US can help facilitate diagnosis and will show thickening of the paratenon. The capillary proliferation and inflammatory cells can be seen within the tendinous tissue histologically. Myofibroblasts in the paratendinous tissue synthesize collagen in response to stress. This may lead to constriction of the paratenon and reduction of the blood supply to the Achilles tendon [7].

Non-insertional Achilles Tendinosis

Achilles tendinopathy is degeneration of the Achilles tendon often associated with pain, swelling, and stiffness. It can be categorized into non-insertional Achilles tendinosis (NIAT) and insertional Achilles tendinosis (IAT).

On physical exam, patients with NIAT will demonstrate thickening of the tendon itself typically proximal to the tendon insertion in the watershed region. Tendinosis can occur as a painless thickening of the Achilles tendon. In symptomatic patients squeezing the thickening area of the tendon may incite pain. Mucoid, myxomatous, and fibrinoid degeneration has been reported pathologically [8–10]. Imaging including radiograph, MRI, or ultrasound can be used to help facilitate diagnosis in determining the type or extent of tendon involved and possible intratendinous calcifications [11].

Insertional Achilles Tendinosis

Insertional Achilles tendinosis (IAT) issues occur at the Achilles attachment site on the posterior aspect of the calcaneus. Degeneration of the tendon and varying degrees of calcification at the insertion site are present. Intrinsic predisposing factors include high BMI, diabetes, seronegative diseases, hypertension, quinolone antibiotics, and lipidemia [11–16]. Ankle equinus shortens the heel cord causing increased Achilles tension. Patients with cavus foot type are prone due to decreased shock absorption and having to work harder to achieve adequate dorsiflexion. Pes planus cause overpronation resulting in altered biomechanics causing micro-tears and tendinopathic changes [17–23].

On examination, both soft tissue and an osseous enlargement may be present just proximal to the Achilles tendon insertional site as coexisting Haglund deformity is often present [24]. Symptoms may include post-static dyskinesia. Periods of prolonged standing, walking, or running may also produce pain.

Lateral radiographs of the ankle often reveal an associated posterior enthesiophyte from the tendon insertion site. Intratendinous calcification may also be appreciated. MRI can further facilitate the investigation of tears to the tendon. Nicholson et al. created an MRI classification based on degenerative changes in patients with insertional Achilles tendinopathy to predict success rates of conservative therapy finding that tendons with greater intrasubstance degeneration on sagittal MRI, specifically grades two and three in this classification, failed conservative therapy and required operative intervention [25]. Although advanced imaging is helpful in operative planning, it is not completely necessary as one can rely on the clinical exam and intraoperative assessment for the appropriate diagnosis and treatment.

Achilles Tendon Trauma

Historically, Paré in 1541 is credited with recognizing an Achilles tendon rupture as a medical condition [26], although his analysis was not recorded in literature until 1633. In the 1920s Abrahamsen and Qeunu [27] advocated surgical repair of the Achilles tendon; therefore, surgical intervention for Achilles tendon ruptures began to be popularized in that decade. Traditionally, surgical repair has been advocated on the basis that it provides for greater strength, endurance, and power with less likelihood of rerupture as compared with nonsurgical management [28–33].

Ruptures of the Achilles tendon often occur in the fourth to fifth decades of life. Males hold a stronger predilection versus females [34]. Injury is often associated with those who live a sedimentary lifestyle but decide to partake in spontaneous athletic activity. Some people refer to such individuals as "weekend warriors." Oftentimes Achilles tendon injuries are associated with an abrupt onset of pain accompanied with an audible "snapping" or "popping" sound. Recent literature suggests that the rate of Achilles tendon ruptures is somewhere in the range of 18 patients per 100,000 patient population annually [35–37]. It is thought roughly a million athletes suffer from acute Achilles tendon ruptures, with an incidence ranging from 6% to 18% each year. Football players are the least likely to suffer from acute Achilles tendon ruptures while compared to higher-risk athletes like gymnasts and tennis players. The most prominent location for Achilles tendon ruptures is circa 2–6 cm from the tendon's insertion into the calcaneus. This is due to the fact that the fibers of the Achilles tendon rotate from medial to lateral in a spiral fashion, with the greatest rotational twist located 2–6 cm from the insertion. Additionally, this particular 2–6 cm region is deemed a zone of hypovascularity, as first described by Lagergren and Lindholm in 1958 [38]. This hypovascular area is widely referred to as a "watershed area."

There are two common theories of Achilles tendon ruptures, the first of which is the mechanical stress theory as described by Inglis and Sculco [39]. They described the malfunction of the inhibitory mechanism within the muscle spindle fibers, which they postulated prevents excessive tension of the Achilles tendon by monitoring forces during sudden muscle overload. Over time this theory has been dismissed as not credible. Furthermore, there are three accepted types of indirect trauma that are believed to cause Achilles tendon ruptures. The mechanisms of indirect trauma were described by Arner and Windholm [40], which are direct push off from a height-bearing forefoot and an extended knee, sudden dorsiflexion of the ankle such as slipping on a stair or ladder, and violent dorsiflexion of a plantarflexed foot that results from jumping or falling from a height and landing with the foot plantarflexed.

Additionally, degenerative theory describes a hypovascular tendon that is exposed to repeated trauma which results in local degenerative changes within the midsubstance of the tendon. According to this theory, the ultimate weakened state of the tendon predisposes it to rupture after an excessive load is applied [41, 42].

There are additional external factors that some believe contribute to Achilles tendon rupture. These include systemic and local steroids, blood type, genetics, renal insufficiency, arteriosclerosis, hyperlipidemia, gout, hypothyroidism, rheumatoid arthritis, and fluoroquinolones. When dealing with Achilles tendon ruptures, it is important to take into consideration systemic and external factors that might influence the chosen approach to treatment [43–49].

Clinical Presentation

Patients will often present with complaints of weakness of the ankle and oftentimes endorse direct trauma to the Achilles tendon. The injury is often only painful during the occurrence of the rupture itself. Additionally, most people do not complain of pain when presenting to the office. The gait pattern is often described as abducted and antalgic.

Clinical Examination

Achilles tendon ruptures are misdiagnosed as an ankle sprain in 20–25% of patients. Upon initial examination there often will be a visually demonstrable deficit known as the hatchet strike defect. This has been described as a physical dell in the posterior ankle compartment when compared to the contralateral side. The Thompson test is performed by placing the patient prone and flexing the leg. With the leg flexed, perform side-to-side compression of the calf; if the tendon is ruptured, there will be no plantarflexion visualized. If no motion is noted, the test is positive. In some cases, there can be false-negative exams. This is seen when the plantaris tendon is intact, resulting in residual plantarflexion. The resulting plantarflexion exam is performed when the patient is prone, and the knee and leg are flexed at 90°. If the Achilles tendon is ruptured, the foot will be visualized resting at 90° or less. The non-affected foot will be slightly plantarflexed. The needle exam is another way to assess if the Achilles tendon is intact. This is accomplished by having the patient prone and placing a needle in the calf muscle belly above the perceived rupture site. With the needle in the place, the plantarflexion of the foot is performed. If the Achilles tendon is intact, the needle will move upon plantarflexion of the foot. If the Achilles tendon is reruptured, the needle will not move upon plantarflexion of the foot [50–52].

Diagnostic Imaging

Whether to conduct diagnostic imaging is the physician's choice. Advanced imaging can be used to assess a rupture or deficit noted between the ruptured ends. If clinical examination provides definitive proof of rupture, then advanced imaging is not indicated. With a delay in treatment, advanced imaging can be more useful for assessed retraction and deficit in the tendon that needs to be repaired. Radiographs are not indicated unless there is a suspicion of tongue-type fracture of the posterior calcaneus.

MRI

MRI is useful to assess the amount of deficit created from the rupture, especially if the clinical exam is nondefinitive. This imaging modality can be used to determine if there is a complete or partial rupture. Sometimes a false-negative exam can occur with MRI. This is due to the fact that after rupturing the tendon lays down into its anatomic position which can give the appearance of partial tear when it is actually fully ruptured. For chronic ruptures, MRI is useful in assessing the deficit in planning surgically.

Ultrasound

Ultrasound has been used successfully to assess acute and chronic injuries, although it can give false-negative results with acute injuries due to hematoma filling the deficit. Astrom compared ultrasound and MRI when assessing chronic Achilles tendinopathy with regard to the nature and severity of the deformity. His results showed that MRI was 98% accurate, with ultrasound at 85% [53].

Treatment of Acute Ruptures

Nonoperative care is utilized for patients who are not good surgical candidates. This includes patients who are immunocompromised, low demand elderly, vascular compromised, and noncompliant [54–57].

Surgical Evaluation and Treatment

The ideal repair time for an acute Achilles rupture is 7–14 days after initial injury due to the fact that the greatest amount of vascularity to the region occurs at that time. This is also consistent with the principles of wound healing. After 7–14 days, the injury is no longer in the inflammatory stage of healing, and vascularity to the area decreases. Surgical repair during the first 7–10 days is also more difficult due to fraying and mop ending of the tendon stumps. After the first 14 days, tendon remodeling allows for easier end-to-end repair. Surgical repair becomes the most challenging when it enters the remodeling phase of healing due to the fact that the tendon becomes avascular. When a rupture becomes chronic, advancement techniques or tendon transfers should be utilized [58]. Although it is easier to repair tendons once they have consolidated, optimal vascularity is seen between 7 and 14 days when the tendon is in the inflammatory stage of healing [59].

Surgical Techniques

There exists a host of techniques utilized for Achilles tendon repairs; furthermore, these surgical techniques can be broadly categorized into open, mini-open, and percutaneous repair [60]. The foundation of all techniques involves end-to-end opposition; many consist of the approximation of the Achilles tendon ruptured ends with supplementary augmentation by the plantaris, flexor hallucis longus, or gastrocsoleus aponeurosis.

Open Repair

Traditionally, the three main suture techniques that have been utilized for the end-to-end open Achilles tendon repair include the Bunnell, Kessler, and Krakow. There are modifications to the aforementioned methods to allow for a four-strand repair and strong construct. The Krakow is described as the strongest of the three techniques because it utilizes a four-strand repair, whereas the Bunnell and Kessler are historically two-strand repairs.

Incisional approaches include posterior midline, posterior medial, and posterior-lateral incisions. Among those stated above, the posteromedial approach is the most frequently used due to hypervascularity on the medial side of the Achilles tendon, as determined from the use of angiography [61]. Once an approach has been chosen, the surgeon should start by making the skin incision. It is also important to remember that care should always be taken to avoid damaging the sural nerve and the saphenous vein which lies in the sura lateral to the Achilles tendon. Following skin incision, dissection is taken through the subcutaneous tissue down to the peritendinous tissue. The epitenon is then split longitudinally and tagged. The epitenon should always be preserved even if it is disrupted, as this facilitates healing and helps to avoid scar adhesions postsurgery. After the peritenon is divided, the "mop ends" of the tendon can be prudently resected. Once debridement is completed, a Krakow-Kessler suture technique is implemented to reapproximate the tendon ends. A nonabsorbable suture, e.g., ethibond, fiber wire, and suture tape, should be utilized. Firstly, the suture should be passed in and through the proximal stump existing superficially. The suture then reenters superficially and is locked in a Krakow ~6-row pattern. The sutures are then passed through the opposing side of the tendon and stitched in the direction of the ruptured end. The same process is completed at the distal end with the two ends approximated and subsequently tied with the foot held at 5–10 degrees of plantarflexion. This technique is used for tendon defects ranging from 2 to 5 cm. To facilitate healing of the paratenon upon wound closure, a flexor hallucis longus fasciotomy can be performed prior to tendon closure. The tendon can also be covered with an autogenous or synthetic tendon graft prior to closure as well. Preferably, this technique is utilized for larger deficits, typically with defects greater than 6 cm. Regardless of the operative approach or technique, care should be taken to restore the proper length of the Achilles tendon while avoiding excessive elongation. If the plantaris is absent, the range of dorsiflexion on the contralateral side can be measured for reference.

Percutaneous Procedure

Literature shows that percutaneous repair with a small incision results in lower wound complication rates and has better cosmesis when compared with open repair. The mini-open repair technique has been proposed to minimize complications typically associated with the percutaneous procedure, e.g., sural nerve injury. This technique is accomplished with a small linear incision that is made over the deficit approximately 1 cm proximal to the distal end of the defect. Care should be taken to avoid injuring the sural nerve. The paratenon is opened and the ruptured ends are grasped with a clamping device. While grasping the proximal stump, a malleable retractor is used to free up the proximal Achilles tendon. The separation of the Achilles tendon from the surrounding paratenon is important for the placement of a percutaneous jig. A locking double-locked suture repair is made within the ruptured site proximally. The instrumentation of a percutaneous jig placement is achieved by advancing the device between the tendon and paratenon. The device is generally designed to have three sutures shuttled through a two-armed jig on either side of the Achilles tendon. This process is then repeated on the distal rupture stump with the addition of two small stab incisions that are made over the calcaneus just proximal to the Achilles insertion. A drill is used through the previous stab incisions to make holes at an angle toward the midline of the calcaneus. The holes are used to anchor the Achilles tendon to the calcaneus via suture material. The device and the suture are pulled out for apposition of the ruptured tendon ends, and the sutures are tied with the ankle in a plantarflexed position [60].

Complications

Complications of operative treatment of acute Achilles tendon rupture include sural nerve injury, infection, rerupture, deep vein thrombosis, and hypertrophic scars. Therefore, operative treatment may not be appropriate for low-demand patients, those with diabetes mellitus, or those with peripheral vascular disease. The most serious complication of open repair is infection. Infection and wound problems mostly occur after surgery with an incidence of 12.5%. Wound healing complications are overall a 5% to 10% risk following surgery. Some of the common risk factors for postoperative infection include smoking, steroid use, open technique versus percutaneous procedures, and female gender. There is an increased risk of infection with the open repair versus the percutaneous technique; however, the risk is relatively small. There is a higher incidence of sural nerve injury with the percutaneous procedure when compared to the open technique [62].

Posterior leg muscle weakness can be a challenge postoperatively. It is not uncommon for patients to be able to walk without complete healing of a ruptured Achilles tendon; therefore the definitive treatment goal for Achilles tendon ruptures is to prevent residual calf muscle weakness [58, 63, 64].

Rerupture can be a debilitating complication of Achilles tendon treatment. Various authors have published have published higher re-rupture rates in younger patients with the majority occurring within 3 months following surgery. Rettig et al. noted a rerupture rate of 16.6% with patients 30 years of age or younger. Reito et al. recorded a rerupture rate of 7.1% in 210 patients with acute Achilles tendon ruptures treated conservatively; the majority of rerupture took place within 3 months after treatment. Young et al. also reported that 75% of rerupture cases were within 3 months after surgery; the study also noted that there was no association between rerupture rate and surgical repair method employed [65–67]. Given abovementioned literature, the correlation between rerupture rates, age, and time should caution clinicians from being too aggressive with early rehabilitation in younger patients.

Neglected or Chronic Achilles Tendon Ruptures

Chronic Achilles tendon ruptures often present as a challenging pathology that usually comprises extended recovery and high morbidity even after surgical repair. Commonly, patients with chronic Achilles complications may have had previous treatment for midsubstance tendinopathy with a conservative treatment course or even immobilization in the past. Repair of chronic Achilles tendon injuries can comprise of tendon transfers, muscle-tendon advancements, and implantation (autograft, allograft, and synthetic) to bridge deficits that occur. Typically, even after surgical repair, there is a loss of one grade of muscle strength to the affected extremity. Prior to surgery, patients should be accurately informed regarding the prolonged recovery and rehabilitation that typically awaits them. There is no official definition for a chronic Achilles tendon rupture, but many physicians consider a chronic rupture to be generally defined as a rupture that has been present greater than 6 to 8 weeks from the initial injury. It is known that tendon fibrils combined with scar tissue do not recreate the proper length of tension in comparison to the natural tendon complex.

Many authors agree that neglected Achilles ruptures should be treated operatively unless there are significant contraindications to surgery or the patient has a low-demand lifestyle [62]. If surgical intervention is planned, advanced imaging is important in assessing the amount of deficit. The surgical goal should be to restore the physiologic length-tension relationship of the Achilles tendon. Chronic ruptures are regularly mended with direct end-to-end repair; usually, this method is limited to tendons with gaps less than 2 cm. A gastrocsoleus recession can be useful to approximate the torn tendon ends. Other options include allograft repair [68, 69], woven gastrocnemius aponeurosis repair [70, 71], gastrocnemius recession, plantaris reinforcement [72], peroneus brevis tendon transfer [73], tendon transfer procedures, and muscle-tendon advancement flaps [74].

The muscle-tendon advancement described by Mendicino et al. [75] allows for the correction of small to large deficits. The procedure consists of a full-thickness inverted V to Y advancement, which does not sacrifice any local tendons and does not include the morbidity of a second surgical site. The amount of correction is dependent on the length of the full-thickness arms of the V. Once the deficit is measured, the lengths of the arms need to be twice the length of the device. This repair can also be reinforced with synthetic grafts and/or local tendon grafts. However, many authors do not recommend V to Y advancement as to poor functional power and cosmesis.

Flexor hallucis longus transfer is generally used for almost all cases, especially when a direct repair is not possible [149–151]. With the use of new technology, the procedure has been simplified, and harvesting of the flexor halluces longus tendon can be performed through a single-incision approach. The use of new interference screws and anchors allows the tendon harvest to be shorter and more secure [76].

Postoperative Protocol

The patient is placed in an Achilles boot immediately after surgery in order to place the foot in 20–30° degrees of plantarflexion. The degree of plantarflexion varies depending on the final position of the postsurgical repair. The amount of wedge placed in the boot corresponds to the angle of the foot in gravity or equinus postsurgically. The patient will remain non-weight-bearing until the surgical incision heals, which typically is 2–3 weeks. Once the incision is healed, the patient is allowed to bear weight in the Achilles boot. This allows for some tension on the repair site which leads to a linear alignment of collagen fibers while avoiding a disorganized alignment. The patient will be followed on a 2-week basis with sequential wedge removal until a neutral position is achieved, which typically takes a total of 6–8 weeks. When a neutral position is achieved, the patient is placed in a stiff-toed shoe with a slight heel lift. Physical therapy is initiated at week 4 to mobilize the scar tissue and to minimize adhesions at the repair site. The first 2 weeks of physical therapy should include a range of motion exercises without resistance. After the first 2 weeks of physical therapy without resistance, exercises broaden to involve progressive strengthening with the use of resistive bands and manual mobilization. Weeks 4–6 include proprioception training, weight-bearing strengthening, and the continuation of manual mobilization. Athletic activities cannot be initiated until a minimum of 10–12 weeks postoperatively. Athletic activities with higher physical demands and movements, such as jumping-type activities, are restricted until 6 months after repair.

It is imperative to avoid Achilles tendon elongation which can be caused by over-aggressive physical therapy. On physical examination, an elongation of the Achilles tendon can be characterized by hyperdorsiflexion of the ankle, plantarflexor weakness, and functional deficit. A period of lengthy immobilization is also not ideal. A patient should not be immobilized in a cast or splint for greater than 3 weeks. Full weight-bearing in an orthosis should last until the 6- to 8-postoperative week mark with it being initiated immediately after surgery or at least within 3 weeks after surgery [77, 78].

Literature Review

There is no current agreement on the best treatment of acute Achilles tendon ruptures. Historically, the literature supports a rerupture rate of the Achilles tendon to be 10–40% when treated with nonoperative management compared to 1–2% with surgical repair. However, new studies have validated the importance of conservative treatment and functional rehabilitation for ruptured Achilles tendons. The accelerated Achilles rehabilitation protocol gained notoriety by Willits et al. in 2010 [79]. More recent literature validates Willits' original findings that there is no significant difference in healing rates of serial casting or functional bracing when compared to surgical repair [54–57, 62, 77, 80]. There are many different Achilles rehabilitation protocols for conservative treatment recorded in the literature, most of which are very similar [79, 81–85]. There is also debate as to whether functional rehabilitation is more important for tendon healing than surgery repair itself. Furthermore, literature has shown that early weight-bearing combined with early ankle motion exercises is more effective for postoperative recovery than conventional immobilization or early ankle motion exercises alone [86]. Brumman et al. underline the importance of functional rehabilitation with an adherence to a specific rehabilitation protocol consisting of full weight-bearing in 30° fixed plantarflexion started immediately after surgery, controlled ankle mobilization in free plantarflexion, and limited dorsiflexion at 0° after the second postoperative week [87].

The importance of early weight-bearing postoperatively has become widely acknowledged; however, the ankle position still remains an area of debate. It is a common practice that the ankle is initially maintained in a plantarflexed position with gradual dorsiflexion after surgery. Some authors advocate placing the ankle in a neutral position immedicably after surgery due to the fact that rerupture occurs frequently with gradual dorsiflexion of the plantarflexed ankle during rehabilitation. A recent study by Ryu et al. recorded that there was no case of rerupture in the total 112 patients who started weight-bearing ambulation in a neutral ankle position immediately after surgery [77]. There is no clear consensus as to the best position of the ankle immediately after surgery; therefore, the physician must use their clinical judgment when determining the position of the ankle. Zhao et al. performed a meta-analysis comparing early functional rehabilitation and traditional immobilization following surgical Achilles tendon repair after acute rupture has been published [88]. The authors performed a comprehensive search using the PubMed and Embase databases and the Cochrane Library with the following keywords that were used: Achilles tendon, or Achilles or TendoAchilles and Rupture or Injury. The references of the included studies were also manually searched, and according to the Jadad decision algorithm, high-quality meta-analysis with a greater number of RCTs was selected [88]. Based on the results, the meta-analysis showed that early functional rehabilitation was superior to cast immobilization in terms of patient satisfaction and the time to return to premorbid sporting levels. The authors also showed there were no differences regarding major complications or the time before return to prior employment and sporting activity.

Historically there was controversy regarding whether to treat acute Achilles tendon ruptures surgically or with cast immobilization. Most literature and studies show slightly better outcomes and decreased rerupture with surgically repaired Achilles tendons. The postoperative recovery time for surgically repaired tendons is usually less than nonsurgically treated tendons as well. One of the problems with cast repairs relates to the Achilles tendon lengthening that results due to the scar tissue formation that bridges the two ruptured ends. This can lead to loss of strength, length, and tension relationship within the tendon-muscle complex. Ochen et al. performed a systematic review and meta-analysis of operative versus nonoperative treatment of Achilles tendon ruptures [89]. The authors compare rerupture rate, complication rate, and functional outcome after operative versus nonoperative treatment of Achilles tendon ruptures; compare rerupture rate after early and late full weight-bearing; evaluate rerupture rate after functional rehabilitation with early range of motion; and compare effect estimates from randomized controlled trials and observational studies. The authors evaluated 29 studies, 10 randomized controlled trials, and 19 observational studies. Based on the study, the authors found that operative treatment of Achilles tendon ruptures reduces the risk of rerupture compared with nonoperative treatment. However, rerupture rates are low and differences between treatment groups are small (risk difference 1.6%). The authors found that operative treatment results in a higher risk of other complications (risk difference 3.3%).

Hurley et al. performed a literature search based on the PRISMA guidelines to identify meta-analysis on Achilles tendon repair [90]. Each meta-analysis was categorized into one of the following subgroupings: (1) Operative versus Non-Operative Treatment (with Conservative Rehabilitation) [OC vs. NOC], (2) Operative versus Non-Operative Treatment (with Functional Rehabilitation) [OF vs. NOF], (3) Conservative Rehabilitation versus Functional Rehabilitation (with Operative Treatment) [OC vs. OF], and (4) Open versus Percutaneous Repair (with Conservative Rehabilitation) [OC vs. POC]. The authors found that the rerupture rates were lower in operative treatment in all studies, even when early functional rehabilitation was used. Also, there was no difference between percutaneous and open repair on the rerupture rate, and there was an overall reduction in wound infection after percutaneous repair.

Seow et al. performed a meta-analysis on the rates of all complications after the treatment of acute Achilles tendon rupture with a "best-case scenario" and "worst-case scenario" analysis for rerupture rates that assumes that all patients lost to follow-up did not or did experience a rerupture, respectively [91]. The authors performed a systematic review of the PubMed and Embase databases according to the PRISMA guideline and demonstrated that surgical treatment was superior to nonsurgical treatment in terms of reruptures. Nonmeaningful values were seen with the number needed to treat analysis for all treatment options, except for surgical versus nonsurgical treatment and minimally invasive surgery versus open repair.

Treatment Algorithm

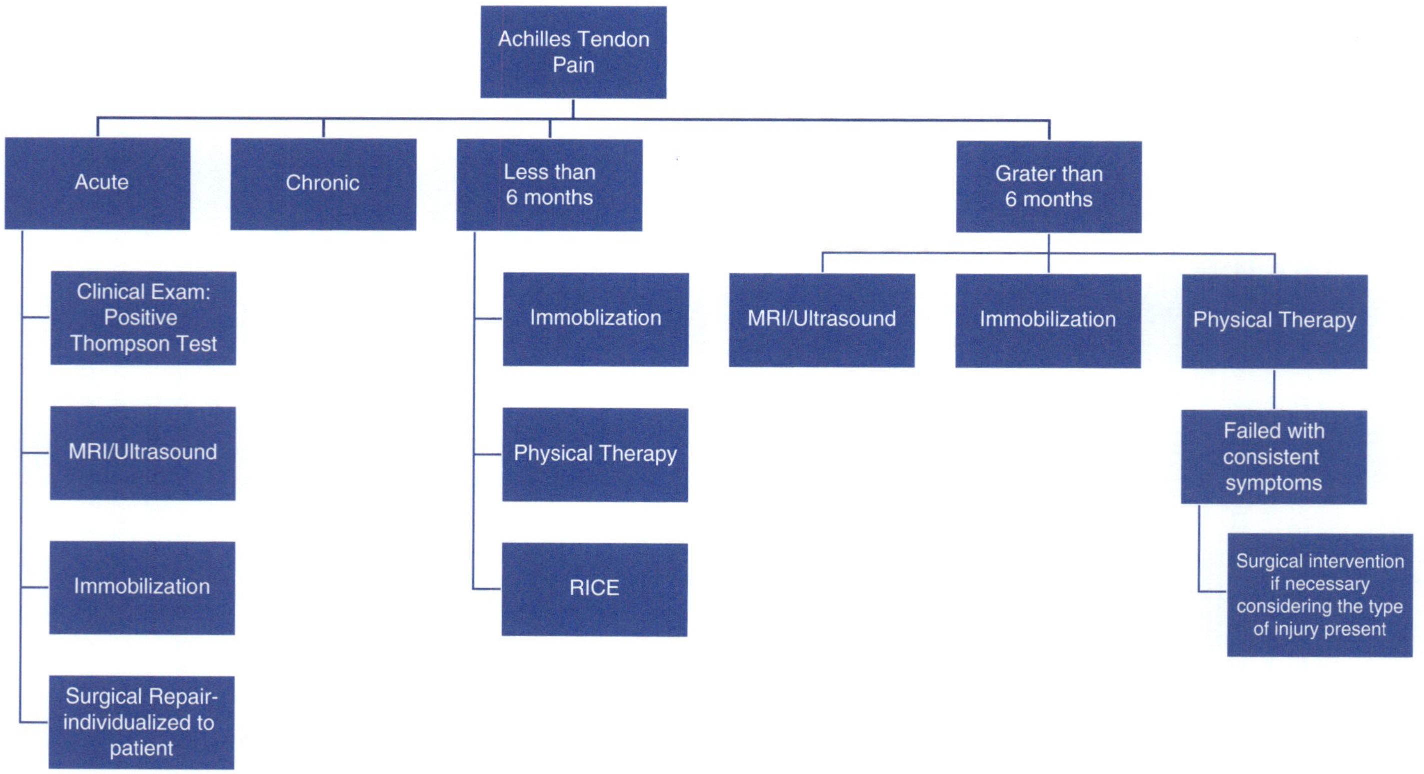

References

1. Demaio M, Paine R, Drez D. Achilles tendinitis. Orthopedics. 1995;18:195–20.
2. Soma CA, Mandelbaum BR. Achilles tendon disorders. Clin Sports Med. 1994;13:811–23.
3. Scott SH, Winter DA. Internal forces of chronic running injury sites. Med Sci Sports Exerc. 1990;22:357–69.
4. Clain MR, Baxter DE. Achilles tendinitis. Foot Ankle. 1992;13:482–7.
5. Chen TM, Rozen WM, Pan WR, et al. The arterial anatomy of the Achilles tendon: anatomical study and clinical implications. Clin Anat. 2009;22(3):377–85.
6. Coughlin MJ, Schon L. Disorders of tendons. In: Mann RA, Coughlin MJ, Saltzman CL, editors. Surgery of the foot and ankle, vol. 1. 8th ed. Philadelphia: Mosby Elsevier; 2007. p. 1149–277.
7. Kvist MH, Lehto MU, Josza L, et al. Chronic Achilles paratenonitis: an immunohistologic study of fibronectin and fibrinogen. Am J Sports Med. 1988;16:616–23.
8. Fox JM, Blazina ME, Jobe FW, et al. Degeneration and rupture of the Achilles tendon. Clin Orthop. 1975;107:221–4.
9. Gould N, Korson R. Stenosing tenosynovitis of the pseudosheath of the tendo Achilles. Foot Ankle. 1980;1:179–87.
10. Lotke PA. Ossification of the Achilles tendon: report of seven cases. J Bone Joint Surg Am. 1970;52:157–60.
11. Paavola M, Kannus P, Jarvinen TA, et al. Achilles tendinopathy. J Bone Joint Surg Am. 2002;84:2062–76.
12. Holmes GB, Lin J. Etiologic factors associated with symptomatic Achilles tendinopathy. Foot Ankle Int. 2006;27:952–9.
13. Fahlström M, Lorentzon R, Alfredson H. Painful conditions in the Achilles tendon region: a common problem in middle-aged competitive badminton players. Knee Surg Sports Traumatol Arthrosc. 2002;10:57–60.
14. Nell EM, van der Merwe L, Cook J, et al. The apoptosis pathway and the genetic predisposition to Achilles tendinopathy. J Orthop Res. 2012;30:1719–24.
15. Posthumus M, Collins M, Cook J, et al. Components of the transforming growth factor-beta family and the pathogenesis of human Achilles tendon pathology: a genetic association study. Rheumatology (Oxford). 2010;49:2090–7.
16. Björklund E, Forsgren S, Alfredson H, Fowler CJ. Increased expression of cannabinoid CB? Receptors in Achilles tendinosis. PLoS One. 2011;6:24731.
17. Johansson C. Injuries in elite orienteers. Am J Sports Med. 1986;14:410–5.
18. Fahlström M, Lorentzon R, Alfredson H. Painful conditions in the Achilles tendon region in elite badminton players. Am J Sports Med. 2002;30:51–4.
19. Reule CA, Alt WW, Lohrer H, Hochwald H. Spatial orientation of the subtalar joint axis is different in subjects with and without Achilles tendon disorders. Br J Sports Med. 2011;45:1029–34.
20. Sharma P, Maffulli N. Tendon injury and tendinopathy: healing and repair. J Bone Joint Surg Am. 2005;87-A:187–202.
21. Järvinen TA, Kannus P, Maffulli N, Khan KM. Achilles tendon disorders: etiology and epidemiology. Foot Ankle Clin. 2005;10:255–66.
22. Munteanu SE, Barton CJ. Lower limb biomechanics during running in individuals with Achilles tendinopathy: a systematic review. J Foot Ankle Res. 2011;4:15.
23. Lysholm J, Wiklander J. Injuries in runners. Am J Sports Med. 1987;15:168–71.
24. McGarvey WC, Palumbo RC, Baxter DE, et al. Insertional Achilles tendinosis: surgical treatment through a central tendon splitting approach. Foot Ankle Int. 2002;23:19–25.
25. Nicholson CW, Berlet GC, Lee TH. Prediction of the success of nonoperative treatment of insertional Achilles tendinosis based on MRI. Foot Ankle Int. 2007;28(4):472–7. https://doi.org/10.3113/FAI.2007.0472.
26. Paré A. Les Oeuvres. 9th ed. Lyon, France: Claude Rigaud et Claude Osbert; 1633.
27. Abrahamsen H. Ruptura tendinis Achillis. Ugeskr Laeger. 1923;85:279–85.
28. Quénu J, Stoianovitch SM. Les Ruptures du tendon d' Achille. Rev Chir. 1929;67:647–78.

29. Christensen I. Rupture of the Achilles tendon. Acta Chir Scand. 1953;106:50–60.
30. Edna TH. Non-operative treatment of Achilles tendon ruptures. Acta Orthop Scand. 1980;51:991–3.
31. Forste RI, Ritter MA, Young R. Rerupture of conservatively treated Achilles tendon rupture. J Bone Joint Surg Am. 1974;56-A:174.
32. Gillesie HS, George AE. Results of surgical repair of spontaneous rupture of the Achilles tendon. J Trauma. 1980;9:247–9.
33. Inglis AE, Scott WN, Sculco TP, et al. Ruptures of the tendo Achillis: an objective assessment of surgical and non-surgical treatment. J Bone Joint Surg Am. 1976;58:990–3.
34. Movin T, Ryberg A, DJ MB, Maffulli N. Acute rupture of the Achilles tendon. Foot Ankle Clin. 2005;10(2):331–56.
35. Gillies H, Chalmers J. The management of fresh ruptures of the tendo achillis. J Bone Joint Surg Am. 1970;52(2):337–43.
36. Houshian S, Tscherning T, Riegels-Nielsen P. The epidemiology of Achilles tendon rupture in a Danish county. Injury. 1998;29(9):651–4.
37. Levi N. The incidence of Achilles tendon rupture in Copenhagen. Injury. 1997;28(4):311–3.
38. Lagergren C, Lindholm A. Vascular distribution in the Achilles tendon. Acta Chir Scand. 1958/1959;116:491–5.
39. Inglis AE, Sculco TP. Surgical repair of ruptures of the tendon Achilles. Clin Orthop. 1981;156:160–9.
40. Arner O, Lindholm A, Orell SR. Histologic changes in subcutaneous rupture of the Achilles tendon. Acta Chir Scand. 1959;116:484–91.
41. Kannus P, Joza I. Histopathological changes preceding spontaneous rupture of a tendon. J Bone Joint Surg Am. 1991;73-A:1507–25.
42. Kvist M, Josza L, Javubeb M. Vascular changes in the ruptured Achilles tendon and local paratenon. Int Orthop. 1992;16:377–82.
43. Melmed EP. Spontaneous rupture of the calcaneal tendon during steroid therapy. J Bone Joint Surg Br. 1965;47:104–5.
44. Mahler F, Fritschy D. Partial and complete ruptures of the Achilles tendon and local corticosteroid injections. Br J Sports Med. 1992;26:7–14.
45. Jozsa L, Kvist M, Balint J, et al. The role of recreational sport activity in Achilles tendon rupture. Am J Sports Med. 1989;17:338–43.
46. Mokone GG, Schwellnus MP, Noakes TD, et al. The COL5A1 gene and Achilles tendon pathology. Scand J Med Sci Sports. 2006;16(10):19–26.
47. Hofmann GO, Weber T, Lob G. Tendon rupture in chronic kidney insufficiency—"uremic tendinopathy"? A literature-supposed documentation of 3 cases. Chirurg. 1990;61(6):434–7.
48. Jávinen T, Kannus P, Maffullo N, et al. Achilles tendon disorders: etiology and epidemiology. Foot Ankle Clin. 2005;10(2):255–66.
49. Movin T, Gad A, Guntner P, et al. Pathology of Achilles tendon in association with ciprofloxacin treatment. Foot Ankle. 1997;18:297.
50. Thompson TC, Dohert JH. Spontaneous rupture of Achilles: a new clinical diagnostic test. J Trauma. 1962;2:126–9.
51. Mates AI. Rupture of tendo Achilles: another diagnostic sign. Bull Hosp Joint Dis. 1975;36(1):48–51.
52. O'Brien T. The needle test for complete rupture of the Achilles tendon. J Bone Joint Surg Am. 1984;66:1099–101.
53. Astrom M, Gentz CF, Nilsson P, et al. Imaging in chronic Achilles tendinopathy: a comparison of ultra-sonography, magnetic resonance imaging and surgical findings in 27 histologically verified cases. Skelet Radiol. 1996;25:615–20.
54. Moller M, Movin T, Granhed H, et al. Acute rupture of tendon Achilles. A prospective randomized study of comparison between surgical and non-surgical treatment. J Bone Joint Surg Br. 2001;83:843–8.
55. Cetti R, Christensen SE, Ejsted R, et al. Operative versus nonoperative treatment of Achilles tendon rupture. A prospective randomized study and review of the literature. Am J Sports Med. 1993;21:791–9.

56. Wong J, Barrass V, et al. Quantitative review of operative and nonoperative management of Achilles tendon ruptures. Am J Sports Med. 2002;30:565–75.
57. Kahn RJ, Fick D, et al. Treatment of acute Achilles tendon ruptures. A meta-analysis of randomized, controlled trials. J Bone Joint Surg Am. 2005;87-A:2202–10.
58. Olsson N, Karlsson J, Eriksson BI, Brorsson A, Lundberg M, Silbernagel KG. Ability to perform a single heel-rise is significantly related to patient-reported outcome after Achilles tendon rupture. Scand J Med Sci Sports. 2014;24(1):152–8.
59. Silvani S. Management of acute tendon trauma. In: McGlamary ED, Banks AS, Downey MS, editors. Comprehensive textbook of foot surgery. 2nd ed. Baltimore, MD: Williams and Wilkins; 1992. p. 1450–63.
60. Hsu AR, Jones CP, Cohen BE, Davis WH, Ellington JK, Anderson RB. Clinical outcomes and complications of percutaneous Achilles repair system versus open technique for acute Achilles tendon ruptures. Foot Ankle Int. 2015;36(11):1279–86.
61. Yepes H, Tang M, Geddes C, Glazebrook M, Morris SF, Stanish WD. Digital vascular mapping of the integument about the Achilles tendon. J Bone Joint Surg Am. 2010;92(5):1215–20.
62. Soroceanu A, Sidhwa F, Aarabi S, Kaufman A, Glazebrook M. Surgical versus nonsurgical treatment of acute Achilles tendon rupture: a meta-analysis of randomized trials. J Bone Joint Surg Am. 2012;94(23):2136–43.
63. Elias I, Besser M, Nazarian LN, Raikin SM. Reconstruction for missed or neglected Achilles tendon rupture with V-Y lengthening and flexor hallucis longus tendon transfer through one incision. Foot Ankle Int. 2007;28(12):1238–48.
64. Yasuda T, Shima H, Mori K, Kizawa M, Neo M. Direct repair of chronic Achilles tendon ruptures using scar tissue located between the tendon stumps. J Bone Joint Surg Am. 2016;98(14):1168–75.
65. Rettig AC, Liotta FJ, Klootwyk TE, Porter DA, Mieling P. Potential risk of rerupture in primary Achilles tendon repair in athletes younger than 30 years of age. Am J Sports Med. 2005;33(1):119–23.
66. Reito A, Logren HL, Ahonen K, Nurmi H, Paloneva J. Risk factors for failed nonoperative treatment and rerupture in acute Achilles tendon rupture. Foot Ankle Int. 2018;39(6):694–7.
67. Young KW, Lee HS, Park SC. Rerupture risk after tenorrhaphy for Achilles tendon rupture. Proceedings of the 32nd annual meeting of Korean orthopedic Society for Sports Medicine; 2018 Sep 15; Seoul, Korea. Daejeon: Korean Orthopaedic Society for Sports Medicine; 2018.
68. Hamish DH, Edwards WH. Neglected ruptures of Achilles tendon. Foot Ankle Clin. 2005;10:357–70.
69. Lepow GM, Green JB. Reconstruction of a neglected Achilles tendon rupture with an Achilles tendon allograft: a case report. J Foot Ankle Surg. 2006;45(5):351–5.
70. Kocabey Y, Nyland J, Nawab A, et al. Reconstruction of neglected Achilles' tendon defect with peroneus brevis tendon allograft: a case report. J Foot Ankle Surg. 2006;45(1):42–6.
71. Bosworth D. Repair of defects in the tendo Achilles. J Bone Joint Surg Am. 1956;38:111.
72. Lindholm A. A new method of operation for subcutaneous rupture of the Achilles tendon. Acta Chir Scand. 1959;117:261–8.
73. Lynn T. Repair of the torn Achilles tendon, using the plantaris tendon as a reinforcing membrane. J Bone Joint Surg Am. 1996;48:268–72.
74. Turco VJ, Spinella AJ. Achilles tendon ruptures-peroneus brevis transfer. Foot Ankle. 1987;7:253–9.
75. Mendicino SS, Reed TS. Repair of neglected Achilles tendon ruptures with a triceps surae muscle tendon advancement. J Foot Ankle Surg. 1996;14(8):443–9.
76. Wapner KL, Pavlock GS, Hecht PJ, et al. Repair of chronic Achilles tendon rupture with flexor halluces longus tendon transfer. Foot Ankle. 1993;35(1):13–8.
77. Ryu CH, Lee HS, Seo SG, Kim HY. Results of tenorrhaphy with early rehabilitation for acute tear of Achilles tendon. J Orthop Surg (Hong Kong). 2018;26(3):2309499018802483.
78. Myerson M. Disorders of the Achilles tendon. In: Myerson M, editor. Reconstructive foot and ankle surgery. Philadelphia: Elsevier; 2005. p. 283–309.
79. Willits K, Amendola A, Bryant D, Mohtadi NG, Giffin JR, Fowler P, Kean CO, Kirkley A. Operative versus nonoperative treatment of acute Achilles tendon ruptures: a

multicenter randomized trial using accelerated functional rehabilitation. J Bone Joint Surg Am. 2010;92(17):2767–75. https://doi.org/10.2106/JBJS.I.01401.

80. Keating JF, Will EM. Operative versus non-operative treatment of acute rupture of tendo Achilles: a prospective randomized evaluation of functional outcome. J Bone Joint Surg Br. 2011;93(8):1071.

81. Young SW, Patel A, Zhu M, van Dijck S, McNair P, Bevan WP, Tomlinson M. Weight-bearing in the nonoperative treatment of acute Achilles tendon ruptures: a randomized controlled trial. J Bone Joint Surg Am. 2014;96(13):1073–9.

82. Hutchison AM, Topliss C, Beard D, Evans RM, Williams P. The treatment of a rupture of the Achilles tendon using a dedicated management programme. Bone Joint J. 2015;97-B(4):510–5.

83. Ecker TM, Bremer AK, Krause FG, Müller T, Weber M. Prospective use of a standardized nonoperative early weightbearing protocol for Achilles tendon rupture: 17 years of experience. Am J Sports Med. 2016;44(4):1004–10.

84. Barfod KW, Bencke J, Lauridsen HB, Ban I, Ebskov L, Troelsen A. Nonoperative dynamic treatment of acute Achilles tendon rupture: the influence of early weight-bearing on clinical outcome: a blinded, randomized controlled trial. J Bone Joint Surg Am. 2014;96(18):1497–503.

85. Kauwe M. Acute Achilles tendon rupture: clinical evaluation, conservative management, and early active rehabilitation. Clin Podiatr Med Surg. 2017;34(2):229–43.

86. Huang J, Wang C, Ma X, Wang X, Zhang C, Chen L. Rehabilitation regimen after surgical treatment of acute Achilles tendon ruptures: a systematic review with meta-analysis. Am J Sports Med. 2015;43(4):1008–16.

87. Brumann M, Baumbach SF, Mutschler W, Polzer H. Accelerated rehabilitation following Achilles tendon repair after acute rupture—development of an evidence-based treatment protocol. Injury. 2014;45(11):1782–90.

88. Zhao J-G, et al. Early functional rehabilitation versus traditional immobilization for surgical Achilles tendon repair after acute rupture: a systematic review of overlapping meta-analyses. Sci Rep. 2017;7:39871. https://doi.org/10.1038/srep39871.

89. Ochen Y, Beks RB, van Heijl M, Hietbrink F, LPH L, van der Velde D, et al. Operative treatment versus nonoperative treatment of Achilles tendon ruptures: systematic review and meta-analysis. BMJ. 2019;364:k5120. https://doi.org/10.1136/bmj.k512.

90. Hurley E, Yasui Y, Gianakos A, et al. Achilles tendon repair—a systematic review of overlapping meta-analyses. Foot Ankle Orthop. 2017; https://doi.org/10.1177/2473011417S000212.

91. Seow D, Yasui Y, Calder JDF, Kennedy JG, Pearce CJ. Treatment of acute Achilles tendon ruptures: a systematic review and meta-analysis of complication rates with best- and worst-case analyses for Rerupture rates. Am J Sports Med. 2021;49(13):3728–48. https://doi.org/10.1177/0363546521998284.

Index

© Springer Nature Switzerland AG 2022

J. D. Cain, M. V. Hogan (eds.), *Tendon and Ligament Injuries of the Foot and Ankle*,
https://doi.org/10.1007/978-3-031-10490-9

MIX
Papier aus verantwortungsvollen Quellen
Paper from responsible sources
FSC® C105338

If you have any concerns about our products,
you can contact us on
ProductSafety@springernature.com

In case Publisher is established outside the EU,
the EU authorized representative is:
Springer Nature Customer Service Center GmbH
Europaplatz 3, 69115 Heidelberg, Germany

Printed by Libri Plureos GmbH
in Hamburg, Germany